The Brain, the Nervous System, and Their Diseases

The Brain, the Nervous System, and Their Diseases

Volume 3: P–Z,
Experiments and Activities

Jennifer L. Hellier, Editor

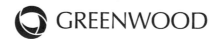

GREENWOOD

AN IMPRINT OF ABC-CLIO, LLC
Santa Barbara, California • Denver, Colorado • Oxford, England

Copyright 2015 by ABC-CLIO, LLC

Library of Congress Cataloging-in-Publication Data

The brain, the nervous system, and their diseases / Jennifer L. Hellier, editor.
　　p. ; cm.
　Includes bibliographical references and index.
　ISBN 978-1-61069-337-0 (hard copy : alk. paper) — ISBN 978-1-61069-338-7 (ebook)
　I. Hellier, Jennifer, editor.
[DNLM: 1. Brain—physiology—Encyclopedias—English.　2. Brain Diseases—Encyclopedias—English.　3. Nervous System—Encyclopedias—English.　4. Nervous System Diseases—Encyclopedias—English.　5. Nervous System Physiological Phenomena—Encyclopedias—
English. WL 13]
　RC334
　612.803—dc23　　　2014019809

ISBN: 978-1-61069-337-0
EISBN: 978-1-61069-338-7

19　18　17　16　15　　1　2　3　4　5

This book is also available on the World Wide Web as an eBook.
Visit www.abc-clio.com for details.

Greenwood
An Imprint of ABC-CLIO, LLC

ABC-CLIO, LLC
130 Cremona Drive, P.O. Box 1911
Santa Barbara, California 93116-1911

This book is printed on acid-free paper (∞)

Manufactured in the United States of America

Contents

Alphabetical List of Entries

Volume 2

Guide to Related Topics

Following are entries in this encyclopedia, arranged under broad topics, for enhanced searching. Readers should also consult the index at the end of the encyclopedia for more specific subjects.

Experiments and Activities

Astrocyte—Building with Clay Activity
Basket Cells—Building with Clay Activity
Behavioral Experiments
Brain Building with Clay Activity: Cerebellum, Cerebral Cortex
Brain Cut-Out Hat Activity
Cell Body (Soma)—Building with Clay Activity
Channel/Receptor—Building with Clay Activity
Circle of Willis and Arterial Supply to the Brain—Building with Clay Activity
Dendrites—Building with Clay Activity
Dendritic Spine—Building with Clay Activity
Discriminative Touch Experiment
Electrophysiology Setup and Experiments
Frog Sciatic Nerve Experiment

Membrane Potential Experiment—Understand Membrane Properties
Myelin Conduction Experiment
Neural Tube—Illustrating Activity
Oligodendrocytes—Building with Clay Activity
Pinched Nerve—Building with Clay Activity
Purkinje Cells—Building with Clay Activity
A Sample Immunohistochemistry Protocol with Thought Questions
Schwann Cells—Building with Clay Activity
Spinal Cord with Vertebra—Building with Clay Activity
Voltage Clamp Experiment

Anatomy

Amygdala
Autonomic Nervous System
Axon
Basal Nuclei (Basal Ganglia)

Auditory

Inferior Colliculus
Musical Memory

Behavior
Addiction
Alcohol and Alcoholism
Behavior
Behavioral Experiments
Behavioral Health
Behavioral Tests
Bipolar Disorder
Circadian Rhythm
Conscious and Consciousness
Depression
Language
Learning and Memory
Limbic System
Neuropsychological
    Assessment/Test
Psychology and Psychiatry
Rapid Eye Movement (REM)
Sleep

Blood Vessels
Aneurysm
Baroreceptors
Beta-Blockers (β-Blockers)
Carotid Body
Cerebrovascular System
Circle of Willis and Arterial
    Supply to the Brain—
    Building with Clay
    Activity (Experiments and
    Activities Section)
Hematoma (Hemorrhage)
Hypoxia
Sinuses
Stroke
Transient Ischemic Attack (TIA)

Brain
Afferent Tracts
Amygdala
Blood-Brain Barrier
Brain Anatomy
Brain Cut-Out Hat Activity
    (Experiments and Activities
    Section)
Brainstem
Brodmann Areas
Caudate Nucleus
Cephalic Disorders
Cerebellum, Cerebral Cortex—
    Building with Clay Activity
    (Experiments and Activities Section)
Cerebrospinal Fluid
Conscious and Consciousness
Diencephalon
Frontal Lobe
Globus Pallidus
Gyrus (Gyri)
Hemispheres
Hydrocephaly (Cerebral
    Hemispheres)
Hypothalamus
Intracranial Pressure
Megalencephaly/Macrencephaly
Microcephaly
Neurotoxicity
Occipital Lobe
Phrenology
Pineal Gland
Pituitary Gland (Hypophysis)
Putamen
Skull
Subconscious
Sulcus (Sulci)
Telencephalon

Dizziness and Vertigo
Encephalitis
Encephalopathy
Epilepsy
Fetal Alcohol Spectrum Disorders
Fibromyalgia
Glasgow Coma Scale
Glioma
Herniated Discs
Huntington's Disease
Hydrocephalus
Hypoxia
Insomnia
Lissencephaly
Lyme Disease
Macular Degeneration
Megalencephaly/Macrencephaly
Meniere's Disease
Meningioma
Meningitis
Microcephaly
Migraine
Multiple Sclerosis
Muscular Dystrophy (Duchenne)
Myasthenia Gravis
Narcolepsy
Parkinson's Disease
Peripheral Neuropathy
Phantom Pain
Poliomyelitis
Post-Traumatic Stress Disorder
Prions
Progressive Multifocal
    Leukencephalopathy
Schizophrenia
Schwannomas
Seizures
Shingles
Spina Bifida
Stroke

Substance Abuse
Tardive Dyskinesia
Taste Aversion
Tay-Sachs Disease
Transient Global Amnesia
Transient Ischemic Attack (TIA)
Trauma
Traumatic Brain Injury (TBI)
Tuberous Sclerosis Complex
Whipple's Disease
Wilson Disease

Drugs
Adrenaline
Anesthesia
Antidepressants
Benzodiazepines
Beta-Blockers (β-Blockers)
Endorphins
Growth Factors
Hormones
Levodopa
Melatonin
Neurotoxicity
Neurotoxins
Noradrenaline
Opiates
Parkinsonism (Drug-Induced)
Phenytoin (Dilantin)
Substance Abuse

Experiments
Behavioral Experiments (Experiments
    and Activities Section)
Brain Stimulators
Discriminative Touch Experiment
    (Experiments and Activities
    Section)
Drosophila

Sensory

Afferent Tracts
Anterolateral Tract (Anterolateral
     System)
Auditory System
Blind Spot
Blink Reflex
Carotid Body
Cochlea
Color Blindness
Cranial Nerves
Diplopia
Discriminative Touch
Facial Nerve
Fibromyalgia
Glossopharyngeal Nerve
Headache
Homunculus
Nystagmus
Olfactory Nerve
Optic Nerve
Prosopagnosia
Ptosis
Retina
Sensory Receptors
Somatosensory Cortex/
     Somatosensory System
Taste Aversion
Taste System
Touch
Trigeminal Nerve
Tunnel Vision
Vagus Nerve
Vestibular System
Vestibulocochlear Nerve
Visual Fields
Visual Perception
     (Visual Processing)
Visual System

Signs and Symptoms

Agnosia
Agraphia
Alexia
Aphasia
Apraxia
Areflexia
Ataxia
Color Blindness
Coma
Congenital Defects
     (Abnormalities)
Deafness
Diplopia
Dysdiadochokinesia
Dyslexia
Dystonia
Foot Drop
Headache
Hemiplegia
Hyperreflexia
Oral Health
Pain
Paralysis
Paresis
Parkinsonism (Drug-
     Induced)
Peripheral Neuropathy
Phantom Pain
Prosopagnosia
Ptosis
Seizures
Spasm
Strabismus
Tremor

Smell

Olfactory Nerve
Olfactory System (Smell)

Tests

Behavioral Tests
Blink Reflex
Computed Tomography (CT or CAT)
Electroencephalogram (EEG)
Electromyelogram (EMG)
Glasgow Coma Scale
Immunohistochemistry
Intracranial Pressure
Lumbar Puncture
Magnetic Resonance Imaging (MRI)
Molecular Biology
Neurological Examination
Neuronal Imaging
Neuropsychological Assessment/Test
Oral Health
Reward and Punishment
Romberg Test

Treatments

Adrenaline
Antidepressants
Brain Stimulators
Cochlear Implants
Depression
Gene Therapy
Opiates
Phenytoin (Dilantin)
Sleep Apnea (CPAP Treatment)
Stem Cell Therapy
Stereotaxic Surgery

Vision

Abducens Nerve
Accommodation
Agnosia
Blind Spot
Blink Reflex
Color Blindness
Diplopia
Macular Degeneration
Muscular Dystrophy (Duchenne)
Nystagmus
Occipital Lobe
Oculomotor Nerve
Optic Nerve
Prosopagnosia
Ptosis
Retina
Saccades
Strabismus
Superior Colliculus
Trochlear Nerve
Tunnel Vision
Visual Fields
Visual Perception (Visual
    Processing)
Visual System

P

Pain

Pain is defined as an unpleasant sensory and emotional experience associated with actual or potential tissue damage. It is a conscious experience involving the interpretation of sensory input that signals a noxious event and is influenced by several factors. One model describes pain in terms of three hierarchical levels: a sensory-discriminative component (location, intensity, and quality), a motivational-affective component (depression and anxiety), and a cognitive-evaluative component (thoughts involving the cause and significance of the pain). This model highlights the reality that the perception of pain is determined by a combination of several components and is very complex to both understand and manage.

Classification of Pain

Acute pain warns an organism of a potentially harmful situation (like a burn) or a disease state (such as appendicitis). Acute pain serves a specific physiologic function and lasts a brief period of time. Unfortunately, if the acute pain is undertreated or severe, it can last longer than its biologic usefulness and may have many harmful effects. Acute pain caused by surgery, acute illness, or trauma is usually nociceptive (a signal from neurons that is usually due to damage to these cell types). The goal of treating acute pain is cure.

Chronic pain results when pain persists for months to years. This type of pain can be nociceptive, neuropathic/functional, or mixed. It is associated with cancer or noncancer etiologies that result in changes to the receptors and nerve fibers within the nervous system. Additionally, chronic pain is often associated with depression, insomnia, and other personal or social problems. The goal of treatment with chronic pain is not cure, but a return to functionality.

Pathophysiology—Nociceptive Pain

Nociceptive pain is "normal" pain resulting from the activation of nociceptive fibers and includes somatic (body) and visceral (gut or abdomen) pains. Sprains and strains produce mild forms of nociceptive pain, while pain of arthritis is much more severe. Nociceptive pain is described as either somatic (arising from skin, bone, joint, muscle, or connective tissue) or visceral (arising from internal organs). Somatic pain presents as a throbbing and well-localized pain, while visceral pain presents localized to the organ from which it originates.

Nociceptive pain occurs as a result of the activation of the sensory system by persistent noxious stimuli, a process involving transduction, transmission, modulation, and perception. Transduction is the process by which noxious stimuli are converted to electrical signals in the nociceptors. Nociceptors have the ability to distinguish between noxious and innocuous stimuli and are activated and sensitized by mechanical, thermal, and chemical impulses. Noxious stimuli may result in the release of naturally occurring chemicals, such as bradykinins, hydrogen and potassium ions, prostaglandins, histamines, interleukins, tumor necrosis factor alfa, serotonin, and substance P. These chemicals sensitize or activate the nociceptors.

When several axons are grouped together and share a similar function, such axons are called *fibers*. In turn, a group of fibers are called a *nerve*. Transmission takes place in two different nerve fiber types: A-delta and C-afferent fibers. A-delta fibers are myelinated (covered with myelin to aid in faster transmission of signals) and have a large diameter. When stimulated, these fibers evoke a sharp, well-localized pain. C-fibers are unmyelinated and have a small diameter. When stimulated, the C-fibers produce a dull, aching, poorly localized pain. For the central nervous system to receive the pain, the signal travels from the affected area toward the brain. This is an *afferent signal*. These afferent nociceptive fibers synapse in various layers of the spinal cord, specifically in the region where most neuronal cell bodies reside in the dorsal horn, the "gray matter of the spinal cord." This, in turn, results in the release of a variety of neurotransmitters (specialized chemicals used by neurons to "talk" to each other) including glutamate, substance P, and aspartate. The role of substance P has been widely studied in pain and how it aids in pain transmission to the brain. Substance P is released from C-fibers in response to tissue injury or to intense stimulation of peripheral nerves.

There are three major classes of nociceptors: thermal, mechanical, and polymodal. Extreme temperatures activate thermal nociceptors, which have a small diameter and are myelinated, sending very rapid signals. Mechanical nociceptors are activated by intensive pressure applied to the skin. They are also thinly myelinated fibers that conduct signals quickly. Polymodal nociceptors are activated by high-intensity mechanical, chemical, or thermal stimuli. These nociceptors have a small diameter and are nonmyelinated, conducting signals much more slowly. The nociceptors transduce signals via specialized proteins—also known as channels—such as transient receptor potential channels or voltage-gated sodium channels (for those nociceptors that are activated by sodium). Depolarization of the primary afferent nerves results in production of substances that are produced by tissues, inflammatory cells, and neurons. These include prostaglandins, bradykinins, protons, and nerve growth factors. Once depolarization occurs, transmission of information continues along the axon to the spinal cord and then on to higher brain centers.

Nociceptive information is transmitted from the spinal cord to the thalamus and cerebral cortex along five ascending pathways: spinothalamic, spinoreticular, spinomesencephalic, cervicothalamic, and spinohypothalamic tracts. The spinothalamic tract is the most prominent ascending nociceptive pathway in the spinal cord. These axons project into the contralateral side of the spinal cord and terminate in the thalamus. The cerebral cortex also contributes to the processing of pain. Neurons in several regions of the cerebral cortex respond selectively to nociceptive input.

At this point, pain becomes a conscious experience that takes place in higher cortical structures. The brain may take in only a limited number of pain signals, allowing cognitive and behavioral functions to modify pain sensation. Variables including relaxation, distraction, and meditation may decrease pain by limiting the number of processed pain signals. On the other hand, depression and anxiety may worsen pain.

Pain is modulated through a number of systems, including the *endogenous opiate system*. This system consists of neurotransmitters including enkephalins, dynorphins, beta endorphins, and mu, delta, and kappa receptors that are found throughout the central nervous system. The poppy plant extract, opium, binds to specialized proteins within the central nervous system. Scientists have expanded on this knowledge and have developed opioids, which are a group of chemicals that bind to one or more of the three opioid receptors in the central nervous system. Endogenous opioids, like exogenous opioids, bind to opioid receptor sites and modulate the transmission of pain impulses. Other receptors, including the *N*-methyl-d-aspartate (NMDA) receptors found in the dorsal horn, also influence the endogenous opiate system. Blockage of NMDA receptors may increase the mu-receptors' responsiveness to opiates. In addition to this mode of modulation, the central nervous system also contains a descending system that controls pain transmission through inhibition of synaptic pain transmission at the level of the dorsal horn in the spinal cord. Neurotransmitters that play an important role in this descending system include endogenous opioids, serotonin, norepinephrine, and gamma-aminobutyric acid (GABA).

Pathophysiology—Neuropathic and Functional Pain

Neuropathic and functional pain are different from nociceptive pain in that they can become disengaged from noxious stimuli or healing and are often described in terms of chronic pain. These types of pain often present as burning, tingling, or shooting sensations. In addition, persons with chronic pain may have exaggerated painful responses to normally noxious stimuli (hyperalgesia) or painful responses to normally nonnoxious stimuli (allodynia).

Neuropathic pain results from direct injury to nerves in the peripheral or central nervous systems. Diabetic neuropathy and phantom limb pain are two examples of neuropathic pain. Phantom limb pain can occur after traumatic or surgical limb amputation. Functional pain syndromes include fibromyalgia, irritable bowel syndrome, tension-type headaches, and sympathetic-induced pain that results from abnormal operation of the nervous system. Both of these types of pain syndromes are complex and can be very difficult to treat, as the pain reported is not evident by examining physical findings.

The exact mechanism of neuropathic or functional pain is complex. Overall, nerve damage or certain disease states may signal changes in inflammatory pain, ectopic excitability, enhanced sensory transmission, nerve structure reorganization, and loss of modulatory pain inhibition. Pain circuits eventually rewire themselves both anatomically and chemically, producing a mismatch between pain stimulation and inhibition. This results in an increase in the discharge of dorsal horn neurons. These changes over time help explain why this type of pain often manifests long after the actual nerve-related injury or when no actual injury is identified.

Pain Management

Successful pain management depends on a comprehensive assessment of the patient including the nature of the pain and how it is impacting the patient's life. Often, numeric rating scales are used to measure pain. A 0 on the scale indicates no pain and a 10 indicates most unbearable pain. Patients should be asked frequently throughout the treatment to rate their pain in order to understand whether they are improving.

There are several classes of agents that can be used for the management of pain. These include nonsteroidal anti-inflammatory drugs (NSAIDs), opioids, anticonvulsants, and antidepressants, among others. Acute and chronic pain states are managed differently. Traditionally, acute pain is managed based on pain scores. A mild pain (score 1–3) is usually treated with a nonopioid medication like acetaminophen (Tylenol) or ibuprofen (Advil). Moderate pain (score 4–6) is treated with an immediate-release, short-acting opioid in addition to a nonopioid if needed. Severe pain (score 7–10) is usually managed with two therapy modalities, including a short-acting opioid that is rapidly titrated in addition to a nonopioid or long-acting opioid.

Opioids are agonists of the mu-opioid receptor and modulate both the transmission of pain at the dorsal horn as well as perception and reaction to pain. Opioids come in several different formulations: immediate and extended release tablets, patches, intravenous solutions, and intramuscular injections. Examples of opioids include morphine, fentanyl, hydrocodone, and oxycodone. Common side effects associated with opioids include nausea, sedation, and constipation.

NSAIDS, including ibuprofen, inhibit prostaglandin synthesis through blockade of enzymes such as cyclooxygenase-1 (COX-1) and cyclooxygenase-2 (COX-2). Typically oral NSAIDS are used for the treatment of mild-to-moderate pain. Two NSAIDS, ketorolac and ibuprofen, are available as an intravenous solution for use in severe postoperation pain. Side effects include gastrointestinal ulceration, increased risk of bleeding, and/or renal (kidney) dysfunction.

Acetaminophen inhibits COX-2 only at sites of central nervous system sensitization. Most commonly, it is administered orally for the management of mild pain. It is also available as an intravenous formulation for more severe pain. The major concern with acetaminophen is *hepatotoxicity,* which is why it must be used with caution in patients with alcoholic liver disease and should not be used when ingesting alcohol.

Local anesthetics block voltage-sensitive sodium channels to interfere with nociceptive transmission. They provide intense, prolonged analgesia and do not have as many side effects as opioids. They can be administered by neuraxial (epidural or spinal) infusion or peripheral nerve block. Side effects include hypotension, neurotoxicity, dizziness, and drowsiness.

Conclusion

Pain is a complex perception that is influenced by emotional states and the environment. Because pain is so dependent on experience and varies from person to person, it is difficult to treat. Nociceptive pain results from direct activation of nociceptors in the skin or soft tissue in response to tissue injury. Neuropathic pain results from direct injury to nerves in the peripheral or central nervous systems. The treatment of pain varies based on the type of pain and duration of pain. NSAIDs, opioids, antidepressants, and anticonvulsant drugs can all be used for the management of pain.

Danielle Stutzman

See also: Depression; Fibromyalgia; Glutamate and Its Receptors; Headache; Migraine; Phantom Pain; Sensory Receptors

Further Reading

Kandel, E. R., Schwartz, J. H., & Jessell, T. M. (Eds.) (2000). *Principles of neural science* (4th ed.). United States: McGraw-Hill.

Medline Plus. (2013). *Pain.* U.S. National Library of Medicine. Retrieved from http://www.nlm.nih.gov/medlineplus/pain.html

National Institute of Neurological Disorders and Stroke (NINDS). (2012). *NINDS chronic pain information page.* Retrieved from http://www.ninds.nih.gov/disorders/chronic_pain/chronic_pain.htm

National Institute of Neurological Disorders and Stroke (NINDS). (2012). *NINDS peripheral neuropathy fact sheet.* Retrieved from http://www.ninds.nih.gov/disorders/peripheralneuropathy/peripheralneuropathy.htm

Paralysis

Paralysis is a condition when the muscles of a body part cannot move or feel. This means there is a disconnection between the central nervous system (the brain, brainstem, and spinal cord), the peripheral nervous system (spinal or cranial nerves that exit the spinal cord or brainstem), and/or the musculature. The word paralysis originated from Greek meaning "disabling of the nerves" with *para* meaning "itself" and *lysis* meaning "to lose." When one or more muscles begin to lose their function, this is a sign of paralysis. In affected areas, paralysis could also cause sensory and motor loss. Persons who are paralyzed show other symptoms such as emotional breakdowns and extreme stress. Studies have shown that about 2 percent of the general population will have some type of paralysis usually due to an accident or neurological disorder (Paralysis Resource Center: Facts and Figures, 2013). It is important to note that paralysis can occur in all animals.

In general, nervous system damage, specifically to the spinal cord, will frequently cause paralysis. Other causes that could trigger paralysis include Parkinson's disease, poliomyelitis, nerve injury, cerebral palsy, peripheral neuropathy, amyotrophic lateral sclerosis, botulism, spina bifida, and strokes, to name a few. During sleep, it is normal for every person to enter REM (rapid eye movement), which includes brief episodes of paralysis. Furthermore, paralysis can also be a side effect from drugs such as curare, which hinders nerve functions.

One of the most famous persons to become paralyzed was Christopher Reeve (1952–2004), an American actor who portrayed the superhero, Superman. Reeve injured his spinal cord after being thrown off a horse in an equestrian competition in 1995. After the accident, Reeve could not breathe without a respirator and became a *quadriplegic* (a person who cannot move any of their four limbs). Reeve had broken his neck particularly fracturing his top two vertebrae (bones that protect the spinal cord). Human necks contain seven vertebrae and in an unfortunate case, if any of the first four were to break along with a spinal cord injury, it will lead to a life of quadriplegia and disrupt the natural ability to breathe. From Christopher Reeve's incident, he and his wife, Dana, formed a foundation dedicated to curing spinal cord injury. For this foundation, Reeve has been titled a real-life hero. The Reeve Foundation funds research and aids in improving the lifestyle for those who had, or currently have, paralysis. One of the rehabilitation strategies that came from the understanding of brains and spinal cord is the *Locomotors Training*. This technique is used to train people who have neurological disorders that occur after injury, such as stroke. Many people who have received Locomotors Training have improved their walking, basic motor skills, and life, after a brain or spinal cord injury. Unfortunately, this is only available in certain locations in the United States, Canada, Germany, and Switzerland.

Types of Paralysis

Vocal Cord Paralysis

Some people experience vocal cord paralysis. This is when the person's larynx (also known as the voice box) is unable to vibrate during speech. Thus, the person will encounter voice problems. In other cases, the person might have difficulty swallowing or breathing. Vocal cord paralysis comes in many different forms. There is the *bilateral vocal cord paralysis* in which the two vocal cords become "stuck" halfway in the paramedian position and are not able to move in any direction. In this situation, a tracheotomy is needed to protect the person from having their food enter their airway. Often, this can be treated medically. If needed, one or both of the vocal cords can be moved surgically to bring it or them closer to the midline.

If only one vocal cord is paralyzed, has very little movement since it cannot vibrate, or vibrates in an abnormal way, it is called *unilateral vocal cord paralysis.* This can be treated medically or by training the individual to use the vocal cord. With medical treatment, substances can be injected into the vocal cord to increase its size, which lowers the chance of having the muscle paralyzed in that area. Muscle-nerve transplant can also be an effective medical treatment for this case. As for training the individual, voice therapy can be taught by a speech-language pathologist. The pathologist will assist the individual on pitch alteration, loudness, breath support, and correct position for optimal voicing. Studies have shown that voice therapy is an effective way in finding a solution to this problem and in diagnosing the individual. Unilateral vocal cord paralysis is more common compared to bilateral paralysis; however; in rare situations the person can be deprived of air and may lose their voice in the process.

People who experience vocal cord paralysis will have swallowing and voice problems depending on the location of the nerve damage. Some symptoms can include inability to speak loudly, coughing or choking while eating, or the possibility of having food and liquid aspirate into the lungs causing pneumonia. This happens while swallowing because the vocal cords cannot close properly to protect the airway.

Vocal cord paralysis can be diagnosed through a few steps. The first step is to insert an endoscope through the mouth or nose. The light from the endoscope is helpful in viewing the pattern of vocal cord while at rest or during phonation. A speech-language pathologist usually evaluates the voice, while the otolaryngologist evaluates the nose, ear, and throat. Head or neck injuries can sometimes be the main cause of vocal cord paralysis. Other cases such as tumors, surgery, stroke, or disease can also cause this paralysis. Any injury that damages the vagus nerve (cranial nerve X) is the main cause of vocal cord paralysis. This is because the vagus nerve arises from the brainstem and its branches innervate the larynx and conduct the displacement of the vocal cords.

Chondrodysplastic

Animals such as dogs that have *chondrodysplasia* are most likely to experience paralysis. These dogs have tiny holes of calcification in their cartilage. This is an inherited disorder that affects the skeletal system, bodily functions, and mental processing. These dogs have shorter body parts and their intervertebral discs are more fragile and break easily. Thus, a broken intervertebral disc can press on the spinal nerve cutting off circulation and killing the spinal cord tissue in less than 24 hours.

Occasionally, dogs that land or jump clumsily can injure their spinal cord along with intense exercises and rough playing. This could lead to *fibrocartilaginous embolism* (a stroke occurring within spinal cord blood vessels), which can also cause paralysis for dogs. This occurs when a small piece of the intervertebral disc material breaks off and falls into the blood vessel of the spinal cord. The nerves in the area become deprived of blood and slowly die. Eventually, the muscles of the hind legs will become weaker and over time the nerves will start to retreat from the posterior part of the spinal cord. Most dogs will usually be able to recover if the pain is resolved within 24 hours.

Paralyzing Toxins

In nature, some carnivorous animals can cause their victims to enter a lethal state of paralysis, while other animal species may use paralyzing toxins as a defense mechanism. For example, the *pufferfish* contains the poison *tetrodotoxin* (a toxin that affects the sodium channel in neurons) and is part of the *Tetraodontidae* family. The pufferfish is believed to be the second most poisonous vertebrate in the world, the *golden poison frog* being the first. The poison tetrodotoxin is contained in some organs such as the skin or the liver of the pufferfish. The pufferfish may use this as a defense mechanism to fend off a predator that would try to eat them. In the nerve cells, the poison binds to the sodium channel, thus blocking it, and starting an immobilizing effect on the muscles. The victim who had encountered the poison in small dosage will temporarily be paralyzed while larger dosages might result in death due to *asphyxiation,* a restriction to breathing. During this time, the victim is fully aware of the situation and will become prey or simply die an immobile death.

Venomous snakes such as the cobra contain *cobratoxin* that blocks the binding of acetylcholine (a natural chemical used to contract muscles) to the nicotinic acetylcholine receptor (specialized proteins within the cell membrane), thus causing respiratory paralysis to victims infected with its venom and eventually death. The venom contains a combination of carbohydrates, proteins, and other materials. The cobra can bite its prey with or without the use (excretion) of its venom. Venom is not always necessary for immobilizing the victim as it costs energy to produce. The cobra has other tactics to immobilize its prey such as constriction, which causes death due to asphyxia (the body is deprived of oxygen).

Insects such as the *digger wasp* may also use toxins to paralyze their victims. The digger wasp is notorious for its stinger, which contains tetrodotoxin to immobilize its prey. Throughout the world, there are about 130 known species of digger wasps. The toxin decreases the nerve activity resulting in decreased muscle contraction. The toxin causes the prey to become paralyzed and the queen wasp lays her eggs within the prey. Eventually, the prey becomes a live meal once the eggs hatch into larvae. The prey's remains may become construction pieces for hives and shelter.

Sleep Paralysis

Lastly, another type of paralysis that does not involve animal toxins or muscle injury is called *sleep paralysis.* This is an experience in which an individual is temporarily unable to move when falling asleep or waking up. Sleep paralysis is a human defense system to warn the body that one is deprived of sleep. Sleep paralysis can be very different depending on the victim. It often occurs before the person falls asleep or immediately after waking up. During sleep paralysis, the individual's mind is awake; however, his or her body is asleep, restricting them from basic motor movements like sitting up. Hallucinations also play a huge part in sleep paralysis. There are three types of hallucinations that humans tend to experience: (1) the individual may experience strong pressure on their chest, (2) they may see an intruder, or (3) have a feeling of levitation.

Every country has a different story about paralysis. Henry Fuseli's (1741–1825) 1781 painting called *The Nightmare* depicts a demon sitting on the chest of a woman was believed to be an example of sleep paralysis. The Western history of sleep paralysis has been documented for the last 300 years; while in China, the earliest occurrence of sleep paralysis dated back to 400 BC. In other countries such as Japan, sleep paralysis is called the "weighing ghost" due to the feeling of a strong pressure on the person's chest. Further, some individuals claim to see demons while they are asleep, while others claim to hear loud high-pitch ringing sounds in their ears. In 1692, during the Salem Witch Trials era, the townspeople of Salem claimed to have been possessed by demons or had people who practiced witchcraft. These descriptions may actually have been about sleep paralysis instead.

The length of sleep paralysis may vary depending on the individual. No cure has been found for sleep paralysis. However, the brain can be trained to shorten the time. People who were able to train their brain have described it to be simple as long as the person is conscious of their condition. Normally, heart rate will increase, as it can be quite frightening to the average person. The individual must keep sending mental signals to their body parts, such as wiggling their toes, moving their fingers, shaking their head, blinking, and twitching, as an incentive of trying to revive and regain mobility again. Eventually, this will work, and the individual will wake up.

Conclusion

Paralysis is quite common in more underdeveloped countries, including Africa and parts of Asia. In Vietnam, civilians will try almost anything that can be believed to cure paralysis, such as consumption of a *black rhinoceros horn*. Black rhinoceros' horns are made of a material called ivory, and were used in ancient Asian medicine as a cure for cancer, fever, and paralysis. Rhinoceros horns were literally worth their weight in gold and sometimes even more. However, scientific research shows that these black rhinoceros horns actually contain no medical properties; making this treatment an expensive and empty promise. Furthermore, black rhinoceros are now considered to be critically endangered, with the Western black rhinoceros being declared extinct in 2011, due to the high demand for their horns.

Nhung T. Nguyen

See also: Amyotrophic Lateral Sclerosis (ALS); Cerebral Palsy; Compression Injury; Hemiplegia; Nerve; Neurotoxins; Parkinson's Disease; Poliomyelitis; Sleep; Spina Bifida; Spinal Cord; Stroke

Further Reading

National Health Services—United Kingdom. (2012). *Paralysis*. Retrieved from http://www.nhs.uk/conditions/paralysis/Pages/Introduction.aspx

Paralysis Resource Center: Facts and Figures. (2013). *Christopher & Dana Reeve Foundation Spinal Cord Injury and Paralysis Resource Center.* Retrieved from http://www.christopherreeve.org/site/c.mtKZKgMWKwG/b.5184189/k.5587/Paralysis_Facts__Figures.htm

Silva, N. A., Sousa, N., Reis, R. L., & Salgado, A. J. (2013). From basics to clinical: A comprehensive review on spinal cord injury. *Progress in Neurobiology.* pii: S0301–0082(13): 00119–6. Retrieved from http://www.ncbi.nlm.nih.gov/pubmed/24269804.

Paresis

Two types of neurons control voluntary muscle movement: upper motor neurons that are located in the cerebral cortex and lower motor neurons that are located in the brainstem and spinal cord. When there is damage to either group of neurons, specific signs or symptoms are seen with voluntary movement, such as *paresis* and *paralysis*. The word *paresis* is derived from Ancient Greek that roughly translates as "letting go." In today's medical terminology, it is defined as general "muscle weakness" while the term *plegia* refers to "paralysis," which is the complete loss of motor movement or function. In general, when damage occurs to the upper motor neurons it produces specific neurological signs including a graded weakness of muscles such as paresis.

Types

Paresis usually refers to muscle weakness of the limbs, but it can include weakness of other body parts such as the eyes (ophthalmoparesis), the stomach (gastroparesis), and the vocal cords (vocal cord paresis, which is different from dysarthria—where the muscles of the throat have difficulty in producing speech). In addition to paresis, the term *myasthenia* also means "muscle weakness" and is also derived from Greek. This type of muscle weakness is due to problems within the skeletal muscles where the muscles have lost strength. Thus, it is different from paresis where the muscle weakness is caused by damage or dysfunction of upper motor neurons.

Muscle weakness is grouped by the location of the muscle in relation to the rest of the body. Distal paresis affects muscles that are farther from the body's midline (such as the lower leg), while proximal paresis affects muscles that are closer to the midline (such as the upper leg). The severity of the muscle weakness is graded by the amount of movement from zero to five. A grade of zero denotes no muscle movement or the inability for the muscle to contract; this would be called paralysis. A grade of one marks a trace of a muscle contraction but not enough to cause a movement of the connecting joint. A grade of two is given when the muscle contracts and moves the joint only if gravity is eliminated from the test. A grade of three denotes movement of the joint against gravity, but not when resistance is added. A grade of four includes movement of the joint against gravity and added resistance, but the movement is decreased compared to normal. Finally, a grade of five is given for normal strength.

If the paresis affects only one limb (an arm or a leg), it is called *monoparesis* where *paraparesis* affects both lower limbs. The term *hemiparesis* is used if an arm and a leg on either side of the body are affected. Lastly, if all four limbs have muscle weakness, it is called *quadriparesis.* All of these terms are usually used to describe muscle weakness caused by multiple sclerosis or stroke, in which both may cause damage to upper motor neurons.

Signs, Symptoms, and Treatments

Certain neurological diseases and disorders can cause paresis such as blunt force trauma, cerebral palsy, migraines, multiple sclerosis, muscular dystrophy, stroke, and tumors. One of the most common types of paresis is hemiparesis, which is less severe than hemiplegia. For example, in patients who are recovering from stroke, they may be able to have some movement of the affected side but they generally have lowered muscular strength in the affected side of the face, arm, and leg. These individuals may also have problems maintaining their balance as well as shifting their weight. The patient may have difficulty sitting because one side is weak and cannot correct the body's position if it begins to slide on the affected and weakened side. Treatment for paresis focuses on alleviating symptoms—like strengthening the muscle via physical therapy—as well as preventing the underlying cause that originally damaged upper motor neurons—like aspirin therapy to reduce the chance of stroke.

Jennifer L. Hellier

See also: Cerebral Palsy; Motor Neurons; Multiple Sclerosis; Muscular Dystrophy (Duchenne); Paralysis; Stroke

Further Reading

Kandel, E. R., Schwartz, J. H., Jessell, T. M., Siegelbaum, S. A., & Hudspeth, A. J. (Eds.). (2012). *Principles of neural science* (5th ed.). New York, NY: McGraw-Hill.

Knierim, J. (1997). Disorders of the motor system. In *Neuroscience Online, an electronic textbook for the neurosciences* (Chap. 6). Open-access educational resource provided by the Department of Neurobiology and Anatomy at the University of Texas Medical School at Houston. Retrieved from http://nba.uth.tmc.edu/neuroscience/m/s3/chapter06.html

Pulman, J., & Buckley, E. (2013). Assessing the efficacy of different upper limb hemiparesis interventions on improving health-related quality of life in stroke patients: a systematic review. *Topics in Stroke Rehabilitation, 20*(2), 171–188.

Yelnik, A. P., Simon, O., Parratte, B., & Gracies, J. M. (2010). How to clinically assess and treat muscle over activity in spastic paresis. *Journal of Rehabilitation Medicine, 42*(9), 801–807.

Parietal Lobe

The mammalian brain (or cerebrum) is made up of *gyri* (plural; *gyrus,* singular) and *sulci* (plural; *sulcus,* singular). Together these make up the bumps and grooves that give the brain a convoluted and unique form. The cerebrum is divided into four major divisions with the *parietal lobe* being located posterior (toward the back)

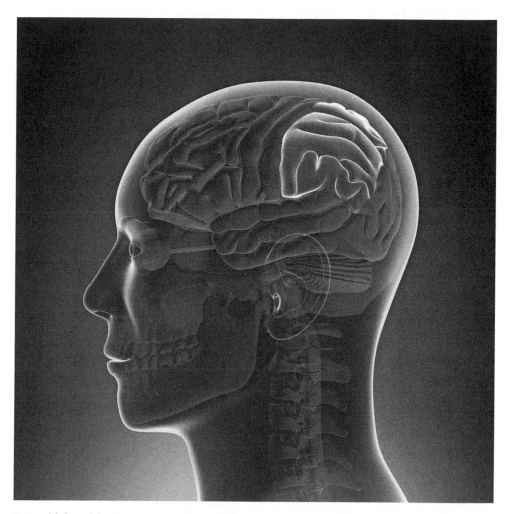

Parietal lobe of the human brain. (Dreamstime.com)

to the frontal lobe, anterior (toward the front) to the occipital lobe, and superior (above) to the temporal lobe. The parietal lobe is generally associated with integrating sensory information as well as spatial orientation. It has also been shown to be important for processing language and spirituality. Because there are two hemispheres of the brain, there are two parietal lobes present, both with the same functions.

Anatomical Divisions

The cerebrum is divided into four lobes that are named after the bones that overlie them: *frontal, parietal, temporal,* and *occipital* lobes. Each lobe has its own distinct function but in general the cerebral cortex of the lobes is organized in a similar way with six horizontal layers. The parietal lobe has three distinct anatomical boundaries. First, the *central sulcus* separates the parietal lobe anteriorly from the frontal lobe. The central sulcus is a prominent landmark in the mammalian brain as it is the longest, uninterrupted, "straight" groove on the lateral aspect of the cerebral hemispheres. Second, the *parieto-occipital sulcus* divides the posterior portion of the parietal lobe from the anterior portion of the occipital lobe. Lastly, the *lateral* or *Sylvian fissure* separates the ventral (toward the chin) region of the parietal lobe from the dorsal (toward the top of the skull) region of the temporal lobe. It is important to note that in humans and monkeys, the directional terms dorsal (back) and ventral (front) are different in the head compared to other mammals. This is because during development, the brain rotates forward. Thus, dorsal is the top of the skull while ventral is under the chin.

The parietal lobe is divided into anterior and posterior portions. The posterior parietal lobe can be further divided into the *superior parietal lobule* and the *inferior parietal lobule.* Within these regions, specific gyri have specific functions. Within the anterior parietal lobe, the narrow strip of brain tissue found just posterior to the central sulcus is called the *postcentral gyrus* and is the *primary somatosensory cortex.* Thus, the somatosensory cortex is the most anterior portion of the parietal lobe. Moving toward the occipital lobe, the somatosensory cortex and the posterior parietal lobe are separated by the *postcentral sulcus.* Lastly, the *intraparietal sulcus* divides the superior parietal lobule and the inferior parietal lobule.

Function

The postcentral gyrus is the somatosensory cortex with the function of integrating and processing all sensory information from the body's surface and the underlying viscera. It is also important for the perception of the senses, particularly of touch, pain, and temperature. The somatosensory cortex is often referred to as *Brodmann areas 3, 1, and 2.* The number order for the somatosensory cortex may seem strange to the reader. This is because when German anatomist Korbinian Brodmann (1868–1918) first sectioned the brain, he did so at an oblique angle. The first area he studied was named *Brodmann area 1*. As he continued his research, he continued to number the regions based on the order he studied them. Today, when looking at the somatosensory cortex from the rostral (toward the nose) to caudal (toward the tail) direction, the somatosensory cortex is numbered 3, 1, and 2.

The superior parietal lobule is a sensory association cortex, meaning it is used to integrate and process additional sensory information such as vision. Its integration of visual signals are used in spatial orientation of where the body is in space (body image) as well as where the body is in comparison to other items. This region is also known as *Brodmann areas 5 and 7*. The main function of Brodmann area 5 is being an association cortex to the somatosensory cortex, while the primary function of Brodmann area 7 is involved with spatial awareness. Most neuroanatomists consider this region the *dorsal stream of vision* (the vision of "where" something is), while the *ventral stream of vision* (the vision of "what" or "how") projects to the temporal lobe.

The inferior parietal lobule is a sensory association cortex that processes auditory information as well as language. It is also known as *Brodmann areas 39 and 40*. In most humans, the function of language is dispersed along the left hemisphere. Thus, the inferior parietal lobule, just around the posterior end of the lateral fissure, is called *Wernicke's area*. This region is not only involved with understanding language but also the ability to read.

When Wernicke's area is injured, most commonly following a stroke, the result is a form of *aphasia*. Aphasia occurs when a person is unable to communicate. This means they cannot be understood by their audience, nor are they able to express themselves through writing. When a person has aphasia resulting from injury to Wernicke's area, a condition known as Wernicke's aphasia, the words spoken by the patient flow freely but they are nonsensical and difficult to interpret.

In the cerebrum, there are two main regions that are important for language: Wernicke's and Broca's areas. As Wernicke's area is found posterior to the lateral fissure and within the parietal lobe, Broca's area is a specialized region of the frontal lobe located adjacent to the temporal lobe and primary motor cortex. Broca's area was first described by French physician Pierre Paul Broca (1824–1880) after he saw two patients that had lost their ability to use language. These patients, Leborgne and Lelong, had severe language deficits in which Leborgne could only say the word "tan" and Lelong could only say the words "yes, no, three, always, and lelo (a variation of his last name)." This type of language deficit is called *Broca's aphasia* or *expressive aphasia*. *Wernicke's aphasia,* or *receptive aphasia,* was originally described by German physician Karl Wernicke (1848–1905). In 1874, Wernicke published his results of studying two patients with profound deficits in their comprehension of the spoken language. Though these patients had no problems forming sounds, the sounds that they formed did not resemble any words in German or any other language. This has been described more recently as "cocktail chatter." Further, the patients did not appear to notice that anything had been disrupted with their speech patterns. Upon examination of one of the patient's brains at autopsy, Wernicke noticed a lesion in the left hemisphere, just posterior to, or behind, the primary auditory cortex. This portion of the brain has been shown to be responsible for sound processing and ultimately hearing.

In addition to being association cortices, recent studies have shown that both the left and right parietal lobes (particularly the inferior parietal lobule) may be involved with a person's understanding of spirituality or self-transcendence. Specifically, an imaging study revealed that the fronto-parieto-temporal network was activated when the person was describing spiritual experiences. This study suggests that there is a neurobiological basis for religious attitudes and behaviors in humans (Urgesi et al., 2010).

Diseases and Disorders

Damage to the parietal lobe can cause devastating consequences. As previously stated, receptive aphasia can occur following damage to Wernicke's area. Aphasia is a language disorder that affects a person's ability to speak, write, read, and listen. Patients with receptive aphasia usually do not know that what they are saying is nonsensical to their audience. In fact, they also lose meanings of words. For example, if the person is asked, "How much does a candy bar cost?" They may answer 100 dollars. They may give that same answer to the question of, "How much do you have to spend to buy a new car?"

Since the right side of the brain controls or receives information for the left side of the body, and vice versa, specific signs or symptoms can be seen when the parietal lobe is injured. Specifically, lesions to the right parietal lobe result in the loss of imagery, problems understanding visual relationships, and spatial neglect of the left side of the body. This neglect of one side of the body is called *hemispatial neglect*. It is often caused by stroke and is characterized by the inability to attend to or interact with people or objects on the opposite side of the affected area. In severe cases, the person may act as if the left side of their body never existed. Treatment for hemispatial neglect includes rehabilitating the patient using visual scanning training, caloric stimulation, neck muscle vibration, and prism adaptation (Striemer et al., 2013). Damage to the left parietal lobe causes problems in understanding: symbols—both written letters and mathematics—and language.

Jennifer L. Hellier

See also: Aphasia; Broca's Area; Brodmann Areas; Cerebral Cortex; Somatosensory Cortex/Somatosensory System; Visual System; Wernicke's Area

Further Reading

Dafny, N. (1997). Overview of the nervous systems. In *Neuroscience Online, an electronic textbook for the neurosciences* (Chap. 1). Open-access educational resource provided by the Department of Neurobiology and Anatomy at the University of Texas Medical School at Houston. Retrieved from http://neuroscience.uth.tmc.edu/s2/chapter01.html

Striemer, C. L., Ferber, S., & Danckert, J. (2013). Spatial working memory deficits represent a core challenge for rehabilitating neglect. *Frontiers in Human Neuroscience, 7,* 334.

Urgesi, C., Aglioti, S. M., Skrap, M., & Fabbro, F. (2010). The spiritual brain: Selective cortical lesions modulate human self-transcendence. *Neuron, 65*(3), 309–319.

Van Vleet, T. M., & DeGutis, J. M. (2013). The nonspatial side of spatial neglect and related approaches to treatment. *Progress in Brain Research, 207,* 327–349.

Vuilleumier, P. (2013). Mapping the functional neuroanatomy of spatial neglect and human parietal lobe functions: Progress and challenges. *Annals of the New York Academy of Sciences, 1296,* 50–74.

Parkinsonism (Drug-Induced)

When a patient presents for the first time with tremor, rigidity, slowness of movement, and balance problems, it is defined as *Parkinsonism symptoms*. Physicians are not always sure that these patients have Parkinson's disease (PD), which is the degeneration of dopamine neurons in the substantia nigra. This is because of all patients that present with these symptoms, only 85 percent actually have PD (Shin and Chung, 2009). In these cases, other causes need to be explored.

Other neurodegenerative diseases and vascular problems can cause Parkinsonism, but with the growing number of the population taking multiple medications, drugs are the second most common cause for these symptoms. The elderly as well as women are more susceptible, but it can affect patients of all age groups. Other risk factors for *drug-induced Parkinsonism* include preexisting extrapyramidal disorder, dementia, human immunodeficiency virus (HIV) infection, and familial PD. Usually symptoms will resolve after discontinuation of the drug, although it may take months and in some cases may persist. In other cases, the symptoms have unmasked PD itself and it is in this case that further treatment would be warranted. The key is for providers to have an understanding of drug-induced Parkinsonism and to use it in a differential diagnosis so that PD is not misdiagnosed.

Traditionally, drug-induced Parkinsonism was thought to be mainly caused by typical antispyschotics (haloperidol) and more recently the atypical antipsychotics (olanzapine, quetiapine, clozapine, etc.). These agents control pychoses in patients by antagonizing dopamine receptors and after years of being on these drugs, symptoms mimicking PD have been seen. PD is diagnosed by the degeneration of dopamine in the striatum nigra, and since these drugs effectively mimic this, parkinonsim is sometimes seen. Other drugs outside of the typical/atypical antipsychotic class also work by blocking dopamine and Parkinsonism is seen in these agents as well. Antiemetics, which help control nausea and vomiting, inhibit dopamine and thus Parkinsonism can be induced. Other medications not directly acting on dopamine receptors, such as calcium channel blockers, antidepressants, and antiepileptics, have been implicated in drug-induced Parkinsonism albeit to a lesser degree. The pathophysiology is not understood in these agents, however they have still occurred and cannot be ruled out as a potential cause in a patient presenting with Parkinsonism symptoms.

Managing these symptoms can be done in several different ways. In general, a simple change to a different medication in the same class is an obvious choice. In the case of schizophrenia, where the only class of treatment presently is using antipsychotic medications, using a drug with the lowest incidence of Parkinsonism symptoms at the lowest effective dose is the best option. Another option is to use anticholinergic agents which have been proven to have benefit, although treating a drug's side effect with another drug is usually a practice providers want to avoid. Anticholinergic medications come with their own array of side effects and they are a class of medications that is not recommended in the elderly, who make up a large percentage of drug-induced Parkinsonism cases.

Jeremy E. Brothers

See also: Parkinson's Disease

Further Reading

Shin, H. W., & Chung, S. J. (2009). Drug-induced Parkinsonism. *Journal of Clinical Neurology, 8*(1), 15–21.

Thanvi, B., & Treadwell, S. (2009). Drug induced Parkinsonism: A common cause of Parkinsonism in older people. *Postgraduate Medical Journal, 85*(1004), 322–326.

Parkinson's Disease

Parkinson's disease is a progressive neurodegenerative disorder that is characterized by the presence of tremor at rest, rigidity, bradykinesia (slowed or decreased motor movement), and postural instability. James Parkinson (1755–1824), an English physician, first described these clinical features in 1817. Nearly 1 million people in the United States suffer from Parkinson's disease and it is the third most common neurological disorder in the elderly. The average age of disease onset is

60 years, with a higher incidence reported among males. While the true cause is not known, it is most likely the result of interactions between aging, genetics, and environmental factors. A key factor is loss of specific neurons located deep in the brain that project to neurons in another part of the brain. Specifically, it is the degeneration of dopaminergic neurons (cells that release dopamine—a neurotransmitter used for activating neurons) in the substantia nigra ("black substance"—a pigmented structure located in the midbrain) that project to the striatum (a mass of striped white and gray matter found in front of the thalamus). These dopaminergic neurons in the substantia nigra naturally die off as a person ages; however, when these neurons die early and in very large numbers, Parkinson's disease develops. While Parkinson's disease cannot be cured, treatment provides patients with improved motor function, which in turn increases a patient's quality of life. Treatment choice will depend on a patient's functional status and age.

Pathophysiology

While the true cause of Parkinson's disease is not known, it is most likely the result of interactions between aging, genetics, and environmental factors. Two important pathological features of Parkinson's disease are depigmentation, or loss of dopamine-producing neurons and the presence of Lewy bodies, which are abnormal collection of proteins within a nerve cell. Many substances are found within Lewy bodies, the most important being a protein called alpha-synuclein, which is found in a clumped form that neurons cannot break down. In the early stages of Parkinson's disease, Lewy bodies are found in different parts of the brainstem—the medulla oblongata (regulates breathing and heart rate), locus coeruleus (assists in stress responses), and raphe nuclei (involved in pain sensation)—and the olfactory bulb (essential for the sense of smell). The presence of these Lewy bodies correlates with symptoms of anxiety, depression, and an impaired sense of smell. As the disease progresses, Lewy bodies spread to the cortex, thus affecting or correlating with cognitive and additional behavior changes.

Clinically detectable symptoms of motor degeneration occur at 70–80 percent loss of dopamine-producing neurons within the substantia nigra. The substantia nigra is an area of the brain where cells produce dopamine, which is an important neurotransmitter that controls muscle movement. This degeneration of neurons may also be present in the basal ganglia, spinal cord, and neocortex. Dopamine neurons project from the substantia nigra to the striatum and synapse on two major populations of dopamine receptor-mediated neurons that control motor activity. In Parkinson's disease, the degeneration of dopaminergic neurons results in reduced activity within these pathways leading to motor deficiencies.

Symptoms

The hallmark features of Parkinson's disease are tremor, bradykinesia, and rigidity. Postural instability occurs much later in the course of the disease. The tremor in Parkinson's disease is described as a "pill-rolling" and a resting tremor. This means that the tremor is most noticeable when the affected body part is supported by gravity and is not engaged in any purposeful activity—at rest. Tremors in other conditions, such as an essential tremor or multiple sclerosis, are referred to as action tremors because the tremor occurs when the affected limb is being used. While a Parkinsonian tremor may occur with action, it is much more severe at rest.

In early stages of the disease, the tremor is most often intermittent and may not be noticeable to others. As the disease progresses, the tremor becomes more evident. Nearly 70 percent of patients will present with tremor being their first symptom. The tremor usually begins unilaterally (to one side) in the hand and then spreads contralaterally (to the other side) several years after the onset of symptoms. While hands are most often affected, the tremor can also involve the legs, lips, jaw, and tongue. Anxiety or stressful situations can exacerbate the tremor.

Bradykinesia is a generalized slowness of movement. It is a major cause of disability in Parkinson's disease and is eventually seen in all patients. A progressive slowing and decline in dexterity (skill or grace of motor movement, generally refers to the use of hands) can impair tasks including hand clapping and handwriting. In the arms, bradykinesia begins distally in the fingers. Tasks like buttoning clothes, tying shoelaces, and typing/keyboarding become difficult to perform. In the legs, patients commonly complain of shuffling while walking. In addition, it may be difficult for patients to stand from a seated position or get out of the car. As the disease progresses, festination may develop, which is the involuntary quickening of a person's gait (walking). James Parkinson defined festination as "an irresistible impulse to take much quicker and shorter steps, and thereby to adopt unwillingly a running pace."

Rigidity occurs in 90 percent of patients with Parkinson's disease and is described as increased resistance to passive movement about a joint. Cogwheel rigidity can be seen in the disease and refers to a ratchety pattern of resistance and relaxation as the doctor moves the limb through its full range of motion. While many patients develop Cogwheel rigidity, not all patients will. Rigidity can affect all parts of the body and ultimately contribute to complaints of stiffness and pain.

Finally, postural instability is an impairment of centrally mediated postural reflexes (along the spine) that cause feelings of imbalance. This symptom leaves patients at significant risk for falls and injury. Postural instability is seen in late progression of the illness. It can be tested clinically with the "pull" test. An examiner stands behind the patient and pulls them by the shoulders. Those with normal postural reflexes are able to maintain balance by stepping backward with one step. A Parkinson's patient with postural instability is likely to fall or take multiple steps backward.

Neuropsychiatric abnormalities may also develop in later stages of the disease. Intellectual deterioration may occur in some patients and can be difficult to distinguish from Alzheimer's disease and other dementia related conditions. Patients with Parkinson's disease are also at increased risk for anxiety and depression, in addition to autonomic and sensory symptoms. These symptoms include bladder disturbances, constipation, and fatigue. Patients may also experience drooling, sweating, and sexual dysfunction.

Diagnosis

Recognizing Parkinson's disease in its early stages can be challenging as patients may present with varying degree and severity of symptoms. The diagnosis of Parkinson's disease is based on clinical impression, as there are no physiological tests or blood work to confirm the diagnosis. The gold standard for diagnosis is neuropathologic examination. Parkinson's disease can be diagnosed when at least two of the following are present: limb muscle rigidity, resting tremor, or bradykinesia. Other clinical features that are generally present are unilateral onset, presence of a tremor at rest, and a persistent asymmetry throughout the course of the disease.

In addition, an excellent response to dopaminergic therapy is an important criterion for diagnosis. A medication challenge test may be recommended if a diagnosis of Parkinson's disease is uncertain and symptoms are bothersome. A medication commonly used to treat the symptoms of Parkinson's, either levodopa or a dopamine agonist, is administered for at least two months. If the patient's symptoms improve, the diagnosis of Parkinson's disease is likely.

Treatment

While there is no known cure for Parkinson's disease, there are many treatment options available to manage symptoms. Most medications work by increasing levels of dopamine in the brain. The goals of treatment are to improve both motor and nonmotor symptoms so that patients are able to maintain a high quality of life. Once a person is diagnosed with Parkinson's disease, it is important to consider both pharmacological (the use of prescription drugs) and nonpharmacological options.

Nonpharmacological options include lifestyle changes that have shown to improve some patient outcomes. Often, it is recommended that patients go through physical therapy, speech therapy, and occupational therapy in order to learn to cope with motor changes characteristic of the disease. Exercise and diet are also important considerations. Many patients with Parkinson's disease are at an increased risk for poor nutrition, weight loss, and loss of muscle mass. All patients should be assessed for physical factors that may interfere with nutrition, such as chewing and swallowing problems, poor dentition (problems with their teeth), and impaired ability to prepare meals. It is important to encourage a balanced diet that includes fiber and fluid to prevent constipation, while taking calcium to maintain bone structure.

First-line medications for symptomatic treatment in early disease stages include levodopa, dopamine agonists, and monoamine oxidase type B inhibitors. Levodopa is a prodrug or a precursor for dopamine. It crosses the blood-brain barrier where it is converted to dopamine. Only about 2 percent of drug enters the brain, while the rest is metabolized by decarboxylation in the gut and other peripheral tissues to dopamine. Once it is converted to dopamine, it cannot cross the blood-brain barrier. For this reason, levodopa is administered in combination with carbidopa. Carbidopa inhibits the peripheral decarboxylation of levodopa, thus increasing the amount of levodopa that reaches the brain and being converted to dopamine. This combination of drugs is very effective in managing the clinical features of Parkinsonism, but is most effective against bradykinesia. It is important to carefully manage a patient's dose in order to minimize adverse reactions that may include dyskinesias and nausea.

Dopamine agonists selectively activate dopamine receptors such as D1, D2, and D3. Bromocriptine is a D2 receptor agonist and partial D1 antagonist and is classified as an ergot derivative (originating from a fungus). Ropinirole is a D2 receptor agonist and pramipexole a D3 receptor agonist, both are classified as nonergot derivatives. Dopamine agonists may cause nausea, hallucinations, or sedation (including sudden sleepiness called sleep attacks). It is important to start at a low dose and increase it gradually to reduce these adverse events.

Monoamine oxidase type B inhibitors decrease the breakdown of dopamine, thus dopamine will remain longer in the extracellular space for neurons to use. Selegeline and rasagiline are two MAO-B inhibitors that are used as adjunct therapy in patients who are not responding well to levodopa therapy. MAO-B inhibitors delay onset of motor complications compared to levodopa, but may be less effective in treating functional impairment and disability.

Other medications for early symptomatic disease include amantadine and anticholinergic drugs. Amantadine is an antiviral drug that is used for the treatment of influenza, but is also related to dopamine release. For this reason, it is thought to be effective in the treatment of Parkinson's disease. Anticholinergic agents, including benztropine mesylate, do not directly act on the dopaminergic system. Instead, they decrease the activity of acetylcholine (a neurotransmitter necessary for muscle movement at the neuromuscular junction) to match the decreased level of dopamine seen in Parkinson's disease. The anticholinergics are the most effective in the control of tremor, but should not be used in older patients as they may cause confusion and hallucinations.

Future

Michael J. Fox, a Canadian-American actor, has Parkinson's disease which was first diagnosed in the early 1990s. He publically announced his illness in 1998 and ever since has been an advocate for Parkinson's disease research and has brought the disease more attention from the general public and the media. Current research for Parkinson's disease focuses on deep brain stimulation, which is implanting a devise in the brain to stimulate dopamine neurons. This treatment is used to control the symptoms of Parkinson's disease, not to cure it. A more controversial therapy is using stem cell transplants to replace the dopaminergic neurons in the substantia nigra. This is ongoing research with clinical trials currently underway.

Conclusion

Parkinson's disease is a disorder that affects the brain's ability to control movement. The disease progressively worsens over time, although the rate of worsening varies from one person to another. The exact cause of Parkinson's disease is not known, but is thought to be related to the degeneration of neurons that produce dopamine. While Parkinson's disease cannot be cured, several treatment options are available to manage symptoms and improve a person's quality of life. Many people with Parkinson's disease who are treated early may be able to live years without serious disability.

Danielle Stutzman

See also: Dopamine and Its Receptors; Levodopa; Multiple Sclerosis; Parkinsonism (Drug-Induced); Tremor

Further Reading

National Institute of Neurological Disorders and Stroke. (2013). *NINDS Parkinson's disease information page.* Retrieved from http://www.ninds.nih.gov/disorders/parkinsons_disease/parkinsons_disease.htm

PubMed Health. (2012). *Parkinson's disease.* Retrieved from http://www.ncbi.nlm.nih.gov/pubmedhealth/PMH0001762/

Pavlov, Ivan (1849–1936)

Ivan Pavlov was a Russian physiologist whose work made an impact in creating behavioral studies still used in neuroscience today. He is most famous for his research in classical conditioning, where he studied dogs and their salivation. This

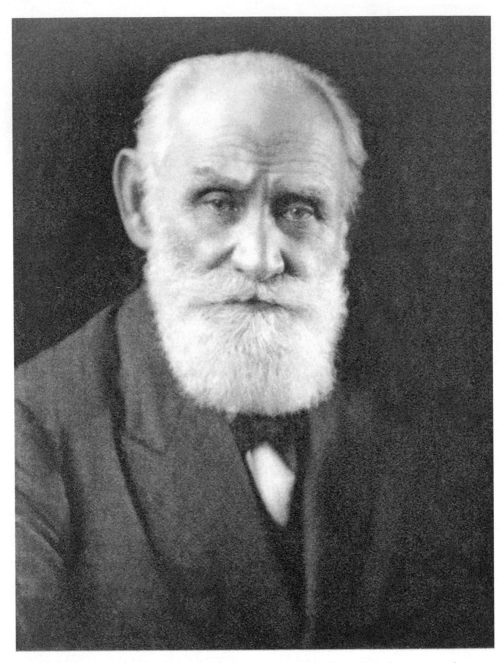

Russian scientist Ivan Pavlov is famous for his experiments with canines that are now known as "Pavlov's Dogs." Not only did his pioneering work on salivation and digestion further the field of physiology, the theory of "conditioned reflexes" played a major role in the development of the discipline of psychology. Pavlov was awarded the Nobel Prize for physiology or medicine in 1904 for his studies of digestion. (Library of Congress)

is commonly called Pavlov's dogs or Pavlovian conditioning. Classical conditioning pairs a condition stimulus with an unconditioned stimulus that results in a form of learning. Specifically, Pavlov noticed that dogs would salivate when they saw food. He called this an unconditioned response (salivating) to a biologically necessary stimulus—or unconditioned stimulus (food). He wondered if he could get the dogs to salivate to another stimulus such as a ringing bell (a conditioned stimulus). Thus, Pavlov was able to pair the two stimuli and conditioned the dogs to salivate whenever a bell was rung, even when food was not present. From his findings, Dr. Pavlov is considered the father of classical conditioning and behavior modification.

Ivan Petrovich Pavlov was born in 1849 in Ryazan, Russia, and was the oldest of 11 children. His father was a priest. Ivan decided to follow in his footsteps and enrolled in the theological seminary in Ryazan as a young man. While he was in seminary, Pavlov became interested in science from Russia's father of physiology, I. M. Secheno. At the age of 21, Pavlov decided to leave the seminary and enrolled in Saint Petersburg University in 1870. As a student, Pavlov won a gold medal for his research on the physiology of the pancreatic nerves. He then continued his education at the Academy of Medical Surgery where he won another gold medal in 1879. Pavlov worked with the famous Russian clinician S. P. Botkin in a physiology lab. There he was able to conduct animal experiments to test his hypotheses that animal behavior is best understood by physiology and not psychology (the study of the mind and its function).

Pavlov met his wife, Seraphima (Sara) Vasilievna Karchevskaya, in 1878 when Sara moved to Saint Petersburg to study education at the Pedagogical Institute. They married in 1881 and were too poor to live together. Once their finances improved, Ivan and Sara started their family. The Pavlovs' first son died as an infant, but they eventually had four surviving children—three boys and one girl.

In 1884, Pavlov moved to Germany where he perfected a dissection on the stomach of dogs called the Pavlov pouch. He then returned to Russia and worked at the Military Medical Academy for the next five years. Pavlov was recruited to the Institute of Experimental Medicine where he raised it to be one of the most important research centers over the 45 years while he was Chair. From 1901 to 1904, Pavlov was nominated for the Nobel Prize in Physiology or Medicine. In 1904, he was awarded the Nobel Prize for his work in the physiology of digestion. In his last days, Pavlov invited one of his students to record his dying days to describe the terminal phase of life from a subjective point of view. Pavlov died in 1936 at the age of 86.

Jennifer L. Hellier

See also: Behavioral Experiments

Further Reading

Saunders, B. R. (2007). *Ivan Pavlov exploring the mysteries of behavior. Berkeley heights.* New Jersey: Enslow Publishers.

Todes, D. P. (2000). *Ivan Pavlov: Exploring the animal machine.* USA: Oxford University Press.

Peduncles

The word *peduncle* means "little foot" in Latin. There are two groups of peduncles within the mammalian central nervous system: the *cerebral* and *cerebellar peduncles*. These are generally large groups of *axons* or *white matter* (named for their color that is caused by the surrounding myelin covering) that connect the different parts of the central nervous system together.

Cerebral Peduncles

The cerebral peduncles, also known as the "crus cerebri" (leg of the cerebrum), are a band of neuronal axons that resemble a stalk and connect various parts of the brain. By classification, the cerebral peduncles are everything in the *mesencephalon* (the midbrain) except for its *tectum* (roof or dorsal portion). There is one peduncle on each side of the brain. They help transmit electrical nerve signals from the higher part of the brain (cortex) and the brainstem to the rest of the central nervous system. Mainly, the cerebral peduncles are necessary for controlling body movement by perfecting the movement; otherwise, these movements would seem erratic and awkward coming directly from the cortex. The cerebral peduncles form a continuation of the *internal capsule* (a large region of white matter deep in the brain) of the cerebral hemispheres. Injury to the cerebral peduncles generally result in symptoms on the opposite side (contralateral) of the body that corresponds to the injured part of the peduncles.

Cerebellar Peduncles

There are three sets or six total cerebellar peduncles—two superior, two middle, and two inferior. The superior cerebellar peduncles are the primary output of the cerebellum. These fibers carry information to the midbrain. The middle cerebellar peduncles transmit inputs from the contralateral cerebral cortex. Finally, the inferior cerebellar peduncles receive proprioceptive information (motion and position of the body) from the ipsilateral (same) side of the body. Overall, the cerebellar peduncles are nerve tracts which permit communication between the cerebellum and other parts of the central nervous system.

Renee Johnson

See also: Cerebellum; Cerebral Cortex; White Matter

Further Reading

Nolte, J. (2009). *The Human Brain: An introduction to its functional anatomy with student consult online access*. 6th Ed. Philadelphia, PA: Mosby-Elsevier.

Penry, J. Kiffin (1929–1996)

J. Kiffin Penry was an American physician whose dedication made an impact in treating epilepsy that is still used today. Epilepsy is a disorder associated with abnormal synchronized neuronal firing (seizure activity), which can be debilitating. He is most famous for his work at the National Institutes of Health and in developing the Antiepileptic Drug Development Program, which he cofounded with Ewart A. Swinyard (1909–1997) and Harvey Kupferberg (ca. 1933–). It is this effort for which Penry is considered one of the fathers of antiepileptic drug development.

Penry was born in Denton, North Carolina, in 1929. He was interested in science and health care and applied to Bowman Gray School of Medicine after completing his degree at Wake Forest College. Penry was an excellent student and became a member of Phi Beta Kappa (the oldest honors society for the liberal arts and sciences) and Alpha Omega Alpha (the medical honor society). In 1955, Penry received his medical degree and began an internship at Pennsylvania Hospital in Philadelphia. He then moved to North Carolina to begin his first residency in internal medicine. His second residency was in neurology at Boston City Hospital. It was during this time when Penry was trained to not only be an excellent clinician and correlate pathology but also to use a humanitarian approach to medicine.

In 1966, Penry moved into a more political position and joined the National Institute of Neurological Diseases and Blindness. He was the Head of the Section on Epilepsy and Chief of Special Projects in the collaborative and field research section. He quickly moved up the ranks and became the Director of the Neurological Disorders Program and the Chief of the Epilepsy Branch at the National Institute of Neurological and Communicative Disorders and Stroke (this Institute has since been renamed). This was the beginning of his work in advancing research in epilepsy.

In 1979, there was a push to include epilepsy research with other neurological diseases in the Institute's new worldwide programs in neurology and neuroscience. Penry headed this effort and both clinical and basic research in epilepsy flourished. In turn, Penry was able to merge academia, biotechnology, and the National Institutes of Health to create the Antiepileptic Drug Development Program. As a clinician, Penry worked tirelessly to improve diagnoses and classifications of seizures and epileptic syndromes. Thus, he became the President of the American Epilepsy Society as well as the International League against Epilepsy.

In his push to improve seizure treatment, Penry realized that for years Europe was using valproate, an American-made antiepileptic drug, to successfully control seizures. However, valproate was not approved by the United States (U.S.) Food and Drug Administration (FDA), meaning clinicians were not able to prescribe this drug in the United States. Penry used his political power and his expertise in epilepsy to have the FDA approve valproate for use in the United States. For this work, Penry won several awards, including the William G. Lennox Award of the American Epilepsy Society, the Distinguished Clinical Investigator Milken Family Foundation Award, and the Epilepsy Foundation of America's 25th Year Anniversary Award. Penry died at the age of 66 from complications of diabetes in 1996. Today, J. Kiffin Penry has several epilepsy mini-fellowships (for clinicians to study seizures and epilepsy) that are named after him.

Jennifer L. Hellier

See also: Epilepsy; Seizures

Further Reading

J. Kiffin Penry Epilepsy Education Programs and Minifellow Network. (2014). Retrieved from http://www.minifellow.net/index.asp

Thomas, Robert McG. (1996, April 3). *Dr. J. Kiffin Penry, 66, leader in search for epilepsy treatments.* Retrieved from http://www.nytimes.com/1996/04/03/us/dr-j-kiffin-penry-66-leader-in-search-for-epilepsy-treatments.html

Peripheral Nervous System

Nerves are bundles of axons that are outside of the central nervous system (CNS) while *ganglia* are groups of neuronal cell bodies that are outside of the CNS. The *peripheral nervous system* (PNS) is made up of both nerves and ganglia and its primary role is to connect the CNS to the organs, limbs, and skin. The nerves of the PNS extend from the CNS to these outermost areas of the body. Axons that originate from neurons located in the CNS make up the PNS and are responsible for delivering signals to the most distant parts of our body. The PNS, unlike the CNS, is not protected by bone or by the blood-brain barrier. This makes it vulnerable to toxins and mechanical injury.

Anatomy and Physiology

The PNS consists of 31 pairs of spinal nerves that originate in the spinal cord and 12 pairs of cranial nerves that originate in the brain. There are two important types of cells within the PNS: *glial cells* and *neurons*. Glial cells of the PNS include Schwann cells which surround nerve fibers and perineuronal satellite cells that surround the cell bodies. Both types of cells produce myelin sheaths around axons and some cell bodies of ganglia. Myelin is essential for fast communication between neurons. Schwann cells also have the ability to become phagocytotic in response to nerve injury and inflammation. Neurons specialize in rapid nerve impulse conduction, allowing for the exchange of signals with other neurons. The body of the neuron, or soma, is located in the CNS while the axon projects and terminates in the skin, organs, or muscles allowing for rapid communication between the CNS and PNS.

Somatic and Autonomic Nervous Systems

The PNS is divided into two parts: the *somatic* and *autonomic nervous systems*. The somatic nervous system conveys and processes conscious and unconscious sensory information including vision, pain, and touch. Additionally, this system is responsible for motor control of voluntary (striated, skeletal) muscles, allowing for coordinated muscle activity that can be adjusted based on an animal's environment. This system contains two major types of neurons: sensory neurons (afferent neurons) that carry information from the nerves in the periphery to the CNS and motor neurons (or efferent neurons) that carry information away from the CNS toward muscle fibers throughout the body.

In addition to controlling voluntary movements, the somatic nervous system is associated with involuntary movements. These involuntary movements are known as reflex arcs, during which muscles move involuntarily without input from the brain through a nerve pathway that connects directly to the spinal cord. Placing one's hand on a hot stove and pulling it away quickly is an example of a reflex arc. A sensory receptor responds to an environmental stimulus (hot stove) and afferent fibers (A-delta and C pain fibers) convey this signal through peripheral nerves to the gray matter of the spinal cord. The afferent root enters the spinal cord and synapses with an interneuron, which synapses with alpha motoneurons. Alpha-motoneurons transmit an impulse to voluntary (striated, skeletal) muscles, causing the person to pull his or her hand away.

The autonomic nervous system conveys and processes sensory input from visceral organs in addition to motor control of the involuntary (smooth) and cardiac musculature. It is responsible for control of involuntary or visceral bodily functions including cardiovascular, respiratory, digestive, urinary, and reproductive systems. Examples of these body functions include heartbeat, digestion, and breathing. Additionally, it plays a key role in the way the body handles stress and recovers from stressful situations.

Sympathetic and Parasympathetic Nervous Systems

The autonomic nervous system is further divided into the sympathetic and parasympathetic nervous systems. The sympathetic nervous system regulates the "fight-or-flight" response, allowing the body to function under stress. A sympathetic response dilates pupils, inhibits salivation, relaxes the bronchi (to ease breathing), decreases digestive activity, and stimulates secretion of epinephrine and norepinephrine from the adrenal medulla. Additionally, stimulation increases blood flow to skeletal muscles, increases chronotropic (heart rate) and inotropic (contraction strength) effects of the heart, and releases glucose stores from the liver. All of these reactions enable a person to respond immediately to an emergent, stressful situation such as avoiding a car accident while driving.

Based on the organization of the sympathetic nervous system, it is also referred to as the *thoracolumbar* or *adrenergic system.* All *preganglionic fibers* within the sympathetic nervous system emerge from the thoracic and upper two lumbar levels of the spinal cord. Norepinephrine and epinephrine are the primary neurotransmitters released by *postganglionic fibers* within this system and are responsible for many effects seen in the fight–or-flight" response. The sympathetic nervous system is designed to exert its effects over widespread body regions for a sustained period of time.

The parasympathetic nervous system regulates the "rest and digest" response, returning one's body to normal function in order to conserve physical resources. A parasympathetic response constricts pupils, stimulates salivation, reduces heart rate, constricts bronchi, stimulates digestive activity, and contracts the bladder. All of these responses allow a person to conserve energy during times of relaxation, preparing them for more stressful situations. The vagus nerve (cranial nerve X) is the main regulator of automatic functions within the parasympathetic nervous system.

The parasympathetic nervous system is also referred to as the *craniosacral* or *cholinergic system.* Preganglionic fibers within the parasympathetic nervous system emerge with several cranial nerve pairs (III—oculomotor, VII—facial, IX—glossopharyngeal, and X—vagus) and at the sacral division (S2–S4) of the spinal cord. Acetylcholine is the neurotransmitter released by postganglionic fibers within the parasympathetic nervous system and is responsible for many effects of "rest and digest." The parasympathetic nervous system is organized to respond transiently to a stimulus in a localized region of the body.

Danielle Stutzman

See also: Afferent Tracts; Autonomic Nervous System; Blood-Brain Barrier; Central Nervous System (CNS); Cranial Nerves; Efferent Tracts; Pain

Further Reading

Kandel, E. R., Schwartz, J. H., Jessell, T. M., Siegelbaum, S., & Hudspeth, A. J. (2013). *Principles of neural science* (5th ed.). United States: McGraw-Hill Companies, Inc.

Kiernan, J. A. (2009). *Barr's the human nervous system: An anatomical viewpoint* (9th ed.). Baltimore, MD: Lippincott Williams & Wilkins.

Noback, C. R., Strominger, N. L., Demarest, R. J., & Ruggiero, D. A. (2005). *The human nervous system structure and function* (6th ed.). Totowa, NJ: Humana Press.

Peripheral Neuropathy

In mammals, there are two distinct nervous systems: the central nervous system (brain, brainstem, and the spinal cord) and the peripheral nervous system (the nerves serving the face, head, and body that send to and receive signals from the central nervous system). The autonomic nervous system is part of the peripheral nervous system and controls involuntary functions that are below the level of consciousness. The term *peripheral neuropathy,* or just *neuropathy,* is a universal expression to describe a myriad of syndromes that cause disease or damage to the peripheral nerves. The nerves that could be affected by peripheral neuropathy are: the *sensory nerves* that receive sensations of heat, pain, or touch; the *motor nerves* that control voluntary motor movements; and, the *autonomic nerves* that control blood pressure, heart rate, digestion, and bladder function. Depending on the severity of the disorder and/or which nerve is damaged, neuropathy can affect sensation, movement, or gland/organ function. This damage results in the nerve's decreased ability to transmit and/or receive its signals to and from the central nervous system. In mild cases of neuropathy, a person may feel a tingling sensation, numbness, or a prickling sensation (*paresthesia*) when using a certain body part for movement. A person with severe neuropathy, however, may experience muscle wasting (*hypotrophy*), paralysis, or organ dysfunction, such as having problems digesting food.

Types

Neuropathies are classified by as *acute, chronic,* or *idiopathic.* Cases of acute peripheral neuropathies have a sudden onset and progress quickly. In these cases, an urgent diagnosis and treatment must be made to ensure that the neuropathy can resolve. An example of acute neuropathy is *Guillain-Barré syndrome.* In chronic neuropathies, the condition is long term and symptoms progress slowly and may be subtle. In fact, a person may not even realize that they are experiencing any signs until it is more severe. Some patients will have bouts of relief, but the symptoms usually return. In other cases, some persons will have a progression of symptoms that eventually plateau. Chronic neuropathies are usually the cause of another disorder such as diabetes. Lastly, idiopathic neuropathies are named as such because the cause is unknown.

Single Nerve Damage

If a single nerve is damaged, it results in a condition called *mononeuropathy.* This is usually caused by localized nerve compression or trauma (such as an infection) to a region supplied by a single nerve. Physical compression of the nerve is the most common cause of mononeuropathy, such as *carpal tunnel syndrome* where the median nerve is compressed as it travels through the wrist; or when a person is sitting with their leg crossed for an extended period of time resulting in the foot "falling asleep." This is a temporary condition and the pins and needles sensation is caused by a compression mononeuropathy. By moving around and adjusting to a better position, a person can be easily relieved from this condition.

An example of damage to a single nerve is seen in *Bell's palsy.* This condition is characterized by unilateral (one sided) temporary weakness or total paralysis of the muscles innervated by the facial nerve (cranial nerve VII). Cranial nerve VII is responsible for controlling the muscles of facial expression and for the sense of taste from the anterior two-thirds of the tongue. It also provides innervation to lacrimal glands (tears), salivary glands, and the stapes (a bone in the middle ear used for hearing). Patients with Bell's palsy suffer a temporary inability to control the muscles of the face that include movements like smiling and raising eyebrows.

Multiple Nerve Damage

It is most common for more than one nerve to be affected. This is a condition called *polyneuropathy* and generally affects more than one limb or several regions of a body. Polyneuropathy is a serious condition because of the large regions it affects as well as the fact that it usually produces symmetrical symptoms on both sides of the body. These may include: muscle weakness; awkward movements; tingling and/

or burning sensations covering large areas; the loss of fine touch like the inability to distinguish between textures; problems feeling temperatures; and difficulty in balance when standing or walking. Most of these symptoms tend to appear first in nerves that are long such as those that supply the feet and hands, and over time progress toward the trunk. Common causes of polyneuropathies are diabetes, Lyme disease, blood disorders, and neurotoxins.

Three types of polyneuropathy include *distal axonopathy, demyelinating poly-neuropathies,* and *neuronopathy.* In distal axonopathy, the axons (or the output of the neurons) are damaged while the cell bodies are normal. This is seen most often in patients with diabetes and presents with a very distinct pattern of progression. The farthest part of the axon is damaged first and the cell death slowly progresses toward the trunk as the disease advances. Thus, a person first loses sensation in their toes and the soles of their feet, then their lower leg, and eventually the entire leg. Next, the hands are affected starting with the fingers, the palms, and then the entire arm. Ultimately, the trunk of the body can be affected.

In demyelinating polyneuropathies, the protective covering of the axon (the myelin) is affected. This results in decreased ability to conduct nerve impulses along the length of the axon. Persons with this type of disease often have muscle weakness and decreased sensation because the nerve impulse is weakened in both motor and sensory nerves. The most common cause of this type of polyneuropathy is multiple sclerosis.

Finally, neuronopathy is a rare polyneuropathy and is the opposite of distal axonopathy. Here the cell body of the neuron is damaged and the axon is relatively fine. Usually only one type of neuron is affected such as motor neurons, which their cell bodies located in the spinal cord and their axons are the peripheral nerves. This would produce a syndrome called motor neuron disease with most sensory function being normal. If the sensory neurons are damaged, then it can disturb pain, temperature, touch sensation and its ability to be perceived by the brain, but motor function may be unchanged.

Two or More Isolated Nerve Damage

Mononeuritis multiplex is a term used to describe two or more isolated nerves that have damage, which causes neuropathies in separate parts of the body. This is a rarer condition compared to polyneuropathy and mononeuropathy. This asymmetric loss of sensation and motor function may occur acutely or subacutely. As the disease process continues, the symptoms become more symmetrical making it similar to polyneuropathy. Thus, it can be difficult for a health care provider to properly diagnose in late-stages of a disease, especially if the symptoms are symmetrical. In general, pain is the first complaint and is described as deep and aching that worsens at night within the lower back, hip joint, or leg. Patients with diabetes often will experience an acute unilateral pain in the thigh that eventually results in loss of the knee reflex (areflexia) and muscle weakness of the quadriceps (anterior muscles of the thigh).

Autonomic Nerve Damage

A form of polyneuropathy that affects the involuntary actions of the body, particularly those of the internal organs, is called *autonomic neuropathy*. Here the functions of the bladder, lungs, digestive track, genitals, and the cardiovascular system may be affected. Within the thorax, abdomen, and pelvis, a large collection of cell bodies (ganglia) and their output fibers are found along the dorsal surfaces and are outside of the spinal cord. These ganglia and nerve fibers are part of the autonomic nervous system and are connected to the spinal cord by the peripheral nerves. If these ganglia or nerves are damaged, it results in autonomic neuropathy. Additionally, some conditions that damage the brain and spinal cord can also produce autonomic neuropathy. Persons who have had diabetes for many years or decades are the typical patients presenting with autonomic neuropathy. Common symptoms include but are not limited to bladder incontinence—where the person is unable to control urine from leaking; urine retention—where a person is unable to urinate; difficulty breathing—especially when asleep called central sleep apnea; abdominal pain, nausea, vomiting, or fecal incontinence; genital impotence; and, tachycardia (abnormal fast heart rate), bradycardia (abnormally slow heart rate at rest), or insufficient increase in heart rate during exertion.

Treatment

As with all medical conditions, the primary cause of the neuropathy must be treated first to best control the disease process. Symptoms are then treated to alleviate pain and to improve muscle control while maintaining muscle strength. Drugs that normally are used for controlling seizures (antiepileptic drugs like valproate or gabapentin) and mood (antidepressants) have shown to be effective in improving neuropathic pain. External electrical stimulation of the affected nerve can improve diabetic-induced neuropathies, especially when continued for several treatments. Nonetheless, symptoms will eventually return after treatment is discontinued. Finally, the temperature of the environment, like living in warmer climates, has shown to improve and manage neuropathies.

Patricia A. Bloomquist

See also: Bell's Palsy (Bell Palsy); Diabetes Mellitus; Guillain-Barré Syndrome; Lyme Disease; Nerves; Pain; Paralysis; Reflex

Further Reading

Donofrio, P. D. (Ed.). (2012). *Textbook of peripheral neuropathy.* New York, NY: Demos Medical Publishing.

The Foundation of Peripheral Neuropathy. (2014). *What is peripheral neuropathy?* Retrieved from https://www.foundationforpn.org/livingwithperipheralneuropathy/

Mayo Clinic Staff. (2013). *Diseases and conditions: Peripheral neuropathy.* Retrieved from http://www.mayoclinic.org/diseases-conditions/peripheral-neuropathy/basics/definition/con-20019948

Morales-Vidal, S., Morgan, C., McCoyd, M., & Hornik, A. (2012). Diabetic peripheral neuropathy and the management of diabetic peripheral neuropathic pain. *Postgraduate Medicine, 124*(4), 145–153.

National Institute of Neurological Disorders and Stroke (NINDS). (2012). *Peripheral neuropathy fact sheet.* Retrieved from http://www.ninds.nih.gov/disorders/peripheralneuropathy/detail_peripheralneuropathy.htm

Phantom Pain

Phantom pain is the pain and sensations that are felt at the location of a missing limb or organ as though that missing body part could still experience sensations. Most of the time, these sensations are felt in an amputated limb or portion of a limb. It is sometimes associated with feelings that the amputated limb is still a part of the body. Phantom pain can also occur in individuals whom were born without limbs. Sensations caused by phantom pain are not limited to only pain; other common sensations are pressure, touch, tingling, burning, and movement, to name a few. American neurologist Silas Weir Mitchell (1829–1914) first coined the term "phantom limb" in 1871. While it is known that phantom pain is neuropathic, the exact mechanism behind the sensations felt is not yet known. One suggested reason for phantom pain is that since the central nervous system suddenly loses its connections to the amputated limb, it acts incorrectly to create the sensations felt by the individual.

Risk Factors and Symptoms

While it is possible for individuals born without limbs to experience phantom pain, the majority of people who feel phantom pain are amputees. There are some risk factors associated with phantom pain, especially in amputees. If an individual experiences preamputation pain, they are more likely to feel pain in the amputated limb after the procedure. In part, this could be due to the nervous system "remembering" the pain and continuing to send pain signals. Stump pain caused by neuromas (abnormal outgrowths of nerve endings resulting in nerve pain) can also have phantom pain or sensations associated with it. An ill-fitting prosthetic replacement can also create phantom pain in the amputated limb. Individuals who have bilateral limb amputations, lower limb amputations, or other pain (e.g., headaches) are at risk for phantom pain.

Phantom pain can happen anywhere from a few days after amputation up to a few weeks after amputation. This disorder is described by the pain felt in amputated limbs postamputation. It is a neuropathic pain, caused by malfunctioning of the nervous system rather than a real injury. This is because the limb in which the pain is felt is no longer connected to the patient's body. *Paraesthesias*—unusual sensations such as tingling or abnormal temperatures (hot or cold) where the limb used to be—are often associated with phantom pain. Patients with phantom pain rarely have persistent pain; rather they feel pain in their phantom limb intermittently. Approximately 50 to 80 percent of amputees experience phantom pain at some point after amputation (Virtual Medical Center, 2009). Persistent pain in the phantom limb only occurs in approximately 5 percent of amputees (Virtual Medical Center, 2009). In most amputees, phantom pain disappears after two years post amputation.

Pathophysiology

Phantom pain is caused by malfunctions of the nervous system rather than actual injury. The mechanisms behind phantom pain are still not well known, but there are multiple ideas about the causes. One known cause of phantom pain is a neurological condition called neuromas, which are abnormal growths of the nerve fibers that results in pain. There are two different types of neuromas that are linked to phantom pain: *tumor* and *traumatic neuromas*. Since the amputation damages the nerve fibers, abnormal nerve growth occurs to try and compensate for the missing portions. This causes extreme pain in patients. Neuromas are not the only cause, however. This is known because individuals born without limbs also experience phantom limb pain and therefore do not have nerve damage due to amputation. Some theories on other causes of phantom pain are based on neurological pathways and mechanisms. There are three broad categories currently being studied: *peripheral mechanisms, spinal mechanisms,* and *central mechanisms.*

Peripheral Mechanisms

Neuromas are considered a disorder of the peripheral nervous system. When nerve fiber growth occurs, neuromas are able to randomly fire abnormal action potentials (nerve impulses) resulting in a pain pathway that the patient experiences as coming from the missing limb. In order to further study how this peripheral mechanism causes phantom limb pain, patients are given a conduction blocking agent to arrest the transduction of action potentials in the damaged nerve tissue. Even when all action potentials are stopped in the nerve fibers, the patient can still experience phantom limb pain, just at a much less intense level. This indicates that the role of neuromas in phantom pain performs more of a modularly function, dampening or intensifying the pain signals being sent to the central nervous system (CNS).

Spinal Mechanisms

Nerve damage in the periphery can lead to degeneration or destruction of nerve fibers in the spinal tract. This degeneration can lead to hyperexcitability of the spinal cord. This means that pain fibers in the spinal cord react to neurotransmitters (natural chemicals that are used to transmit nerve impulses) and other neural signals that would not normally result in a pain pathway. However, even patients with complete spinal cord injury experience phantom pains, so this still does not provide the complete picture as to what occurs in the nervous system.

Central Mechanisms

The brain is capable of reorganizing its connections and developing new connections. This is called *neuroplasticity*. In amputees, it is thought that the brain undergoes various degrees of motor cortical remapping. Sometimes the pathways that the amputated limb used are shifted to the cortical region for the mouth. The amount that this shift has occurred has been correlated with the magnitude of the pain that the individual experiences. The process for cortical remapping is still not completely understood. However, in amputee patients, it is known that the cortical network for the hand and for the lips/mouth are remapped within each other in individuals experiencing phantom limb pain.

Management

Since the causes of phantom limb pain are still not completely understood, it is difficult to treat phantom pain. Additionally, each individual reacts differently to the pain and to the various treatments available, so there is no cure-all for phantom pain. Multiple types of treatments can be used to manage phantom pain, including medicine, surgical therapies, and alternative therapies. Analgesics, a broad class of pain killer that works with the peripheral nervous system and CNS, can be used to treat this disorder, but they do not ease pain in most patients. Anticonvulsants and tricyclic antidepressants have proven to work more effectively at relieving phantom pain and neuropathic pain in general.

Drug therapies are not the most effective way of treating phantom pain, especially chronic phantom pain. One surgical therapy that has been used to treat the pain is deep-brain stimulation. In deep-brain stimulation, the location of the misfiring neurons involved with phantom pain within the brain is determined using positron emission tomography (PET) scans and magnetic resonance imaging (MRI). Once the location has been determined, surgeons open the skull and stimulate this region on the brain with electrodes until the patient feels the most relief from their pain. The electrode is then left in the brain and secured so that the patient continues to get relief as they go about their life. A pulse-generator is connected to continue the stimulation and is implanted below the skin above the collar bone.

There are also a variety of alternative therapies available to treat phantom limb pain with various results. Mirror-box therapy is one of the most well-known alternative treatments for phantom limb pain. In mirror-box therapy, the stump from the amputated limb and the intact limb are placed in a box with a mirror that reflects the intact limb as though it was the phantom limb. The patient then undergoes various exercises while watching the mirrored image. This can trick the brain into believing that the phantom limb is unclenching or a variety of other things.

Another alternative treatment that can be used to treat phantom limb pain is acupuncture. In acupuncture, very small, fine, sterilized needles are stuck into the skin at certain locations. Acupuncture is thought to stimulate the CNS to release endorphins which often act as natural pain relievers. This relief of endorphins helps to counteract the pain felt at the amputated limb. Transcutaneous electrical nerve stimulation (TENS) is another type of nerve stimulation which can help manage the pain felt by patients. Adhesive patches are placed around the site of pain and small electrical signals are sent through them. TENS is thought to disrupt the pain signals incorrectly sent to the brain, preventing the patient from feeling pain from the phantom limb.

Finally, the use of an electric prosthetic limb, termed a *myoelectric prosthetic,* can help relieve the symptoms of phantom limb pain. The prosthetic is linked to the intact limb and has motors that respond to the signals sent when the patient is voluntarily moving muscles in the intact limb. One thing that is important to recognize with phantom pain is that most amputees will experience this type of pain. Unfortunately, many patients that develop phantom pain or phantom limb sensations think that the sensations they are experiencing are all in their heads and will not seek out treatment to manage the pain that they feel.

Riannon C. Atwater

See also: Brain Stimulators; Central Nervous System (CNS); Homunculus; Pain; Sensory Receptors; Somatosensory Cortex/Somatosensory System; Transduction and Membrane Properties

Further Reading

Amputee Coalition. (n.d.). *Managing phantom pain.* Retrieved from http://www.ampu tee-coalition.org/limb-loss-resource-center/resources-for-pain-management/managing-phantom-pain/index.html

Mayo Clinic Staff. (2011). *Diseases and conditions: Phantom pain.* Retrieved from http://www.mayoclinic.org/diseases-conditions/phantom-pain/basics/symptoms/con-20023268

Virtual Medical Center. (2009). *Phantom limb pain.* Retrieved from http://www.myvmc.com/diseases/phantom-limb-pain/#Symptoms

Phenytoin (Dilantin)

Under the brand name *Dilantin, phenytoin* is an anticonvulsant medication used to treat seizures. Phenytoin was first synthesized by Heinrich Biltz (1865–1943) in 1908 but it was not used experimentally until the late 1930s by Merritt and Putnam. At this point in the history of epilepsy, anticonvulsants had a sedative component and it was thought that the sedation aided the anitconvulsant's ultimate effect on controlling seizures. It was not until phenytoin was introduced, however, that a medication was able to control seizures by stabilizing electrical activity in the brain without the side effect of sleepiness. Phenytoin was used as the first-line choice for treatment of epileptic seizures until the 1980s when other agents such as carbamazepine and valproate were introduced.

The Food and Drug Administration approved phenytoin for use in generalized tonic-clinic and complex partial seizures as well as treatment and prophylaxis of seizures during or after neurosurgery. Scientists have shown that a possible mechanism of action for phenytoin is that it depresses the sodium action potential. It is thought to "filter out" excessive and abnormal neuronal activity. For instance, it may block specialized proteins (sodium channels) located within the cell membrane that are responsible for producing an action potential—the signal used by neurons to "talk" to each other. By obstructing this action, it may reduce the abnormal positive feedback that underlies the development of maximal seizure activity.

Phenytoin has a narrow therapeutic index (the difference between efficacy and toxicity is small) and the drug can accumulate in the body easily. Therefore, the effective level of phenytoin for most patients is between 10 and 20 mcg/mL (micrograms per milliliter). In general, levels that are less than 10 mcg/ml potentially do not control seizures while levels greater than 20 mcg/ml indicate toxicity. Thus, patients taking phenytoin must have their drug levels measured frequently to avoid adverse effects. The manner in which phenytoin is eliminated from the body is very unique because unlike the majority of medications, it is cleared from the body via zero-order, or nonlinear kinetics. This means that phenytoin is eliminated at a constant rate that is independent of the amount of drug in the body.

Phenytoin has many side effects that have limited its use over the years because safer anticonvulsants have taken its place and have been shown to work just as well. The side effects increase with higher levels of drug in the body, which is why it is important to have blood levels checked. Some of the side effects are nystagmus, ataxia, blurred vision, slurred speech, dizziness, and at very high levels, coma and death can occur. In addition to side effects, phenytoin induces the CYP 3A4 hepatic enzyme, which is the most common enzyme responsible for metabolizing drugs. This means phenytoin can decrease the effectiveness of other drugs the patient is taking via this mechanism. Thus, clinicians must be aware of the potential interaction.

Although phenytoin's use has declined over the last few decades, it was a novel drug that paved the way for the many anticonvulsant medications that patients use today.

Jeremy E. Brothers

See also: Ataxia; Epilepsy; Nystagmus; Seizures; Sodium Channels

Further Reading

Medline Plus. (2013). *Phenytoin.* Retrieved from http://www.nlm.nih.gov/medlineplus /druginfo/meds/a682022.html

Shorvon, S. D. (2009). Drug treatment of epilepsy in the century of the ILAE: The first 50 years, 1909–1958. *Epilepsia, 50*(Suppl. 3), 69–92.

Phrenology

Phrenology is a pseudoscience (not a true science but a collection of beliefs collected by mistake as being based on the scientific method) that uses the morphology of the skull to predict the personality of a person. The term *phrenology* comes from Greek meaning the study of knowledge or the study of the mind.

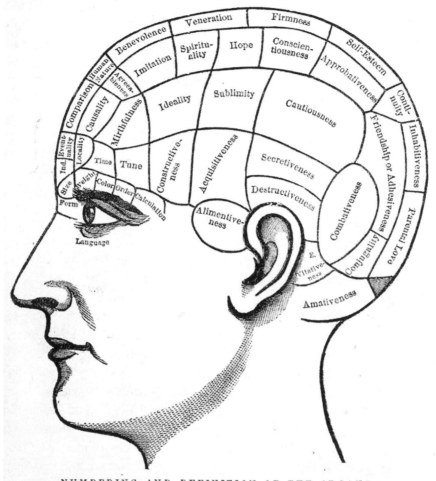

NUMBERING AND DEFINITION OF THE ORGANS.

1. AMATIVENESS, Love between the sexes.
A. CONJUGALITY, Matrimony—love of one. [etc.
2. PARENTAL LOVE, Regard for offspring, pets,
3. FRIENDSHIP, Adhesiveness—sociability.
4. INHABITIVENESS, Love of home
5. CONTINUITY, One thing at a time.
E. VITATIVENESS, Love of life.
6. COMBATIVENESS, Resistance—defense.
7. DESTRUCTIVENESS, Executiveness—force.
8. ALIMENTIVENESS, Appetite—hunger.
9. ACQUISITIVENESS, Accumulation.
10. SECRETIVENESS, Policy—management.
11. CAUTIOUSNESS, Prudence—provision.
12. APPROBATIVENESS, Ambition—display.
13. SELF-ESTEEM, Self-respect—dignity.
14. FIRMNESS, Decision—perseverance.
15. CONSCIENTIOUSNESS, Justice, equity.
16. HOPE, Expectation—enterprise.
17. SPIRITUALITY, Intuition—faith—credulity.
18. VENERATION, Devotion—respect.
19. BENEVOLENCE, Kindness—goodness.
20. CONSTRUCTIVENESS, Mechanical ingenuity
21. IDEALITY, Refinement—taste—purity.
B. SUBLIMITY, Love of grandeur—infinitude.
22. IMITATION, Copying—patterning.
23. MIRTHFULNESS, Jocoseness—wit—fun.
24. INDIVIDUALITY, Observation.
25. FORM, Recollection of shape.
26. SIZE, Measuring by the eye.
27. WEIGHT, Balancing—climbing.
28. COLOR, Judgment of colors.
29. ORDER, Method—system—arrangement
30. CALCULATION, Mental arithmetic.
31. LOCALITY, Recollection of places.
32. EVENTUALITY, Memory of facts.
33. TIME, Cognizance of duration.
34. TUNE, Sense of harmony and melody.
35. LANGUAGE, Expression of ideas.
36. CAUSALITY, Applying causes to effect. [tion.
37. COMPARISON, Inductive reasoning—illustra-
C. HUMAN NATURE, Perception of motives.
D. AGREEABLENESS, Pleasantness—suavity.

19th century phrenological diagram with definitions of the various areas of the human skull. Now considered a pseudoscience, phrenology was an area of study where individuals believed that the personality traits of a person could be derived from the bumps and shape of the skull. (iStockPhoto)

This pseudoscience is based on the premise that the natural bumps and indents on the skull reflect the morphology of the brain below. Specifically, the protuberances on the skull were thought to indicate regions where the brain was enlarged underneath the skull; and conversely, indents on the skull indicated places where the brain was less developed. The regions of enlargements and indentations correspond with a phrenological map, which represents organs responsible for personality traits. Even though it was, for the most part, discredited by the late 1840s, phrenology advanced modern-day neurology by first suggesting that mental faculties resided in the brain.

History

The brain has not always been known as the seat of control for the body. Hippocrates (ca. 460–370 BC) and his colleagues were the first to suggest that control over the human body originated from the brain rather than the heart. The study of phrenology was founded by the German scientist, Franz Joseph Gall (1758–1828), in a publication from 1819, *The Anatomy and Physiology of the Nervous System in General, and of the Brain in Particular,* and was popularized by his colleague and collaborator, Johann Gaspar Spurzheim (1776–1832). In the late 18th century and the beginning 19th century, phrenology was mostly confined to practice by Gall and Spurzheim. However, in 1815, a publication in the *Edinburgh Review* created a craze over the science of phrenology. It became the average middle-class man's occupation. By the 1850s, phrenology had mostly died away. In the United States, American phrenologist Lorenzo Niles Fowlers (1811–1896) reintroduced the pseudoscience in the 1860s and 1870s. This later movement contributed heavily to the *anthropometric* movement in the later 19th century. Anthropometrics was the pseudoscience of head reading and was primarily concerned with racial profiling. Currently, phrenology is largely discredited as a pseudoscience.

Phrenology was one of the first ideas to bring about the attempt to rehabilitate criminals. It was thought that by studying the morphology of the skull, and thus the brain, criminal tendencies could be diagnosed. Once diagnosed, rehabilitators would be able to create a plan to help patients control their urges. For example, if a patient had a tendency for violence (as determined through phrenology), a useful and beneficial occupation could be found that would harness this violent personality such as becoming a butcher.

The Phrenological System

The theory of phrenology is based on the underlying idea that the contours of one's head are indicative of the underlying cerebral contours. By measuring these contours, the intelligence, personality, strengths, weaknesses, and abilities of an individual were determined. The science of phrenology is based on a few basic principles that govern it. The most important of these principles is the idea that the brain is the center of all mental faculties. Gall also hypothesized that the brain was not one single organ, but a multitude of organs each responsible for one aspect of human personality and intelligence. Finally, in order for phrenology to be true, the relative size of each "organ" determined which innate abilities were more predominant and this could be measured based on the cranial bumps in the skull since the skull reflected the underlying brain.

There are anywhere between 27 and 43 organs of the brain depending on which text is referenced. Nineteen of these exist in animals as well as humans and the final eight exist only in human brains. Each of these organs was responsible for one aspect of the human personality. These organs were organized into a phrenological map of the skull that could be used when examining patients. Some of the phrenological organs are listed in the following:

1. Amativeness (sex drive)
2. Philprogenitiveness (ability to produce offspring)
3. Concentrativeness/Inhabitiveness (to stay in one place)
4. Adhesiveness
5. Combativeness
6. Destructiveness/Alimentiveness (appetite for food)
7. Secretiveness
8. Aquisitiveness (the desire to possess things)
9. Constructiveness
10. Self-esteem
11. Love of approbation (love of praise)
12. Cautiousness
13. Benevolence (to do good)
14. Veneration (great respect)
15. Firmness
16. Conscientiousness (concerned with doing something correctly)
17. Hope
18. Wonder
19. Ideality (the state of being ideal)
20. Wit
21. Imitation
22. Individuality
23. Form
24. Size
25. Weight

26. Coloring
27. Locality
28. Number
29. Order
30. Eventuality
31. Time
32. Tune
33. Language
34. Comparison
35. Causality

Phrenologists would run their hands and fingertips over their patients' heads to determine where the bumps and indentations were. Sometimes calipers were used to take measurements of the skull. The practiced phrenologist would have each of the faculties memorized and what the pros and cons in the personality for each faculty. In reading the bumps on the skull of a patient, a phrenologist would be able to tell any defects in an individual's character. It was thought that a phrenologist could help an individual find the perfect job based on their personality and even find true love.

Impact on the Modern Study of Brain and Behavior

Phrenology played a huge role in establishing the brain as the mental faculty of the human body. Even though the many organs proposed by phrenologists are not accurate, the idea that regions within the brain which were utilized more often would be enlarged holds some truth. Enlargement of the brain in certain regions can indicate that the connections made in that region are used frequently. It also introduced the idea that there is localization of functions within the brain. Magnetic resonance imaging (MRI) studies show that certain regions of the brain are active during different emotions or actions. In Gall's initial phrenological map of the organs, his faculty for words and speech was closely located to the region of skull overlaying *Wernicke's area* and *Broca's area*.

Riannon C. Atwater

See also: Brain Anatomy; Broca's Area; Wernicke's Area

Further Reading

LHOON. (1998). *The history of phrenology*. Retrieved from http://www.phrenology.org /intro.html

van Wyhe, J. (2000). *The history of phrenology*. Victorian Web. Retrieved from http:// www.victorianweb.org/science/phrenology/intro.html

van Wyhe, J. (1999–2011). *The history of phrenology on the web: Overview*. Retrieved from http://www.historyofphrenology.org.uk/overview.htm

van Wyhe, J. (1999–2011). *The phrenological organs (the "bumps")*. Retrieved from http://www.historyofphrenology.org.uk/organs.html

Pineal Gland

The *pineal gland* is a single structure located in the midline of the mammalian brain. It receives information about light intensity and light duration from the retina, which is located at the back of the eye. In mammals, there is a distinct and direct neural connection from the eye to the brain and autonomic nervous system. This information is passed through the nervous system, ultimately resulting in the stimulation of pinealocytes, which are specialized cells found in the pineal gland. This stimulation of pinealocytes results in the synthesis and release of melatonin, a hormone that is important in sleep-wake cycles and regulation of the mammalian reproductive system.

History

Throughout history, the pineal gland has been studied for its anatomy and function in the human brain. In ancient times, it was often called the "third eye" by philosophers of the day as they had observed the relationship between light and the function of this gland. The French philosopher René Descartes (1596–1650) went so far as to declare the pineal gland as the seat of the human soul. Today, fossil evidence shows that several extinct species including ostracoderms (members of the Phylum Agnatha or boneless fishes), placoderms (extinct bony fishes), and the crossopterygians (bony fishes hypothesized to be ancestral to current day amphibians) had a "socket" or foramen (opening) located on the midline between the two parietal bones of the skull. Today this foramen is still found in modern-day amphibians and reptiles but not in modern-day birds or mammals. For some time, scientists thought the pineal gland was simply a vestigial organ with no important function. Through more recent experiments in the past 25 years, the function and importance of the pineal gland have been identified in mammals.

Anatomy of the Mammalian Pineal Gland

The pineal gland in humans is a single organ located in the brain along the midline that is shaped much like a pinecone, hence its name. It is situated dorsal or behind the thalamus (part of the diencephalon) and dorsal to the superior colliculi, which are paired structures that play an important role in the visual systems of most mammals. In humans, the pineal gland is approximately 1 centimeter in size. However, the size of the pineal gland among other mammals is quite variable ranging from 1 millimeter in dogs to 1 centimeter or larger in other primates. It is composed primarily of neuroendocrine cells called *pinealocytes* that secrete melatonin, a natural brain hormone. In addition, the pineal gland has *glial cells* that are hypothesized to provide support for the pinealocytes. Embryologically, the pineal gland is derived from the ectoderm of the roof of the developing diencephalon. It develops within the first two months into gestation of the growing fetus.

Functional Anatomy

Fishes, amphibians, and most reptiles have a "third eye," more commonly known today as a parietal eye or organ that is located just below the epidermal and dermal layers of skin in the parietal bone of the skull. Within this tissue, there are *photo-receptor cells* that receive light from the external environment. Light penetrates through these dermal layers because of a thin layer of clear cells that forms a primitive lens, which in turn directs light from the external environment onto the cornea of the organism. This light then stimulates the pineal gland through stimulation of the nervous system.

In contrast to fishes, amphibians, and reptiles, birds and mammals do not have cells that directly receive light stimulation. In these more derived species, stimulation of the pineal gland is accomplished through a very specific pathway that connects the retina of the eye to the pineal gland. In this system, light first strikes the photoreceptors cells (cones and rods) of the retina generating action potentials. These action potentials then activate bipolar cells and ganglion cells of the retina and enter into the optic nerve or cranial nerve II (CN II). From CN II, the action potential enters the suprachiasmatic nucleus of the hypothalamus and then onto the superior cervical ganglia, which are part of the *autonomic nervous system* (ANS). These ganglia send axons out that innervate the pineal gland, inducing pinealocytes to secrete melatonin in response to the action potentials first generated in the retina. This pathway is very similar to how the adrenal medulla (part of the adrenal gland located near the kidney) is stimulated. In both instances, nervous system impulses through the sympathetic pathway of the ANS are transduced from electrical signals to hormonal signals.

More recent research has identified two receptors located in the cell membrane of both pinealocytes and cells in the suprachiasmatic nucleus of humans. These two receptors are known as the Mel 1A and Mel 1B receptors and they are both G protein–coupled receptors. These receptors are *adrenergic* receptors and respond very rapidly to melatonin binding. It is hypothesized that these receptors are important for the light-dependent function of the pineal gland.

Tumors of the Pineal Gland

While tumors of the pineal gland are not very common, they do occur and more frequently occur in prepubescent children than adults. Pineal gland tumors make up approximately 1 percent of all brain tumors and are visualized most often using *magnetic resonance imaging* (MRI) or computerized axial tomography (CAT) scans. When found early, these tumors are easily treated via surgery. In advanced cases, chemotherapy or radiation therapy may be needed to help decrease the size of the tumor. Pineal gland tumors are most often found when young children start to exhibit precocious puberty (enter puberty earlier than normal). Tumors of the pineal gland often result in a decrease in melatonin, which causes a decrease in the inhibition of gonadotropin releasing hormone from the hypothalamus. This results in an increase in the sex hormones and the stimulation of early puberty.

Charles A. Ferguson

See also: Action Potential; Autonomic Nervous System; Diencephalon; Melatonin; Optic Nerve; Retina

Further Reading

Bowen, R. (2003). *The pineal gland and melatonin.* Retrieved from http://www.vivo.colo state.edu/hbooks/pathphys/endocrine/otherendo/pineal.html

Maronde, E., & Stehle, J. (2007). The mammalian pineal gland: Known facts, unknown facets. *TRENDS in Endocrinology and Metabolism, 18*(4), 142–149.

Moller, M., & Baeres, F.M.M. (2002). The anatomy and innervation of the mammalian pineal gland. *Cell and Tissue Research, 309,* 139–150.

Nolte, J. (1993). *The human brain: An introduction to its functional anatomy* (pp. 246–248). St. Louis, MI. Mosby Yearbook Inc.

Romer, A.S., & Parsons, T.S. (1977). *The vertebrate body* (pp. 471–473). Philadelphia, PA.: Holt-Saunders International.

Pituitary Gland (Hypophysis)

The *pituitary gland* or *hypophysis* is a single midline structure located deep within the brain of humans and mammals and is directly connected to the hypothalamus via a structure called the *pituitary stalk* or *infundibulum.* It is one of many endocrine glands in the human body. Endocrine glands are "ductless" and secrete hormones directly into the environment around them through either *paracrine* (the biological action of synthesizing and releasing a hormone that binds to a nearby receptor on another organ) or *autocrine* (the biological action of synthesizing and releasing a hormone that binds to a receptor on the gland that produced it) release of hormones. The hypophysis is necessary to support hormone secretion throughout the body as well as secrete neurohormones within the brain. These hormones assist in maintaining homeostasis.

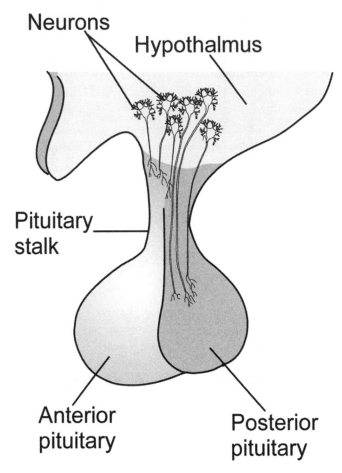

The anatomy of the pituitary gland. Here hypothalamic neurons are shown terminating in the pituitary gland. (Sandy Windelspecht)

Anatomy and Physiology

The pituitary gland resides in a bony structure known as the *sella turcica,* which is a saddled-shaped depression in the sphenoid bone, one of the eight cranial bones in humans. It is composed of two lobes known as the *anterior pituitary lobe* or *adenohypophysis* (glandular part) and the *posterior pituitary lobe* or the *neurohypophysis* (neural part). The pituitary gland was often called the master gland because of its wide-ranging regulation of many other endocrine glands in the body. Today, scientists have shown that while the pituitary gland is very critical for the proper functioning of most other endocrine glands, it is not the single point of regulation of these other glands.

Hormones that are released by the pituitary gland are hormones that either stimulate release of a second hormone from another gland, or prevent secretion of hormones from another gland. For these releasing or inhibiting hormones to get to other glands in the endocrine system, they must travel in the body via the vascular system (veins and arteries). For example, the *thyroid gland* is an important gland for maintaining the use of energy (metabolism) in mammals. The pituitary gland secretes *thyroid stimulating hormone,* which enters the vascular system, travels to the thyroid gland located in the anterior aspect of the neck, and stimulates the cells of the thyroid gland to secrete the appropriate hormones. There is no duct or tube that makes a direct connection between the pituitary gland and the thyroid gland. This is true of all the endocrine organs in the body.

Releasing or inhibiting hormones from the pituitary gland regulate other endocrine glands by binding to a specific location on a cell called a *receptor.* These receptors are most often composed of proteins that have a very unique and specific three-dimensional shape. This shape will allow only one specific molecule to bind or interact with the receptor. This "lock and key" system is what allows hormones to be found in a mammal's body at any point but only act on specific cells associated with a specific endocrine organ. The anterior pituitary gland secretes six known hormones, while the posterior pituitary gland secretes two known hormones.

Development of the Pituitary Gland

The pituitary gland is a very unique gland in that the two lobes of the hypophysis—the anterior and posterior lobes—have very different embryologic origins. This is reflected in the alternative names for the pituitary gland and accounts for the very different histological structures of each lobe, that is the cell and tissue composition.

The anterior pituitary lobe begins to develop approximately five weeks into embryological development in humans. Tissues of a structure called the *stoma,* which is part of the early digestive system, begin to differentiate. As this differentiation occurs, these tissues begin to form the *oral ectoderm* (the outermost layer of the developing embryo that forms the oral cavity). Cells from the oral ectoderm then begin to migrate in a *superior* or upward direction toward the developing nervous system. This migration upward will eventually become what is called the anterior pituitary or adeno-(glandular)-hypophysis. This anterior pituitary lobe is composed of several different types of cells, all of which, when mature, synthesize and secrete various hormones under the control of the hypothalamus.

The posterior pituitary lobe also begins to develop approximately five weeks into embryological development. The posterior pituitary lobe is derived from the developing brain, specifically a region of the brain called the *diencephalon,* which will eventually mature into the thalamus and hypothalamus. Cells that make up the floor of the developing diencephalon will begin to migrate in an *inferior* or downward direction at the same time that cells from the oral ectoderm are migrating superiorly. As each of these cell types migrate, the cells of the floor of the diencephalon will move behind (posterior) the cells of the oral ectoderm (moving anteriorly) and will ultimately form the mature pituitary gland. As these cells are migrating, bone cells that will make up the bony portion of the sphenoid bone and the sella turcica will form around the maturing pituitary gland, enclosing it in its protective bony chamber. The posterior pituitary lobe has no cells within it. Instead, it is composed of *axon terminals* that migrated downward into the gland from the diencephalon. The cells that synthesize and secrete hormones from the posterior pituitary lobe are the *supraoptic nucleus and the paraventricular nucleus* (a group of cell bodies). These nuclei are located deep within the hypothalamus.

Hormones of the Adenohypophysis

The anterior pituitary gland secretes six known hormones.

- *Thyroid stimulating hormone (TSH)* regulates the synthesis and secretion of two hormones needed for the regulation of metabolism. These two hormones include tri-iodo-thyronine (T3) and thyroxine (T4), both of which are synthesized and secreted by the thyroid gland.
- *Adrenocorticotropic hormone or corticotropin (ACTH)* regulates the synthesis and secretion of glucocorticoid hormones such as cortisol from the cortical layer of the adrenal gland. This hormone is important in regulating stress responses and helping with the regulation of glucose metabolism.
- *Prolactin (PRL)* stimulates breast milk production in a pregnant female and continues to do this postpartum.
- *Follicle stimulating hormone (FSH)* is one of two gonadotropin hormones released by the anterior pituitary lobe. In females, FSH plays a very important role in regulating the menstrual cycle and is critical for the proper release of estrogen, an important steroid hormone responsible for the secondary sexual characteristics in postpubertal females. In males, FSH is important for the development and maturation of sperm cells.
- *Luteinizing hormone (LH)* is the second gonadotropin hormone. In females, LH is also important in the menstrual cycle. It is the hormone that is thought

to be critical for the ovulation process to occur in females (release of an egg). In males, LH is important in the maturation process for sperm.

- *Growth hormone or somatotropin (GH)* is critical for the growth and development of humans. GH has a wide range of functions. It is important in childhood growth and development for the increase in muscle mass, protein synthesis, lipid synthesis, and increased calcium retention. GH has also been shown to be very important in the development and maintenance of a healthy immune system.

Hormones of the Neurohypophysis

The posterior pituitary gland secretes two known hormones.

- *Oxytocin (OXY)* plays a critical role in both females and males. In females, OXY is essential in the process of labor and delivery. The uterus is composed of smooth muscle called the myometrium and is under the control of the autonomic nervous system. In labor and delivery, this muscle tissue undergoes contractions to expel the fetus during labor. OXY is the hormone that is critical for the stimulation of the uterine muscle and causes it to contract. It is also very important in the process of cervical dilation and effacement in preparation for labor and delivery. For breast-feeding, OXY binds to receptors in breast tissues to stimulate the "let-down" reflex. This reflex causes milk to collect in the subareolar sinuses of the breast (ducts around the nipple), allowing for more successful breast-feeding. The role of OXY in males is much less understood. Some studies suggest that OXY is important in sperm motility and transport. However, the relationship between OXY and male reproductive success is still very unclear.
- *Vasopressin or antidiuretic hormone (ADH)* plays an important role in the regulation of water content in the body and is important in the regulation of blood pressure. Vasopressin acts on cells located within the tubular portion of the kidney to regulate how much water is removed from blood as waste and excreted as urine.

Vascular System of the Pituitary Gland

As discussed previously, the pituitary gland is an endocrine gland and therefore does not have any tubes or ducts associated with it to transport hormones to the rest of the body. All endocrine glands, including the pituitary gland, require a direct association with the vascular system to accomplish the transport of hormones throughout the body. Transport of pituitary hormones is accomplished through a very specialized vascular system called the *hypothalamic-hypophyseal portal system.*

To begin, it is important to define a portal system in the vascular system. The normal pathway blood would follow in the vascular system would be from an artery, to an arteriole, to a capillary bed, to a venule, and then to a vein and back to a point of origin. In this system, there is only one capillary bed or system. A portal system incorporates a second capillary bed in the pathway before blood is returned to a starting point. There are three known portal systems in humans: one in the kidneys, one in the liver (the hepatic portal system), and one in the pituitary gland.

The hypothalamic-hypophyseal portal system is formed by a vessel called the superior hypophyseal artery which branches off the internal carotid artery coming up through the neck and into the cranium. This artery then forms the first capillary bed (called the *primary plexus*) which surrounds the infundibulum of the pituitary gland. This is where hormones from the hypothalamus would enter the vascular system to get to the cells of the pituitary gland. The primary plexus is then connected to the *secondary plexus,* which is a capillary bed around the anterior and posterior pituitary lobes by the *hypophyseal portal vein.* Releasing hormones from the hypothalamus then exit the secondary plexus to stimulate cells of the pituitary, which in turn secrete their hormones back into the secondary plexus and exit the portal system via the inferior hypophyseal vein and into the body.

Pathology

There are many types of pathology that involve the pituitary gland. Two of the most common include *acromegaly* and *Cushing's disease.* Acromegaly occurs when the anterior pituitary lobe secretes excess amounts of growth hormone after puberty has been completed. The excess in growth hormone results in enlargement of the hands and feet, and often causes increased skull growth as well as an enlargement of the mandible (jaw). This increased secretion of growth hormone is most often a result of a benign tumor known as a *pituitary adenoma.* This type of tumor, in addition to causing an increase in growth hormone, can put pressure on the optic nerve and create visual disturbances, such as blindness.

Cushing's disease is also caused by a pituitary adenoma. In this instance, the tumor causes an increase in the secretion of adrenocorticotropic hormone (ACTH) resulting in increased levels of cortisol in the vascular system. Symptoms of this disease include unexplained and rapid weight gain, and the formation of fat pads along the clavicle and the top of the shoulders (buffalo hump). One of the most common presenting symptoms is swelling of the face or the appearance of a "moon face." Lesser symptoms include increased swelling, peripheral capillary dilation (telangiectasia), and thinning of the skin which results in bruising and bleeding.

In both illnesses, acromegaly and Cushing's disease, treatment usually consists of either a surgical removal of the tumor and/or the use of steroids to reduce the size of the tumor.

Summary

The pituitary gland, one of several endocrine glands in the body, is located midline in the brain, and is composed of two lobes. These lobes make up the anterior and posterior pituitary lobes. The anterior pituitary gland synthesizes and secretes six different hormones that regulate body functions such as metabolism, stress, and reproductive functions. The posterior pituitary lobe synthesizes and secretes two hormones that help with water balance and also play a role in reproduction.

Charles A. Ferguson

See also: Cushing Syndrome; Diencephalon; Homeostasis; Hormones; Hypothalamus

Further Reading

Campbell, I. (2011). Hypothalamic and pituitary function. *Anesthesia and Intensive Care Medicine, 12*(10), 458–460.

Donald, R. A. (1990). The assessment of pituitary function. *Clinical Biochemistry, 23,* 23–30.

Jones, T. H., & Kennedy, R. L. (1993). Cytokines and hypothalamic-pituitary function. *Cytokine, 5*(6), 531–538.

Kandel, E. R., Schwartz, J. H., & Jessell, T. M. (1995). *Essentials of neural science and behavior.* Norwalk, CT: Appleton and Lange.

Nolte, J. (1993). *The human brain: An introduction to its functional anatomy.* St. Louis, MI: Mosby Yearbook Inc.

Widmaier, E. P., Raff, H., & Strang, K. (2004). *Human physiology: The mechanisms of body functions.* New York, NY: McGraw-Hill Press.

Poliomyelitis

Poliomyelitis (polio) is a viral disease that affects humans by destroying motor neurons (specialized cells used for movement) causing lifelong paralysis and death. Since there is no treatment for polio, doctors attempt to prevent further infections through vaccination. Polio incidence peaked in the United States in the 1950s, and has since been eradicated in the United Sates due to successful vaccination campaigns. Polio was eliminated from the Western Hemisphere in the 1990s, but in 2012 three countries still had endemic polio (naturally occurring levels of polio infections). As long as there are cases of polio in the world, international travel could reintroduce polio to unvaccinated citizens in countries where it has been eradicated. Additionally, in areas where polio has been eradicated, people who have had past polio infection may still suffer from the lifelong effects of the virus.

History

Polio has been a disease of humans since before written history and is documented in the medical literature as early as the 1700s (Sass, 1996). In 1840, a German orthopedist named Jacob von Heine described the deformities that result from polio and proposed that a spinal lesion (damage to the spinal cord) could be the cause. At that point, the infectious nature of polio was unknown. In the late 1800s, however, Oskar Medin described the epidemic nature of polio, suggesting an infectious agent.

By the early 1900s, many researchers suspected that polio was a result of an infectious agent; and in 1949, John Franklin Enders, Frederick Chapman Robbins, and Thomas H. Weller cultured the virus that causes polio. The team received the 1954 Nobel Prize for their culture methods, which are still used today to culture many other viruses.

Classification

The virus that causes polio is a member of the Picornaviridae family and belongs in the enterovirus subgroup. All picornaviruses carry genetic information in the form of RNA and have a nonenveloped structure (nonenveloped viruses have a viral protein coat on the outside). Several human diseases are caused by picornaviruses including the common cold.

Enteroviruses, subgroup of the picornavirus family, are unique in that all of these virus types replicate in the gastrointestinal (GI) tract. Enteroviruses are often spread to other people through fecal contamination. This is why hand washing is important to prevent the spread of such viruses. Several enteroviruses infect humans and cause varied diseases including polio; the common cold; and hand, foot, and mouth disease. Although the virus replicates in the GI tract, the damage is caused due to the virus entering the central nervous system (CNS; brain and spinal cord) damaging motor neurons.

Infection

Poliovirus infection takes place in several steps; the virus must travel from initial exposure in the mouth to the motor neurons where the virus causes damage. Exposure to the poliovirus occurs primarily via the fecal-oral route. It is also possible to be exposed by oral contact with infected mucous, such as uncovered sneezing or coughing. Once the virus enters the body it multiplies in the pharynx (throat), then travels to the small intestine. The virus is not destroyed by the acidic conditions in the stomach and moves through the GI tract until it reaches the small intestine and starts replicating. From the intestine the virus enters the blood stream and ultimately travels to the CNS.

Once the virus enters the brain, the replication cycle in the CNS is responsible for permanently damaging the motor neurons, resulting in paralysis, a hallmark of the disease. When the virus enters a motor neuron, it takes over the machinery of the cell, turning the cell into a viral factory. After new viral particles are manufactured, the neuron is destroyed when the viruses burst out. A destroyed neuron can no longer "talk" to its corresponding sections of muscles. When muscles do not receive acetylcholine, the chemical necessary for muscle contraction, from the motor neuron, they are no longer controlled by the brain and spinal cord. Adjacent motor neurons may be able to compensate for the lost motor function and the patient may experience only muscle weakness. However, lost motor neurons do not regenerate and severe motor neuron damage leads to paralysis in most cases.

Disease

Poliomyelitis is the disease caused by infection with the poliovirus. Infection can have several outcomes including subclinical infection, nonparalytic infection, and paralytic infection.

Approximately 95 percent of poliovirus infections cause a subclinical infection. This infection may go unnoticed by the patient or the patient may mistake the viral infection for a cold and/or other upper respiratory viral infection. The danger of having a subclinical infection is that the infected patient is still contagious and can pass on the virus to healthy individuals.

The second type of infection that can result from exposure to the poliovirus is a nonparalytic infection. Symptoms last 1 to 10 days and then resolve. Symptoms of nonparalytic polio include fever, sore throat, headache and fatigue, as well as pain and stiffness in the back, neck, arms, and legs. Nonparalytic infection does not cause motor nerve damage or paralysis, but unlike a subclinical infection, patients are aware that they have been ill.

The third type of infection resulting from poliovirus exposure is paralytic polio. Paralytic polio is the most serious type, but affects less than 1 percent of polio patients. Symptoms include bloating in the GI tract from viral replication, muscle aches and spasms, and abnormal sensations due to nerve damage during active infection. The motor neuron damage also causes loss of reflex responses. The course of the disease is rapid with paralysis occurring 1 to 10 days after onset of illness.

The paralysis often occurs on one side of the body only and may be accompanied by extreme sensitivity to touch. Once the patient's fever decreases, paralysis rarely progresses. Recovery from paralysis is possible, but paralysis present one year after infection is unlikely to resolve.

Paralytic polio is further divided into three types: spinal polio, bulbar polio, and bulbospinal polio. Spinal polio is the most common. Damage to the spinal cord causes asymmetric paralysis, often in the legs. This damage is a direct result of the virus infecting and destroying the part of the spinal cord where the cell bodies of the motor neurons are found. These motor neurons innervate muscles and cannot be regenerated, so paralysis is permanent. Bulbar polio is more severe because the poliovirus infects and destroys the motor neurons in the brainstem. Destruction of motor neurons in the brainstem can interfere with the ability to breathe, speak, and swallow. Lastly, bulbospinal polio is characterized by infection of both the spinal cord and the brainstem.

Prognosis

The prognoses of patients infected with poliovirus vary based on the type of infection. Patients with subclinical infection have an excellent prognosis for complete recovery and no damage that could lead to post-polio syndrome (see the following text). Patients with nonparalytic infection also have a good prognosis for complete recovery and a very low risk of lifelong problems caused by post-polio syndrome. The prognosis is worse for patients with paralytic polio. These patients may suffer from lifelong paralysis as well as from post-polio syndrome later in life. CNS involvement resulting from paralytic polio can cause death, often from respiratory problems, or lifelong reliance on a respirator.

Transmission

Although polio can be contracted at any time of the year, the peak number of infections occurs during the summer. Exposure to contaminated water is a primary mechanism of spread. The virus is stable in acid, but can be destroyed (inactivated) with heat treatment, formaldehyde, chlorine, and ultraviolet light.

Once a patient has the virus, the patient is highly contagious. It has been estimated that 90 percent of adults living in the same house as a patient with polio will also contract the virus, and nearly 100 percent of children living in the same house with a polio patient will contract the virus.

Incubation times for the virus vary but average incubation is 7 to 14 days. Patients shed infectious viral particles in their feces before they realize they have the virus. After symptoms clear, patients continue to shed viral particles in their feces for an additional three to six weeks.

Diagnosis

Polio may be recognized by symptoms in an area where there is a polio outbreak. Definitive diagnosis involves collecting a sample from the patient's throat or stool and confirming presence of the poliovirus. If paralytic polio is suspected, the virus will be sent to a lab for sequencing and fingerprinting to verify whether the virus is wild type (naturally occurring in the wild) or vaccine acquired (infected by a vaccine). Acquiring polio from the oral polio vaccine is rare but still monitored in areas where the vaccine is in use.

Treatment

There is no known cure for polio. Instead, patients are given supportive therapy and are treated based on their symptoms. Supportive treatment includes rest and hydration. Treatment of symptoms may include pain relievers, heating pads, and physical therapy. By treating the symptoms, physicians aim to decrease pain and increase function of weakened muscles. In patients with respiratory involvement, an artificial respirator may be necessary. The most well-known artificial respirator used by polio patients is the iron lung, a type of negative pressure ventilator encasing the patient.

Vaccines

Because there is no cure for polio, researchers have focused on prevention. Two effective vaccines are currently used worldwide for polio prevention, an inactivated vaccine that is injected and a live attenuated (weakened) oral vaccine. Humans are the only reservoir for the poliovirus, so elimination of the virus is possible if human-to-human transmission can be stopped.

The inactivated polio vaccine was developed by Jonas Salk and introduced nationwide in the United States in 1955. The inactivated polio vaccine is given by intramuscular injection. When the inactivated viral strains are injected, they induce immunity by stimulating the patients' immune system to produce antibodies. If a patient were later exposed to the poliovirus, these antibodies would inactivate the virus, stopping viral invasion of the neurons and the resulting damage. An enhanced-potency version of Salk's inactivated polio vaccine is still used in the United States.

In 1961, Albert Sabin introduced a second polio vaccine, the live attenuated oral vaccine, which works by a different mechanism. The oral polio vaccine consists of several strains of live poliovirus that are weakened by growing the viruses in harsh conditions. The resulting attenuated viruses can replicate in the GI tract and induce immunity to the virus but cannot enter the bloodstream or infect the neurons. There is a slight risk that the virus can revert to an infectious form and cause vaccine associated paralytic polio. This vaccine is appropriate for use in regions with active polio outbreaks because people make a response to this vaccine in the intestine (rather than the blood) and are more likely to fight off polio if exposed. The oral polio vaccine also has the advantage of being easy to administer, and is shed in the feces, so others living near people who are vaccinated are exposed to the viruses and receive protection, too. Use of the oral polio vaccine was stopped in the United States in 2000 because of the low risk of exposure and the risk of vaccine associated paralytic polio.

Post-Polio Syndrome

Decades after a poliovirus infection, 25–40 percent of patients will experience post-polio syndrome (www.post-polio.org). Symptoms of post-polio syndrome include new pain, increased muscle weakness, and possible new paralysis. Patients experiencing post-polio syndrome are not contagious and there is no risk of contracting polio from a person with post-polio syndrome.

Post-polio syndrome primarily affects people who have had paralytic polio infections. During infection, motor nerve cells are destroyed. After infection, new branches (called sprouts) of undamaged motor nerve cells are formed to make new synapses (re-innervate) with the muscle. Patients who have had polio have larger sections of muscle innervated by each nerve, forming larger motor units. Weichers and Hubbell (1981) hypothesized that these new sprouts are not as stable as the original, undamaged nerve cell connections. Perhaps it is the loss of the rebuilt sprouts that cause the post-polio patients to have new weakness and paralysis.

Future

Polio has been eradicated in many parts of the world due to vaccination. In 2012, three countries had endemic polio: Afghanistan, Nigeria, and Pakistan. Due to these areas with polio, there is still a worldwide risk of polio outbreaks. In 2011, for example, polio was reintroduced in Angola, Chad, and the Democratic Republic of the Congo. Officials are optimistic that polio can be eradicated with proper vaccination campaigns because humans are the only reservoir for the virus. Weekly updates on the status of global polio eradication can be found at http://www.polioeradication.org/Dataandmonitoring/Poliothisweek.aspx

Lisa A. Rabe

See also: Neuromuscular Junction; Paralysis; Retrovirus

Further Reading

CDC. (2011). Tracking progress toward global polio eradication—Worldwide, 2009–2010. *Morbidity and Mortality Weekly Report, 60*(14), 441–445.

The Global Polio Eradication Initiative. (2012, October 31). *Polio this week.* Retrieved from http://www.polioeradication.org/Dataandmonitoring/Poliothisweek.aspx

Post Polio. (2012, March 23). Retrieved from www.postpolio.org.

Sass, E. J. (Ed.). (1996). *Polio's legacy: An oral history.* Lantham, MD: University Press of America.

Wiechers, D., & Hubbell, S. L. (1981). Late changes in the motor unit after acute poliomyelitis. *Muscle & Nerve, 4,* 524–528.

Pons

In vertebrates, the brainstem connects the spinal cord to the brain. From caudal to rostral, the brainstem is made up of the medulla oblongata, pons, and midbrain. The *pons* is a bulging structure of the brainstem connecting the cerebrum to the cerebellum. From an evolutionary standpoint, the pons is a relatively old structure and existed in the first agnathans, which are jawless fish. The pons is located just ventral to the cerebellum, rostral to the medulla oblongata, and caudal to the midbrain and thalamus. The pons functions primarily to relay information to and from the cerebrum and between the two hemispheres of the brain. It also functions to help regulate arousal and sleep. The pons contains the anterior and

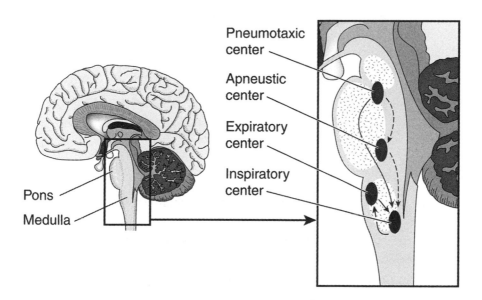

Drawing of the brain and brainstem, showing areas of the pons that control respiration. (Dreamstime.com)

posterior pontine nuclei, which are distinct clusters of neuronal cell bodies (gray matter). The anterior nuclei relay information from the cerebrum to the cerebellum, while the posterior nuclei are termination points for several cranial nerves. Located within the pons are also centers for sleep and respiration (breathing), which work in conjunction with the medulla oblongata to regulate respiratory movements and arousal.

Pontine Nuclei and Its Diseases

The posterior pons contains nuclei for the trigeminal (cranial nerve V), abducens (cranial nerve VI), facial (cranial nerve VII), vestibulocochlear (cranial nerve VIII), and glossopharyngeal nerves (cranial nerve IX). Central pontine myelinosis is a disease of the pons in which the nervous tissue becomes demyelinated—resulting in slower impulses between neurons. Central pontine myelinosis causes motor problems particularly impairments in balance, sensation, walking, swallowing, and speaking.

Kevin Lee

See also: Brainstem; Cranial Nerves; Medulla Oblongata

Further Reading

Blumenfeld, H. (Ed.). (2010). *Neuroanatomy through clinical cases* (2nd ed.). Sunderland, MA: Sinauer Associates, Incorporated.

Jasmin, L. (2012). *Central pontine myelinosis.* MedlinePlus. Retrieved from http://www.nlm.nih.gov/medlineplus/ency/article/000775.htm

Kandel, E. R., Schwartz, J. H., Jessell, T. M., Siegelbaum, S. A., & Hudspeth, A. J. (Eds.). (2012). *Principles of neural science* (5th ed.). New York, NY: McGraw Hill Companies.

Patestas, M. A. & Gartner, L. P. (Eds.). (2006). *A textbook of neuroanatomy.* Malden, MA: Blackwell Science Ltd.

Postsynaptic Potentials

Brain cells, or neurons, are unique in that they use chemicals called neurotransmitters to "talk" to each other. There is a small space between the two neurons called the *synaptic cleft*. The presynaptic neuron releases a chemical into this space and the postsynaptic neuron receives the chemical. This action results in a voltage change across the postsynaptic neuron's membrane. Specifically, *postsynaptic potentials* (PSPs) represent *graded voltage changes* in the electrical membrane potential of the postsynaptic neuron in a chemical synapse. Functionally, PSPs are the result of either (1) an increase in the net positive current (*depolarization*) to the membrane potential, which increases the likelihood of *action potential* (neural signal) firing; or (2) a net negative current (*hyperpolarization*) of the membrane potential, which decreases the likelihood of an action potential being fired. For a PSP to occur at a chemical synapse, the presynaptic neuron must release neurotransmitter-containing vesicles from its axonal terminal into the synaptic cleft. These neurotransmitters then bind to corresponding receptors on the postsynaptic neuronal membrane to illicit a response typically by either (1) opening *ion channels* and allowing current flow, affecting the electrical potential of the membrane; or (2) stimulating a response from *intracellular chemical second messengers,* which can affect the characteristics of postsynaptic responses.

History

Early ideas about how the nervous system was organized involved the existence of a large, single, cellular mass with multiple nuclei. In the early 1900s, using the Golgi stain technique, Santiago Ramon y Cajal (1852–1934) demonstrated that the nervous system was rather composed of a vast collection of individual neurons. This demonstration led to the description of the "synapse," a term derived from the Greek word meaning "connect," which was introduced at the end of the 19th century by the British physiologist Charles Scott Sherrington (1857–1952). During the beginning of the 20th century, there were two schools of thought on how the synapse functioned. One idea heralded by Sir John Carew Eccles (1903–1997) was that communication at the synapse between the "presynaptic" neuron and the "postsynaptic" neuron was electrical in nature and resulted from ion movement during direct physical connections between the neurons. The second view, put forth by Sir Henry Hallett Dale (1875–1968), was that synaptic transmission was mediated by chemicals from the terminal of the presynaptic neuron that interacted with the postsynaptic neuron. It is now known that in fact both electrical and chemical types of synapses exist, each producing different types of responses and serving distinct functions within the nervous system. The earliest explanations of how the synapse worked came from studying the *neuromuscular junction* in a frog where motor nerve endings control muscle movement by releasing the neurotransmitter, *acetylcholine,* across the synaptic cleft causing a change in the postsynaptic membrane potential. When applied to the connections between neurons themselves, the same principles of chemical synaptic communication remained consistent.

Mechanisms of Postsynaptic Responses

PSPs are visualized and studied using the techniques of electrophysiology which allow for the recording of membrane potential changes and current flow across a neuronal membrane as well as of individual ion channels embedded within a membrane. When an action potential is activated, spreads, and reaches the axonal terminal of a presynaptic neuron, it stimulates the release of vesicles containing neurotransmitter molecules. These neurotransmitters then diffuse across the synaptic cleft and bind to a corresponding receptor on the postsynaptic neuronal membrane. Often, there exists a region known as the *postsynaptic density,* which is associated with the postsynaptic membrane directly across from the density of vesicles on the presynaptic side of a synapse. This region may aid in securing neurotransmitter receptors in the membrane and contain molecules used in the conversion of the chemical signal into an electrical response in the postsynaptic neuron. PSPs are produced locally at areas where neurotransmitter receptors are present and then spread electrotonically. Depending on where the receptors are located on a neuron, either near the axons' trigger zone or on a distal dendrite, will determine whether it produces a powerful response or one that decays while electronically spreading toward the trigger zone, respectively. Often, synapses that occur on a neuron's cell body or initial axonal segment produce inhibitory responses, which allows for a means of controlling the effects of excitatory responses generated further away. Once a neurotransmitter is bound to a receptor on the postsynaptic neuronal membrane, it can stimulate the transient opening or closing of an ion channel which permits the entrance and exit of current carrying ions such as sodium (Na^+), potassium (K^+), chloride (Cl^-), and calcium (Ca^{2+}). The flow of ionic current changes the electrical potential of the neuronal membrane in either a positive direction which depolarizes the membrane, or a negative direction which hyperpolarizes the membrane.

Types of Postsynaptic Responses

Neurons typically have a negative resting membrane potential of approximately −70 mV. If ion flow produces a net increase in positive charge across the membrane and depolarizes it, the voltage of the membrane will approach its threshold for firing an action potential. This type of graded postsynaptic response is known as an *excitatory postsynaptic potential* (EPSP). On the other hand, if ion flow produces a net gain of negative charge across the membrane and hyperpolarizes it, the voltage will move further away from its threshold for firing an action potential. This type of graded response is knows as an *inhibitory postsynaptic potential* (IPSP).

An EPSP is the "go" signal which produces an excitatory response in the nervous system. The opening of ion channels selective for monovalent cations (having a single positive charge), such as Na^+, typically results in an EPSP. An IPSP is the "stop" signal, which can potentially decrease or prevent further neuronal circuits from being activated. Typically, opening of ion channels selective for Cl^- produces an IPSP. There also exist PSPs that produce an electrically silent change in the membrane polarization, but these are less common. Neurotransmitters themselves are not inherently excitatory or inhibitory, rather it is the receptor to which they bind that plays a significant role in determining the type of postsynaptic response. For example, different receptors for the same neurotransmitter may open different types of ion channels and produce either an EPSP or IPSP. The termination of either type of PSP is the result of the detachment of a neurotransmitter from its receptor on the postsynaptic membrane. As a result, the receptor returns to its unbound state, ion channels close, and ion levels return to their state of equilibrium.

Graded Postsynaptic Responses

Both EPSPs and IPSPs can either be large or small and fast or slow in their response. A small magnitude postsynaptic response occurs when a single or a small number of vesicles containing neurotransmitter are released from the presynaptic neuron and bind to receptors on the postsynaptic neuron. This produces a postsynaptic response that only allows for a small amount of current flow through ion channels that are stimulated to open. Although this may produce an EPSP depending on the corresponding neurotransmitter and receptor, it will not be large enough to elicit an action potential in the postsynaptic neuron. Large magnitude postsynaptic responses are the result of large numbers of neurotransmitter containing vesicles being released from a presynaptic neuron or neurons and binding to receptors on the postsynaptic neuron allowing for a large current flow through the membrane and potentially producing an EPSP large enough to elicit an action potential. Postsynaptic neurons can receive a multitude of simultaneous synaptic inputs from different presynaptic neurons producing a collective response strong enough to produce significant shifts, either depolarizing or hyperpolarizing, in the postsynaptic membrane potential. Typically, fast synaptic transmission occurs via the opening and closing of ion channels, while slow synaptic transmission involves postsynaptic receptors coupled to intracellular chemical *second messengers.* One such type of second messenger, called a *G protein,* can stimulate a multistep process whereby a subunit dissociates from the receptor and moves laterally in the postsynaptic membrane to influence the functional state of other ion channels. Although this type of postsynaptic response is relatively slower, it allows for the amplification of synaptic inputs and for a broader set of postsynaptic effects.

Summation of Postsynaptic Potentials

EPSPs and IPSPs that are the result of neurotransmitter-containing vesicle release across a synapse from a single presynaptic neuron are not capable of producing enough of a postsynaptic membrane potential response to produce any significant changes. However, more than one PSP, excitatory or inhibitory, can be added together if received in close proximity to each other, a phenomenon known as *spatial summation.* This may also occur with an excitatory and inhibitory response being added together to potentially cancel each other out or result in the difference between the two. Secondly, if a neuron received PSPs close together in time, they too can be added together, whether received from the same or different synapses. This phenomenon is known as *temporal summation.*

Although in order to produce a postsynaptic response the presynaptic neuron must be activated, the same postsynaptic response is not always produced based on the recent activity history of the specific synapse. For example, the presynaptic neuronal terminal could release excess neurotransmitter when stimulated, producing a phenomenon known as *potentiation* in the postsynaptic neuron. Alternatively, the presynaptic neuronal terminal could release depleted amounts of neurotransmitter, a phenomenon known as *depression* in the postsynaptic neuron. Although these types of responses can last for seconds, longer lasting effects that can last up to days at a time and known as *long term potentiation* and *long term depression* may also occur, and in the case of the former, contribute to the process of *learning and memory* in the central nervous system.

Simon Waldbaum

See also: Action Potential; G Proteins; Ion Channels; Learning and Memory; Neuromuscular Junction; Presynaptic Terminals; Secondary Messengers; Synaptic Cleft

Further Reading

Levitan, I. B., & Kaczmarek, L. K. (1997). *The Neuron.* New York, NY: Oxford University Press.

Takamori, M. (2012). Structure of the neuromuscular junction: Function and cooperative mechanisms in the synapse. *Annals of the New York Academy of Sciences, 1274,* 14–23.

Yamashita, T., Pala, A., Pedrido, L., Kremer, Y., Welker, E., & Petersen, C. C. (2013). Membrane potential dynamics of neocortical projection neurons driving target specific signals. *Neuron, 80,* 1477–1490.

Yang, Y., & Calakos, N. (2013). Presynaptic long term plasticity. *Frontiers in Synaptic Neuroscience, 5,* 8.

Post-Traumatic Stress Disorder

Post-traumatic stress disorder (PTSD) is a complex, multisystem disorder that develops in individuals who have experienced a catastrophic life event and has a prevalence of nearly 7 percent in the general population (National Institute of Mental

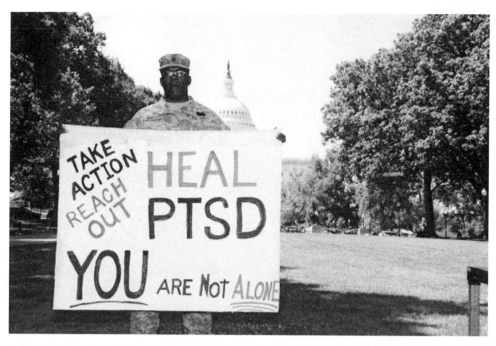

Soldier holds a sign with a message to heal post-traumatic stress disorder (PTSD). (U.S. Army)

Health, 2013). PTSD can occur at any age and can affect war veterans, survivors of accidents, abuse, assault, natural disasters, and other extreme stressors. Traumatic events are the major cause of PTSD and by definition must be severe enough to be outside the range of a normal human experience. It is thought that the more severe the trauma, the greater the risk of developing PTSD.

A person's age, level of social and emotional support, history of other emotional disturbance, and proximity to the stressor are all factors that play a role in the development of PTSD. Those who have received previous psychiatric treatment are more likely to develop PTSD, as they may be more vulnerable to stress. On the other hand, those who have a strong support system are less likely to develop PTSD.

Scientists have tried to determine why some individuals are more likely to develop PTSD than others and how it can best be treated. Research has focused on alterations within the hypothalamic-pituitary-adrenal axis indicative of low cortisol and increased glucocorticoid sensitivity, which are both naturally occurring steroids. Brain imaging studies have found reduced hippocampal volume and increased metabolic activity in the amygdala in patients with PTSD. Other studies have shown decreased rapid eye movement latency in stage IV sleep and this is thought to play a role in its development. The noradrenergic and serotonergic pathways in the central nervous system have also been implicated in the development of PTSD.

Signs and Symptoms

There are three major elements of PTSD: reliving the trauma through dreams or intrusive thoughts, emotional numbing and feeling detached from others, and symptoms of autonomic hyperarousal (an exaggerated response of fear to a normal stimulus). If these symptoms have lasted less than three months, it is referred to as acute PTSD, and chronic PTSD if symptoms last three months or longer. Symptoms usually begin soon after experiencing the stressor, but the onset can be delayed from months to years.

Patients with PTSD often experience symptoms of increased arousal. These can include severe anxiety, irritability, insomnia, and poor concentration. Severe anxiety can manifest as panic attacks and episodes of aggression. Avoidance and dissociative symptoms are also common. These symptoms include detachment, an inability to feel emotion, and a diminished interest in activities. Intrusions refer to memories of the traumatic event that appears suddenly in the form of a flash back or nightmare. Depressive symptoms are also common. Unfortunately, many patients develop maladaptive coping responses, which may include excessive use of alcohol or drugs.

Treatment

Cognitive behavioral therapy (CBT) is an important PTSD treatment strategy. There are three components of CBT: recalling and sequencing memories of the traumatic event, correcting misinterpretations (the idea that the individual could have done more to help or that flashbacks are a sign of insanity), and confronting any situations that trigger memories of the event, referred to as controlled exposure. As PTSD is often associated with comorbid depression, it is important to always consider CBT and other types of support.

Selective serotonin inhibitors (SSRIs) are the most commonly prescribed medications for the treatment of PTSD. Both paroxetine (Paxil) and sertraline (Zoloft) are FDA approved for the treatment of PTSD, but other SSRIs are likely effective as well. By increasing the amount of serotonin in the synaptic cleft, SSRIs help to decrease depressive symptoms, reduce intrusive thoughts and anxiety, and normalize sleep. Other classes of medications including serotonin-norepinephrine reuptake inhibitors (SNRIs), tricyclic antidepressants (TCAs), and monoamine oxidase inhibitors (MAOIs) have shown some benefit.

Danielle Stutzman

See also: Amygdala; Behavioral Health; Depression; Hypothalamus; Pituitary Gland (Hypophysis); Rapid Eye Movement (REM); Sleep; Trauma; Traumatic Brain Injury (TBI)

Further Reading

Black, D. W., & Andreasen, N. C. (2011). *Introductory textbook of psychiatry* (5th ed.). United States: American Psychiatric Publishing, Inc.

National Institute of Mental Health. (2013). *Post-traumatic stress disorder (PTSD)*. Retrieved from http://www.nimh.nih.gov/health/topics/post-traumatic-stress-disorder-ptsd/index.shtml

U.S. Department of Veterans Affairs. (2013). *PTSD: National Center for PTSD*. Retrieved from http://www.ptsd.va.gov/public/

Wounded Warrior Project. (2013). Retrieved from http://www.woundedwarriorproject.org

Potassium Channels

Potassium (K^+) is a positively charged ion. In the central nervous system, it is essential for the falling phase of an action potential (a neuronal signal or impulse), where sodium (Na^+) ions are responsible for the rising phase of an action potential. Potassium ions are highly concentrated in the intracellular fluid of a neuron, which is a specialized cell found only in the nervous system.

When neurons send neural impulses between each other, specifically at the junction of where two neurons are located (the synaptic cleft), it causes a significant change in the receiving neuron (or postsynaptic neuron). Within the postsynaptic neuron, certain integral membrane proteins, called receptors or ion channels, will open allowing sodium ions to rush through. Because these ion channels conduct sodium through the plasma membrane, they are generically called *sodium channels*. Sodium will flow down its concentration gradient and enter the postsynaptic neuron. This results in a change in the resting membrane potential (voltage difference across the membrane at rest, which is typically around −70 mV) of the postsynaptic neuron such that it is depolarized (becomes more positive and closer to 0 mV). If a cell depolarizes enough (to about −55 or −40 mV), it may result in the production of an action potential. However, a neuron can only flux so much sodium resulting in a peak of depolarization. At that peak, sodium channels will inactivate and *potassium channels* will open. Because these ion channels conduct only potassium through the plasma membrane, they are generically called potassium channels. Potassium ions will flow down its concentration and electrochemical gradients and exit the postsynaptic neuron. This results in hyperpolarizing the membrane potential of the neuron and helps restore it to its normal resting membrane potential.

Types of Potassium Channels

Potassium channels are named based on the way the protein is activated to allow potassium to flow. To date, there are five main classifications: (1) *calcium-activated potassium channels;* (2) *inwardly rectifying potassium channels;* (3) *tandem pore domain potassium channels;* (4) *voltage-gated potassium channels;* and, (5) *G protein-coupled inwardly rectifying potassium channels.* As suggested by its name, calcium-activated potassium channels will open when calcium ions (Ca^{2+}) or similarly charged signaling molecules concentrations are increased in the neuron; while inwardly rectifying potassium channels will move potassium into the cell creating a positive inward current. Inwardly rectifying potassium channels are commonly denoted as Kir or IRK channels.

It is important that the membrane potential return to rest and with the fast activation of sodium and potassium channels, some channels must be open all the time (called constitutively open). These are the tandem pore domain potassium channels, which are often called "leak channels" or "resting potassium channels." They are essential to help maintain the negative membrane potential of neurons. As seen with voltage-gated sodium channels, the voltage-change receptors are activated when the voltage of the membrane is altered. These receptors are also called voltage-dependent, voltage-sensitive, and voltage-gated potassium channels. They are universally designated as Kv to denote the voltage requirement. Finally, G protein-coupled inwardly rectifying potassium channels, or muscarinic potassium channels are opened when a muscarinic receptor (part of the acetylcholine receptor family) is activated. They are denoted as IKACh, as they represent an outward current. These potassium channels are generally found in the cardiac muscles to slow down heart rate. The remainder of this entry will focus on the first four types of potassium channels, as these are found in the central nervous system.

Structure and Function

The complex structure of the potassium channel was determined by X-ray crystallography by American biophysicist Roderick MacKinnon (1956–) and colleagues in 1998. For his discovery and contribution to science, MacKinnon shared the 2003 Nobel Prize in Chemistry with American molecular biologist and physician Peter Agre (1949–), who discovered aquaporins (water channels). The unique structure of potassium channels allows them to be selective for only potassium. This means that smaller ions, like sodium, do not pass through these channels. This is counterintuitive in nature, which made it difficult to determine its structure until MacKinnon worked on the problem.

In general, potassium channels consist of four protein subunits with each subunit spanning the plasma membrane six times, thus integrating them within the membrane. When four subunits come together, they form a common, symmetric pore. This pore is specialized as it conducts only potassium ions, either out of or into the neuron. If the four subunits are identical, the potassium channel is called a *homotetrameric complex;* if the subunits are related but different, the resulting channel is called a *heterotetrameric complex.* Nonetheless, all potassium channel subunits have an extracellular protein domain called a pore-loop, or P-loop, structure. This means it projects into the extracellular side of the plasma membrane. Together, these four P-loop structures line the top of the pore and are the part of the channel that determines its selective permeability.

Calcium-Activated Potassium Channels

There are three main types of calcium-activated potassium channels: BK, IK, and SK channels. Big potassium channels (BK), or Maxi-K, are noted for their large conductance of potassium through the plasma membrane. These have four alpha subunits that are encoded by the *KCNMA1* gene. Additionally, these alpha subunits are modulated by beta subunits, which are encoded by *KCNMB1, KCNMB2, KCNMB3,* or *KCNMB4* genes. This modulation will alter the kinetics of the BK channel, meaning how quickly it will conduct potassium through the cell and how long it will be in an open or closed state. Similarly, the small conductance potassium channel, or SK, is made up of four alpha subunits that are encoded by four different genes, *KCNN1, KCNN2, KCNN3,* and *KCNN4.* The protein subunit made by the *KCNN4* gene, however, will conduct potassium more than the other three SK subunits but less than the BK subunits, hence they are the intermediate potassium channels (IK).

Inwardly Rectifying Potassium Channels

There are seven known subfamilies of inwardly rectifying potassium channels that are called ROMK1 (or $K_{ir}1.1$), IRK1 through IRK4, GIRK1 through GIRK4, $K_{ir}1.2$ through $K_{ir}1.4$, K_{ATP}, and BIR9. These proteins are encoded by 15 different genes from *KCNJ1* through *KCNJ6,* then *KCNJ8* through *KCNJ16.* Four alpha subunits will combine to form these channels.

Tandem Pore Domain Potassium Channels

There are 15 known members of the tandem pore domain potassium channel family. Their name is derived from the fact that each channel is made up of two alpha subunits with both subunits having two P-loop domains. Thus, these channels are dimers. It is important to not confuse the tandem pore domain potassium channels with another family called the two-pore channel family. Tandem pore channels are also called leak channels and follow the Goldman-Hodgkin-Katz rectification of the neuron. This helps keep the correct electrochemical gradient needed when an action potential or postsynaptic potential arrives in the neuron. Although these channels are constitutively open, their activation can be altered depending on mechanical stretch, pH, oxygen tension, and G protein activation. The following genes encode the alpha-subunit proteins: *KCNK1* through *KCNK7, KCNK9, KCNK10, KCNK12, KCNK13,* and *KCNK15* through *KCNK18*. The channels are denoted for their two pores by K_{2P}.

Voltage-Gated Potassium Channels

There are 12 known alpha subunits that make up the voltage-gated potassium channel family. Within these 12 alpha subunits (called Kvalpha1 through Kvalpha12, there about 40 different channels based on how the alpha subunits combine. Additionally, beta subunits (encoded by the *KCNAB1–3, KCNE1–4, KCNIP1–4,* and the *KCNE1L* genes) will associate with the four alpha subunits to modulate the activity of the channel. Though all of these channels open when a specific change in the transmembrane potential occurs, they each have slightly different functions. These include (1) delayed rectifiers, either slowly inactivating or noninactivating; (2) A-type potassium channels, or rapidly inactivating; (3) outward or inward rectifying (meaning the direction of the flow of potassium ions); (4) slowly activating; and (5) modifier/silencer. Most of these describe the state of the potassium channel, activating (open), deactivating (closed), or inactivating (closed). The difference between deactivating and inactivating is that when a channel is in the deactivating state, the channel can easily move into the activating or open state. In inactivating states, the channel is blocked so that it cannot open even if the transmembrane voltage is favorable. Instead it must move into the deactivating state first. This is a protective mechanism for the cell. Specifically, it regulates the flux of potassium ions so that not too much will leave or enter the cell, thus maintaining homeostasis and the resting membrane potential.

Diseases and Disorders

There are many different types of potassium alpha and beta subunits and the genes that encode for them; if a mutation occurs it can result in significant neurological diseases and/or disorders. In fact, studying these disease states, such as epilepsy, helped researchers better understand the role and function of potassium channels. Since potassium channels are essential to terminate action potentials, when the proteins are mutated these channels may not work correctly and continue to allow action potentials to persist. Thus, potassium channels are associated with seizures and inherited epilepsies. There is a therapeutic attempt to stabilize the activation state of these potassium channels so that membrane excitability can be regulated. Thus, specific potassium channel agonists have shown some success in reducing the chances of seizures. It is important to note, however, that antiepileptic drugs do not cure the epilepsy. Instead, they just lessen the chances for future seizures.

Jennifer L. Hellier

See also: Epilepsy; Ion Channels; Membrane; Membrane Potential: Depolarization and Hyperpolarization; Membrane Potential Experiment—Understand Membrane Properties; Postsynaptic Potentials; Presynaptic Terminals; Seizures; Sodium Channels

Further Reading

Doyle, D. A., Morais, C. J., Pfuetzner, R. A., Kuo, A., Gulbis, J. M., Cohen, S. L., . . . MacKinnon, R. (1998). The structure of the potassium channel: Molecular basis of K+ conduction and selectivity. *Science, 280*(5360), 69–77.

Hillel, B. (2001). *Ion channels of excitable membranes* (3rd ed.). Sunderland, MA: Sinauer Associates.

Kandel, E. R., Schwartz, J. H., Jessell, T. M., Siegelbaum, S. A., & Hudspeth, A. J. (Eds.). (2012). *Principles of neural science* (5th ed.). New York, NY: McGraw-Hill.

MacKinnon, R., Cohen, S. L., Kuo, A., Lee, A., & Chait, B. T. (1998). Structural conservation in prokaryotic and eukaryotic potassium channels. *Science, 280*(5360), 106–109.

Maljevic, S., & Lerche, H. (2013). Potassium channels: A review of broadening therapeutic possibilities for neurological diseases. *Journal of Neurology, 260*(9), 2201–2211.

Premotor Cortex

The cerebral cortex of the mammalian brain consists of gyri (bumps) and sulci (valleys) that are divided into different lobes as well as different regions. Regions of the cerebral cortex have been defined according to structure and organization of the neurons that they contain. These regions are called *Brodmann areas.* Within the frontal lobe, the *primary motor cortex, supplementary motor area,* and *premotor cortex* are found. Specifically, the supplementary motor area and premotor cortex are just rostral (toward the nose) to the primary motor cortex (the precentral gyrus, Brodmann area 4) and are called Brodmann area 6. The premotor cortex is important for integrating sensory information into initiating motor movements that are appropriate for the intended voluntary action.

Anatomy and Physiology

The premotor cortex is located in the frontal lobe and is surrounded by the supplementary motor area (dorsal and medial to the premotor cortex); primary motor cortex (caudal—toward the back of the brain); and the prefrontal areas (rostral). The neurons (brain cells that transmit nerve impulses) located within the premotor cortex receive direct input from the supplementary motor area, primary motor cortex, posterior parietal cortex (sensory information about location in space), and nuclei of the thalamus (a deep brain structure that modulates motor and sensory information). Indirect inputs are received from (1) the somatosensory cortex—postcentral gyrus, Brodmann areas 3, 1, and 2—via the primary motor cortex; (2) the cerebellum—the "little brain" that modulates and coordinates voluntary movements—via the thalamus; and (3) the basal ganglia—deep brain structure that modulates and controls voluntary movements—via the thalamus. The premotor cortex projects its outputs to the primary motor cortex, supplementary motor area, and thalamus. Based on the numerous direct and indirect inputs into the premotor cortex as well as its direct outputs, it is apparent how complex and integrated voluntary movements are.

The functions of the premotor cortex differ depending on where the intended action originated, either the lateral (to the side) or medial (toward the midline) part of the premotor cortex. The lateral region is mainly responsible for learned movements in specific directions (such as skipping or writing the number "2") as well as timing those movements. The movements are generated in response to external cues, such as visual signs. Additionally, this area will be activated prior to that expected movement, showing its importance for the needed intention of the specific movement as well as selecting the planned/learned movement for the intended action.

The medial premotor cortex is also responsible for selecting movements, but those movements in response to internal cues. For example, a person is walking to the store but gets an itchy nose. The person will continue to walk—based on learned activity from the lateral premotor cortex—and scratch their nose—based on medial premotor cortex function. The person will not have to stop walking to scratch their nose as both can occur at the same time; scratching is an automatic or spontaneous response to the internal cue. These are self-initiated actions that are also learned.

Lesions and Symptoms

Damage to the lateral premotor cortex results in severe inability to perform a movement based on an external cue. For example, a person would have difficulty in moving to the left if they see a blinking arrow pointing traffic to move to the left.

However, the person understands what the visual cue means and can move to the left on their own without the visual cue. Similarly, a person with damage to the frontal lobe will have difficulty selecting certain movements based on an external cue, even though they understand the meaning of the cue. For example, if the person is asked to raise their right hand, the premotor cortex will not be able to select that learned movement to perform the action. Nonetheless, the person can raise their right hand for other movements without being verbally asked. Finally, lesions to the medial premotor cortex result in a person having decreased spontaneous movements (like scratching or stretching) but will have no problems in producing movements based on external cues.

Jennifer L. Hellier

See also: Brain Anatomy; Brodmann Areas; Motor Cortex

Further Reading

Purves, D., Augustine, G. J., Fitzpatrick, D., Hall, W. C., LaMantia, A.-S., McNamara, J. O., & Williams, S. M. (Eds.). (2004). *Neuroscience* (3rd ed.). Sunderland, MA: Sinauer Associates.

Presynaptic Terminals

A primary function of the nervous system is communication, and it is this transfer of information that sets it apart from other organ systems. The nervous system achieves its complex forms of communication by the structure of specialized portions of the neurons themselves and through *chemical synapses.* These chemical synapses are specialized junctions that are made up of: a *presynaptic terminal,* a *synaptic cleft,* and a *postsynaptic neuron.* The presynaptic terminal is a specialized area at the end of the neuron's axon, which stores neurotransmitter chemicals in small membrane-bound *synaptic vesicles.* The presynaptic terminal is separated from the postsynaptic neuron by the synaptic cleft, which is a small extracellular space. Upon receiving an *action potential,* the presynaptic neuron is stimulated to release its synaptic vesicles that contain neurotransmitters (or chemicals) into the synaptic cleft that then bind to receptors on the postsynaptic neuron. This action can produce either an excitatory or inhibitory *postsynaptic response.* The maintenance and release of different kinds of synaptic vesicles and their contents from the presynaptic terminal is controlled by (1) various functional proteins, and (2) by the influx of calcium ions (Ca^{2+}) through ion channels in the neuronal plasma membrane.

Presynaptic Terminal Morphology

The presynaptic portion of a synapse is typically formed from the terminal expansion of an axon. However, they can also be formed from dendrites or portions of the neuronal cell body. The use of high powered electron microscopy has allowed visualization of the presynaptic terminal and revealed insights into its unique morphology. A specific area of the presynaptic terminal membrane appears relatively thickened compared to other areas. Furthermore, it is characterized by the presence of a large number of membrane-bound synaptic vesicles that contain neurotransmitters. These synaptic vesicles are often clustered together close to the neuronal membrane at its point of closest contact with the postsynaptic neuron. The synaptic vesicles appear "docked" at these sites called *active zones*. Synaptic vesicles appear to have different shapes and colors when visualized with electron microscopy depending on which types of neurotransmitters they contain. Asymmetrically shaped synapses are characterized (1) by rounded vesicles in the presynaptic neuron, and (2) by a prominent postsynaptic density. These asymmetrical synapses are typically excitatory, meaning they "turn on" the postsynaptic neuron. On the other hand, symmetrically shaped synapses have flattened or elongated vesicles and lack a prominent postsynaptic density. Moreover, symmetrical synapses are typically inhibitory, meaning they "turn off" the postsynaptic neuron.

The majority of both cell body and dendrite surfaces in the central nervous system synapse with a large number of presynaptic terminals, producing a *convergence* of input onto a single neuron from potentially thousands of presynaptic cells. Additionally, a presynaptic axon may branch a large number of times providing input to many postsynaptic targets producing a *divergence*. The release of a single or a small number of synaptic vesicles only produces a small effect on the postsynaptic neuron which may not elicit a significant response. In order to produce a more significant response, there needs to be a concerted vesicle release from many presynaptic terminals onto a single postsynaptic neuron, which is achieved through divergent synaptic connections.

Neurons typically contain two types of synaptic vesicles docked at their active zones. The first type is *large dense core* vesicles approximately 100 nm (nanometers or 10^{-9}) in diameter that contains mainly peptide neurotransmitters. The second type is *small synaptic vesicles* approximately 40 nm in diameter that contain nonpeptide neurotransmitters. Small synaptic vesicles tend to be homogeneous in size and are assembled within the presynaptic terminal itself. Because they are small in shape, these synaptic vesicles are associated with a rapid release of neurotransmitters. Small synaptic vesicles have the ability to be recycled and refilled many times at the presynaptic terminal when retrieved through *endocytosis*. However, large dense core vesicles are capable of releasing their contents only once before the membrane proteins of the vesicle are degraded and/or returned to the cell body.

Presynaptic Terminal Vesicle Release

The release of neurotransmitters from the presynaptic terminal takes place through a type of *exocytosis* called *vesicle secretion*. When stimulated by an action potential that travels down the axon and reaches the presynaptic terminal, the synaptic vesicles docked there are triggered to fuse with the neuronal membrane. This fusion allows the synaptic vesicles to release their neurotransmitters into the synaptic cleft. The origins of this process are likely rooted in a cell's need to both (1) extricate proteins and molecules that do not easily cross through the phospholipid membrane; and (2) to insert proteins into its plasma membrane, such as in the case of ion channels. It is often difficult to study neurotransmitter release due to the small size of the majority of presynaptic terminals. However, this challenge can be circumvented when studying the giant synapse present in the stellate ganglion of the squid. This giant synapse is stimulated in escape behavior and its size allows for the placement of several recording electrodes at the synapse. *Patch clamp recording,* a type of electrophysiological technique, can be used to study the means of synaptic vesicle fusion with the neuronal membrane. Specifically, when a synaptic vesicle releases its contents, neuroscientists can record the electrical changes that occur during exocytosis. Because the neuronal membrane has the ability to store electrical charge, its electrical *capacitance,* a measure of its stored charge, can be determined. The neuronal membrane's capacitance is directly correlated to its surface area. When a synaptic vesicle fuses with the membrane, there is an increase in the measured capacitance, which is used to detect the exocytosis of vesicles. On the other hand, a decrease in capacitance indicates retrieval of vesicles by endocytosis. This type of recording technique has supplied evidence for the *kiss and run* mode of exocytosis. A vesicle "kiss" and "run" occurs when a vesicle fuses with the membrane temporarily to releases its neurotransmitter then reseals without losing any of its physical integrity. The appropriate location for the fusion between synaptic vesicles and the presynaptic neuronal membrane is controlled by specialized molecules on the surface of each to allow docking at exact locations. *Synaptobrevin* is a synaptic vesicle protein and *syntaxin* is a plasma membrane protein that match together similar to a lock and key. This lock and key mechanism ensures the appropriate location of exocytosis from the presynaptic terminal. Additionally, Synaptosomal Associated Protein (SNAP-25) is another plasma membrane protein that regulates the fusion of the two membranes.

Calcium-Dependent Vesicle Secretion

A presynaptic neuron is excited by an action potential, which spreads toward its axonal terminal and causes ion channels in the membrane to open in response to voltage changes. These open ion channels allow calcium ions, Ca^{2+}, to enter the terminal and raise their intracellular concentrations approximately 1,000 times at the active zone. Imaging techniques have revealed that calcium channels in the presynaptic terminal membrane are clustered near sites of neurotransmitter release producing higher concentrations of Ca^{2+} there. These high concentrations of Ca^{2+} within the terminal subsequently activate protein receptors on docked synaptic vesicles, changing their shape and driving the vesicles to fuse with the neuronal membrane. This process eventually allows the synaptic vesicles to release their neurotransmitters into the synaptic cleft. The time from action potential arrival at the terminal to the release of small vesicle's contents can take place in as little as 100 μs (microseconds or 10^{-6}). In order to stimulate the release of larger synaptic vesicles that are docked further away from the active zone, repetitive action potentials need to be received causing the opening of additional voltage-gated Ca^{2+} channels for longer periods. This extended signaling produces a corresponding further increase in Ca^{2+} concentration. This process can take as long as tens of milliseconds (or 10^{-3}).

Synapses are often thought of as a one-way street from pre- to postsynaptic neuron. However, there are instances when presynaptic terminals also possess the same kinds of receptors that postsynaptic neurons contain, which can influence the amount of transmitter released by the presynaptic terminal. These types of presynaptic terminal receptors, called *autoreceptors,* typically inhibit further transmitter release when bound by small amounts of released neurotransmitter. The inhibition of presynaptic neurons can also occur when a presynaptic terminal receives an axoaxonic (axon-to-axon) synaptic input that works to decrease Ca^{2+} entry and subsequently the amount of transmitter released when an action potential arrives at the terminal. Presynaptic *depression* describes the situation when a progressive decrease in neurotransmitter is released during repetitive action potentials and is likely the result of transmitter depletion during a high rate of stimulation. These effects can decrease the likelihood that the postsynaptic neuron will fire an action potential. In turn, it produces an inhibition of the synaptic connection and allows for the selective suppression of certain inputs to a postsynaptic neuron, thus effecting broader circuit communication. Alternatively, presynaptic *facilitation* occurs when axoaxonic synapses act to increase the entry of Ca^{2+} into a presynaptic terminal and promote an excess release of neurotransmitter containing vesicles. Facilitation occurs during a brief and repetitive activation of action potentials and is likely caused by residual Ca^{2+} remaining at the release site that does not have time to return to baseline levels between action potentials. Presynaptic *potentiation* describes the situation when an increase in neurotransmitter release occurs following successive stimulation at a presynaptic terminal. Potentiation differs from facilitation by being long lasting and slow to onset and is likely caused by an increase in sodium concentrations. Although calcium-dependent exocytosis of presynaptic vesicles is used widely in the nervous system, there also exists instances of alternative mechanisms. One such example occurs in the retina with photoreceptors and horizontal cells that do not contain synaptic vesicles and do not require an influx of calcium. Rather, in response to depolarization of the presynaptic membrane and without changing calcium concentrations, these neurons utilize carrier proteins to move neurotransmitters from the intracellular to extracellular space producing a graded release of chemical.

Simon Waldbaum

See also: Action Potential; Ion Channels; Membrane; Membrane Potential: Depolarization and Hyperpolarization; Neuromuscular Junction; Postsynaptic Potentials; Retina; Synaptic Cleft; Voltage Clamp Experiment

Further Reading

Li, L., & Chin, L. S. (2003). The molecular machinery of synaptic vesicle exocytosis. *Cellular and Molecular Life Sciences, 60*, 942–960.

Meldolesi, J., & Chieregatti, E. (2004). Fusion has found its calcium sensor. *Nature Cell Biology, 6*, 476–478.

Mendoza Schulz, A., Jing, Z., María Sánchez Caro, J., Wetzel, F., Dresbach, T., Strenzke, N., . . . Moser, T. (2014). Bassoon-disruption slows vesicle replenishment and induces homeostatic plasticity at a CNS synapse. *The EMBO Journal.* Epub ahead of print. PMID 24442636.

Sudhof, T. C. (2004). The synaptic vesicle cycle. *Annual Review of Neuroscience, 27*, 509–547.

Wolfel, M., & Schneggenburger, R. (2003). Presynaptic capacitance measurements and Ca^{2+} uncaging reveal submillisecond exocytosis kinetics and characterize the Ca^{2+} sensitivity of vesicle pool depletion at a fast CNS synapse. *Journal of Neuroscience, 23*, 7059–7068.

Prions

The term *prion* stands for proteinacious infectious particle, and is therefore considered a new type of infectious disease among parasites, viruses, and bacteria. They do not contain nucleic acids, and cannot be destroyed through means used to kill bacteria and viruses. Prions are a neurodegenerative agent that affect both humans and animals alike, and are commonly known as transmissible spongiform encephalopathies (TSE). A prion is an altered protein that essentially recruits proteins of similar types to wreak havoc on the nervous system. These proteins do not function as they normally should, due to configuration, and lead

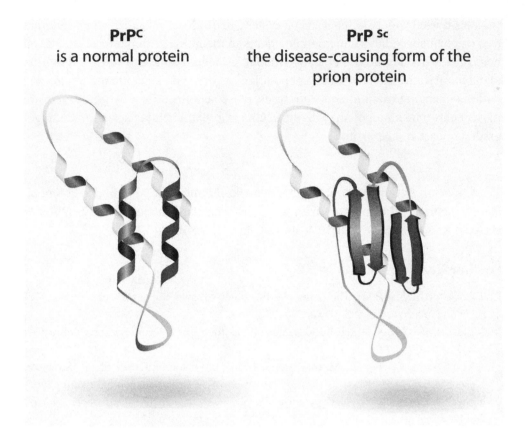

PrP^C
is a normal protein

PrP ^{Sc}
the disease-causing form of the prion protein

Prions are composed of proteins that are misfolded and are responsible for the transmissible mad cow disease, Creutzfeldt-Jakob disease. All known prion diseases are currently untreatable and fatal. (Dreamstime.com)

to the creation of tiny holes in the brain. This is the "spongy" appearance of the brain, hence the term "spongiform encephalopathies" (NINDS, 2011). Well-known human prion diseases include Creutzfeldt-Jakob Disease (CJD), as well as CJD's newer cousin, Variant Creutzfeldt-Jakob disease (vCJD), fatal familial insomnia (FFI), Kuru, and Gerstmann-Sträussler-Scheinker disease (GSS). As mentioned earlier, prions appear in animals more so than they do in humans. The diseases for animals include bovine spongiform encephalopathy (BSE), commonly known as "Mad Cow" disease, scrapie, chronic wasting disease (CWD), and transmissible mink encephalopathy (TME). Human TSEs occur in three ways: sporadic, hereditary, or through transmission from infected brain matter. As of yet, there is no cure for any form of prions disease, which usually end in the afflicted individual dying. There are, however, forms of prevention that will be explained in the following, as well as some limited treatments for the symptoms, which include fatigue, dementia (loss of mental ability that causes the inability to perform normal daily activities), headaches, cerebellar ataxia (inability to control movement), and cognitive degeneration, which can take anywhere from 3 to 15 years to appear.

History

The term scrapie is often associated with prions, and is the name for the TSE that affects sheep. In the 18th century, some sheep in France were noticed to be trembling while sheep in Germany were characterized with an itching or trotting disease. The Scottish term "scrapie" now commonly refers to these diseases, and originated for animals that had a habit of scraping their feces against hard objects. In 1922, CJD was coined to describe a human TSE that was known for symptoms of dementia and ataxia in the hosts, as observed and researched by Hans Gerhard Creutzfeldt (1885–1964) in 1920, and then by Alfans Maria Jakob (1884–1931) in 1921. Major outbreaks of prions disease include the spread of Kuru in the South Fore tribe of New Guinea in the 1950s, where it was custom to eat the brain of the deceased. Women, children, and the elderly would mainly partake in this form of cannibalism. The Kuru epidemic is now under control. The other well-known outbreak is the BSE epidemic in British cows in the 1980s, where the incidence of bovines with prions disease increased rapidly due to the bone meal and meat infected with prions that were fed to the cattle. Ten to 20 years later, there was an increase in the incidence of various forms of TSE that was seen in humans. BSE is not yet completely eradicated from cattle, and can be seen in at least 50 countries outside of England.

Causes, Transmission, Types, and Symptoms

Normal prion proteins, generally located in the central nervous system, are referred to as PrP^C, which is the common form. The infectious form of prion proteins that causes disease is the PrP^{Sc} protein. The "Sc" in the infectious form refers to scrapie disease, which was seen in sheep. The biggest difference between the two forms is that PrP^C proteins have an α-helix structure, which can visually be thought of as a spring. On the other hand, the PrP^{Sc} protein is primarily composed of β-sheets, which is similar to straightening the spring out and layering it. The interesting aspect is that once the PrP^{Sc} protein is introduced to the central nervous system, it converts PrP^C proteins into more PrP^{Sc} proteins. The exact mechanisms behind this action are still being researched, but essentially there is a self-perpetuating process in which more of the pathogenic forms of the prion are formed, and therefore leads to an increase in symptoms. Current research has identified a protein known as Mot3 that may lead to prionogensis, but it is suspected that there are more proteins that aid in prion creation (Wrighton, 2009).

The introduction of the prion can be noted to have three different forms of manifestation. The misfolded, infectious PrP^{Sc} protein can arise spontaneously, occur as a result of mutation (familial), or come from an external infective source. Spontaneous cases are usually seen as random occurrences with no known links to genetics or to a source of infection. As with mutation, there have been several forms of prions disease that can be hereditary in the sense that the coding within genes can show autosomal dominance of the PrP^{Sc} form to occur. Therefore, prions disease can travel through families. Infective sources vary widely, but generally, prion disease is transmitted to people through contact with infected brain matter and spinal cord, from bovine, minks, deer, elk, and other humans. There have been cases where prions disease has occurred from cornea transplants and surgical equipment, where the autoclave used to clean the equipment did not eradicate prions.

CJD, a sporadic and the most common form of transmissible spongiform encephalopathy, only occurs in 1 out of 1 million people per year worldwide; it occurs most commonly among the older adult population near the age of 65. Associated symptoms include progressive dementia, myoclonus (abnormal contractions of muscle), fatigue, headaches, cognitive degeneration, and a change in behavior. These symptoms can fit into a very broad set of diseases, and currently, there is no single diagnostic test for determining if someone has CJD or another prions disease. Most often, the only test to identify prions disease properly in a person is to perform a brain biopsy. Due to the risk, brain biopsies are often performed on deceased individuals, and are the best way to confirm the disease. Magnetic resonance imaging (MRI), spinal taps (tests of the cerebrospinal fluid that bathes the central nervous system), and partial brain biopsies can be used to help narrow the gap in determining if the afflicted individual has prions disease or not. The outcome for people with CJD is death, which occurs on average within four months from when symptoms first start to present; however, the incubation period from when the first PrP^{Sc} is present in the central nervous system until symptoms begin is still unknown.

Kuru and vCJD are two forms of the infectious TSE, where the former occurs from contact with human brain matter and the latter with bovine brain matter. The period from the onset of symptoms until death is, on average, 14 months long. vCJD is often widespread throughout the body, leading to concern as to whether some PrP^{Sc} proteins can make it into and survive in blood. Three cases were identified where PrP^{Sc} proteins may have infected blood donation recipients with nonleucodepleted blood, meaning that the proteins can be found in white blood cells (Ironside, 2010). Symptoms are similar to those of CJD, but the progression of symptoms is slower. Kuru, as discussed previously, occurs due to cannibalism. Both of these TSE have symptoms similar to those with CJD, but patients also have dysarthria (difficulty in speaking due to damage of the muscle used for speech), dysphagia (problems with swallowing), trembling, emotional outburst, and toward the final stages, lack of control of sphincters.

GSS is the first human TSE that was discovered to be autosomal, or genetic. Mutations within the prion protein can cause changes from PrP^C to PrP^{Sc}. There are over seven mutations in codons that can occur to bring on symptoms of this disease, which generally occur with an α-helix to β-sheet conformation. Symptoms are similar to other TSE. Identification of genetic diseases can be done through immunohistochemistry. However, since identification of the codons that mutate is still ongoing, this is not a precise diagnostic technique.

All these neurodegenerative symptoms that prions present are caused by literal holes in the brain from the PrP^{Sc} protein. Vacuoles (fluid-filled cavities) form in the areas with the misfolded protein. These vacuoles start to multiply and increase in size, giving the brain a somewhat spongy appearance. This process of vacuolization can take years, to the point where the incubation period has been estimated to be 2 months to 20 years. The locations of the vacuoles vary, but generally they are seen in the basal ganglia (consisting of the caudate nucleus, putamen, and globus pallidus all located near the base of the brain) and cerebellar cortex. This process cannot be reversed, as of yet, so afflicted individuals are certain to die with or because of the disease. The prion is not attacked by the immune system, as it is not a foreign body. It is also not destroyed by proteases because it is a functional protein. The blood-brain barrier (a physical barrier that separates circulating blood from the brain and spinal cord) has shown to prevent antiviral and antibiotic medications from reaching the prion, so there are limited treatment options as delivery is a problem.

Prevention

Prions are mysterious and terrifying to research scientists and to health care providers because it is difficult to kill prions as well as to synthesize a cure. Therefore, preventative techniques are a current focus. Countries do take precautions on protecting their citizens from prions, such as the United States, as they ask blood donors if they have been in Britain during a certain time frame, generally from 1980 to 1990. The reason for this is because of the BSE outbreak in British cows due to cattle feed that contained cow meat and bone meal. The beef from these cows, if the cow had prions disease, can only infect other cows or people if it had brain or spinal cord tissue on it, which can happen from bad butcher practices. Britain, in response to the rise of vCJD and BSE, had a mass slaughter of their cattle in order to decrease the odds of infection. They also stopped the practice of adding cattle meal into their cattle feed.

Education is the primary tool in prevention of spreading prion diseases. Specifically, hunters need to be educated about prions disease in deer and elk, as well as what parts of the wild game are safe to ingest. CWD, found in deer and elk in the United States, is related to BSE. This means that, similar to BSE, people who eat infected elk or deer brain tissue may become infected, but evidence of this possibility is still under scrutiny. Individuals should also be careful to not ingest cow brain or glands as a form of prevention. This is important as cowherds across the world, not just those in the United Kingdom, have cattle with BSE. Another safe practice would be to decrease the consumption of beef.

The hunt for a reliable test of prions disease on live patients is making headway, but these tests are not at the level of complete accuracy that brain biopsies postmortem. There are several ways of testing, which include tonsil biopsies, urine tests, MRI, electroencephalogram (EEG), and blood assays. However, there are problems with each. For example, although tonsil biopsies are relatively reliable tests, they do require the individual to have intact tonsils. Urine tests can show possible PrP^{Sc} proteins in it, but are not very reliable assays. MRI can show some forms of neurodegeneration, but it is not a definitive diagnosis technique and not all forms of prions disease will show heavy vacuolization in the brain. EEG can show abnormal brain activity, but this test is not definitive either. Blood assays and codon testing can be used, but they require specific regions for investigation, are expensive, and can report false readings, meaning that another test may need to be performed. However, an assay known as RT-QUIC has been useful in identifying 83 percent of patients that have CJD, making it a fairly accurate test. Although there is no cure currently for prion diseases, researchers are focusing on identifying medications that can pass the blood-brain barrier that can attack both the PrP^{C} and PrP^{Sc} forms.

Joshua R. Skeggs

See also: Creutzfeldt-Jakob Disease

Further Reading

Introduction to prion diseases. (n.d.). Retrieved from http://mjlprionsdiseases.wordpress .com/

Ironside, J.W. (2010). Variant Creutzfeldt-Jakob disease. *Haemophilia, 16,*175–180. doi:10.1111/j.1365–2516.2010.02317.x.

National Institute of Neurological Disorders and Stroke (NINDS). (2011). *Transmissible spongiform encephalopathies information page.* Retrieved from http://www.ninds.nih .gov/disorders/tse/tse.htm

National Institute of Neurological Disorders and Stroke (NINDS) (2012). *Creutzfeldt-Jakob disease fact sheet*. Retrieved from http://www.ninds.nih.gov/disorders/cjd/detail_cjd .htm#186483058.

Wrighton, K. H. (2009). Prions: Prying into prions. *Nature Reviews Molecular Cell Biology, 10*, 372. doi:10.1038/nrm2692.

Progressive Multifocal Leukencephalopathy

Myelin is an insulating sheath that surrounds axons of neurons, and is necessary for fast conduction of signals between neurons. When the myelin is damaged by disease, it is called a *demyelinating disorder*. *Progressive multifocal leukencephalopathy* (PML), also known as multifocal leukencephalitis, is a virally mediated demyelinating disorder of the central nervous system that occurs in people with suppressed immune function. The presentation of PML is variable, and depends on the locations in the brain that are damaged. Among others, PML occurs in patients with AIDS (acquired immunodeficiency syndrome) and in patients with diseases that require treatment that suppresses the immune system, such as multiple sclerosis (MS). Currently there are no treatments for PML, and it is considered a progressive and fatal disease. Research is ongoing, but has been hampered by the fact that an animal model for PML does not exist at the time of the release of this encyclopedia.

History

Astrom and colleagues first described PML in 1958. They noticed that patients suffering from *lymphoproliferative disorders* frequently presented with progressive neurologic symptoms and exhibited signs of white matter (myelin) loss upon autopsy. Lymphoproliferative disorders occur when cells of the immune response are abnormal and produced in excessive amounts. In 1971, the causative agent was first identified. In a patient that had Hodgkin's disease but ultimately died of PML, a virus was isolated from his brain. This virus, known as the JC virus (named for the initials of the patient from which it was first identified), is now known to cause the demyelinating lesions of PML. Over the next few decades, the understanding of the disease processes behind PML evolved. Until the 1980s, PML was largely associated with lymphoproliferative disorders, in which the disease was originally identified. The AIDS epidemic that took place in the 1980s saw a dramatic increase in the number of PML cases, as the patients' immune systems were dramatically weakened by the HIV virus, allowing for the JC virus to wreak havoc on their brains. Prior to the advent of more effective antiviral treatments, 4–5 percent of patients with AIDS contracted PML (Koralnik, 2013). These cases were frequently fatal. The next increase in the number of PML cases came at the beginning of the 21st century, with the advent of monoclonal antibody treatments for diseases such as MS and Crohn's disease. These antibodies purposefully reduced the function of the immune system, which is thought to play a part in the pathophysiology of those diseases. Unfortunately, the dampened immune system that was both the goal and the result of these new treatments allowed for the JC virus to attack the brains of these patients, causing a spike in the number of PML cases. PML is still a significant concern for people that are immunosuppressed, as no treatment currently exists.

Types and Symptoms, Treatments and Outcomes

The JC virus that causes PML is from the polyoma family of viruses. It is a double-stranded DNA virus. Typically acquired during childhood or adolescence, it is thought that up to 90 percent of adults are seropositive for the virus (Koralnik, 2013). Because PML only occurs in the setting of a suppressed immune system, the JC virus is not a problem for the general population. It is unknown how JC virus initially infects its host. It is thought that the virus replicates in the kidney and bone marrow, and then stays latent in the kidneys, spleen, or lymph nodes until immunosuppression allows for its reactivation. It is also believed that a mutation in the viral genome needs to take place for it to become "neurotropic," which allows it to enter the brain.

As the name "multifocal" suggests, multiple regions of the brain are typically affected in PML. The virus commonly attacks the myelinating cells of the central nervous system, called oligodendrocytes. Though white matter is typically affected, gray matter can be attacked as well. The virus has also been shown to attack support cells (astrocytes) and even the neurons themselves. Common areas of the brain that are affected in PML include the parietal and the occipital lobes, as well as the cerebellum. Typically, the optic nerve and the spinal cord are spared in PML. The result of these attacks is a loss of myelin similar to that seen in MS, but PML progresses much more quickly and attacks different parts of the nervous system than those affected in MS.

As previously stated, PML is typically seen in the setting of immunosuppression. Common conditions that are associated with PML include AIDS, in which the human immunodeficiency virus (HIV) attacks the host immune response, thereby increasing the likelihood of JC activation. Diseases with an immunologic component such as MS, Crohn's disease, rheumatoid arthritis, lupus, or psoriasis often require pharmacologic suppression of the immune system for control of the disease. This unfortunately opens the door for JC reactivation and PML. One notable drug that is associated with PML is Tysabri, or natalizumab, which is used to treat MS and Crohn's disease. Tysabri is a monoclonal antibody that binds to a protein class called integrins, thereby inhibiting the movement of immune cells called leukocytes. There was such concern about the association of Tysabri treatment with PML that it was briefly removed from the market. PML is also seen following organ transplant, in which immunosuppressive drugs aid in the acceptance of the foreign body part. Finally, there have been reports of PML in the context of immunosuppression, such as old age, liver, or kidney diseases.

Because the regions of the brain that are effected in PML are quite variable, so too are the symptoms. Common features of PML include progressive limb weakness, problems with balance and coordination, difficulty speaking (aphasia), visual disturbances, memory loss, headaches, and personality changes. Seizure is a presenting feature in approximately 18 percent of PML cases (Lima et al., 2006). A rapid and progressive course in the setting of immunosuppression such as AIDS typically heightens the clinical suspicion for a case of PML.

There are several tests that can be used to diagnose PML. The "gold standard" for diagnosis is a biopsy of the brain that shows the JC virus to be present in the myelinating oligodendrocytes. Another common method is to sample the cerebrospinal fluid (CSF) and perform a polymerase chain reaction (PCR) to detect the DNA of the JC virus. These demonstrations of the virus will be accompanied by imaging studies, such as computed tomography (CT) or magnetic resonance imaging (MRI) that will typically show multiple sites of demyelination in the white matter of the brain. However, lesions can be seen in the gray matter as well. Unfortunately, because of the progressive nature of the disease, a diagnosis is sometimes made in a postmortem setting.

As the name suggests, PML is typically progressive. The mortality rate is believed to be between 30 and 50 percent, and the median survival of patients with PML is 2.6 months (NINDS, 2011). Patients that do survive frequently have severe neurologic deficits for the rest of their lives. There are no definitive predictive factors of prognosis, though the amount of JC virus in the CSF has been correlated with the severity of disease and outcome. Interestingly, a robust inflammatory response that frequently increases the severity of symptoms is paradoxically associated with a better outcome.

There are currently no treatments for PML. Because it almost always occurs in the setting of immunosuppression, therapies should be aimed at boosting the immune response of the patient to allow attack of the JC virus. For example, doctors will aggressively treat the HIV virus with what is called highly active antiretroviral therapy (HAART). HAART in AIDS patients has dramatically increased the survival of PML. Furthermore, patients with PML may benefit from discontinuing or decreasing the dose of immunosuppressive medicines. In other studies, there have been case reports of an antimalarial drug called mefloquine successfully attacking the JC virus in the setting of PML. However in a large-scale test, mefloquine showed no statistically significant efficacy in PML.

Future

PML is a severe disease. Its course is rapid, it is frequently fatal, and survivors are often fraught with neurologic sequelae. A major issue in the research of the PML is that there does not exist an animal model for the disease, which could be used for testing of drugs and therapeutic treatments. The JC virus has not been shown to cause demyelinating lesions in a laboratory animal setting. Further, with the continual advent of new immunosuppressive therapies to control other disease processes and to aid in transplants, PML cases likely will not decline. Care must be taken in the immunosuppressed population to recognize the signs of PML. Revitalizing the host immune response is currently the best way to attack the JC virus and combat PML. Development of an animal model would allow researchers to identify compounds that preferentially attack the JC virus. Further, better control of diseases like AIDS or cures for diseases like MS would likely decrease the incidence of PML, as fewer patients would have the immunosuppression that can lead to PML.

Christopher Knoeckel

See also: Acquired Immunodeficiency Syndrome (AIDS); Multiple Sclerosis; Myelin

Further Reading

Astrom, K. E., Mancall, E. L., & Richardson, E. P., Jr. (1958). Progressive multifocal leukoencephalopathy; a hitherto unrecognized complication of chronic lymphatic leukaemia and Hodgkin's disease. *Brain, 81,* 93–111.

Jasmin, L. (2012). *Progressive multifocal leukoencephalopathy.* Retrieved from http://www.nlm.nih.gov/medlineplus/ency/article/000674.htm

Koralnik, I. J. (2013). Progressive multifocal leukoencephalopathy: Prognosis and treatment. *UpToDate.* Wolters Kluwer Health. Retrieved from http://www.uptodate.com/contents/progressive-multifocal-leukoencephalopathy-prognosis-and-treatment

Lima, M. A., Drislane F. W., & Koralnik I. J. (2006). Seizures and their outcome in progressive multifocal leukencephalopathy. *Neurology, 66*(2), 262. *UpToDate.* Wolters Kluwer Health. Retrieved from http://www.uptodate.com/contents/progressive-multifocal-leukoencephalopathy-epidemiology-clinical-manifestations-and-diagnosis

National Institute of Neurological Disorders and Stroke (NINDS). (2011). *NINDS progressive multifocal leukoencephalopathy information page.* Retrieved from http://www.ninds.nih.gov/disorders/pml/pml.htm

Prosopagnosia

Prosopagnosia (from Greek; *prosopon* meaning "face" and *agnosia* meaning "not knowing"), also known as face-blindness, is a *visual agnosia* in which one has a deficit in the ability to recognize a person by looking at their face. Individuals with prosopagnosia have trouble distinguishing familiar people from unfamiliar people in pictures and in person, can have trouble recognizing close friends and family, and even themselves in pictures and mirrors. They know when they are looking at a face, can describe its features, and the ability to interpret facial expressions remains preserved; however, the ability to naturally piece together the unique features of an individual's face into a overt, coherent image is impaired. The disorder can be acquired due to brain injury or inherited. Prosopagnosia has provided some of the strongest evidence for a face-selective visual processing system.

History

Case studies of patients with face-blindness date back to the 19th century; however, the term prosopagnosia was not coined until 1947 by German neurologist Joachim Bodamer (1910–1985). These were mostly cases of prosopagnosia *acquired* in adulthood due to brain tissue damage. A case of *congenital* (born with) prosopagnosia was recorded in 1844; however, it seems congenital face-blindness was overlooked for a long time until another case was reported in 1976 and one after that in 1996. By 2002, less than a dozen cases of congenital prosopagnosia had been published worldwide. Around 2002, public interest increased when several websites about the disorder were made. Ken Nakayama (n.d.) and Brad Duchaine (n.d.) of the University of London started one such website and have received feedback from thousands of people with lifelong face-blindness, ranging from mild to severe (visit their website at www.faceblind.org). It appears that in brain damage cases, acquiring prosopagnosia is extremely rare, whereas congenital cases are quite common, but less reported.

Causes

There are congenital cases and acquired cases of prosopagnosia. In almost all cases of acquired prosopagnosia, the person obtained bilateral lesions from a stroke, head trauma, encephalitis, or poisoning to the visual association cortex on the ventromedial region of the occipitotemporal cortex. This region includes the *fusiform, lingual, and parahippocampal gyri*. Functional imaging studies of unaffected persons highlight the importance of the fusiform gyrus, particularly a region referred to as the fusiform face area, in processing and recognizing faces. Abnormal activity in this area has even been correlated with hallucinations of faces. Some prosopagnosics have lesions to this region in the right hemisphere only, and functional imaging studies, split brain studies, and the Wada test also indicate the right hemisphere to be more important in face recognition.

In developmental (congenital) cases, a genetic aspect is suspected, for prosopagnosia can run in families; however, no specific gene has been identified. Pedigree analysis of prosopagnosic families indicates a simple autosomal-dominant inheritance. Since symptoms are so similar between people with congenital prosopagnosia, it could be a simple point mutation of one or more genes as the source of the defect. The mutation most likely results in prosopagnosia due to defective neural development. In congenital prosopagnosia, functionally independent but anatomically adjacent brain structures are never affected, suggesting that a blood vessel malformation or birth trauma is not the cause. Prosopagnosics that acquired damage in utero or early infancy are often referred to as developmental prosopagnosics as well.

It is estimated that about 2.5 percent of the world's population suffers from severe congential prosopagnosia (Duchaine et al., 2007; Kennerknecht et al., 2006). These individuals may not realize that there is anything abnormal about their facial processing until someone points it out or they learn about the disorder (visit faceblind.org/facetests to test your face recognition abilities). Developmental prosopagnosia has been associated with diminished activation of the fusiform gyrus and reduced white matter connectivity in the ventral occipitotemporal cortex. One study by Behrman and colleagues (2007) showed the anterior fusiform gyrus to be significantly smaller in his face-blind patients. Some studies, however, show no anatomical or functional abnormalities of the fusiform gyrus of congenital prosopagnosics.

Diagnosis

The diagnoses of prosopagnosia are usually achieved through tests in which the individual is asked to identify faces. Commonly used ones are the *Warrington Recognition Memory for Faces* and the *Benton Facial Recognition Test.* Some tests require the identification of famous faces, and persons with prosopagnosia will fail this test. Other tests have pictures of familiar and unfamiliar people and require the individual to decide if the face is familiar or unfamiliar. Congenital prosopagnosics lack confidence about familiarity. They might have a sense of familiarity when they see a face, but are unable to identify the face and unable to distinguish if it is a face they have seen before. They can falsely recognize an unfamiliar face as familiar. This is in contrast to people who have acquired prosopagnosia; no faces can generate a feeling of familiarity. One commonly noted side affect/symptom of congenital prosopagnosia is *abnormal gazing patterns,* where the person with prosopagnosia does not feel the need to make gaze contact in social interactions.

To be considered prosopagnosic, the defect in recognition of familiar faces must not be associated with linguistic or general intellectual impairment. Prosopagnosics often rely on unique characteristics of a person to visually identify them such as hair and skin color, gait, height and weight, or facial hair. They often rely heavily on recognizing voices to identify someone. The majority of prosopagnosics do not have difficulty assessing the emotional expressions of faces, nor do they seem to have any trouble judging facial attractiveness or gender compared to control groups. They also have no trouble remembering semantic information about people. The condition can be emotionally stressful and embarrassing for those who have it. There are no treatments or cures for the disorder other than learning compensatory strategies, such as the ones listed earlier, to identify people. The increasing awareness of the disorder by the general public will hopefully relieve some of the social and emotional stress prosopagnosics experience.

People with face-blindness sometimes have other visual perception deficits. Acquired prosopagnosia is sometimes associated with deficits of adjacent brain regions, such as *bilateral upper visual field deficits* and *achromatopsia* (a deficit in color perception). *Topographagnosia* (difficulty navigating familiar places) and some object agnosia are frequently present in congenital prosopagnosia. In Farah and colleagues research (1995), the object agnosia of prosopagnosics is intracategory. That is, they can identify the category of object (such as fruit, dogs) but not if it is an apple or pear, Beagle or Labrador. Some theorize that prosopagnosia is a general impairment of visual recognition and the ability to distinguish items within categories, with deficits in faces being the most prominent. Some believe that the common co-occurrence of face blindness with object agnosia is evidence that the system that processes faces is not distinct from the one that processes other objects. However, many prosopagnosics have no object agnosia, and many people with object agnosia have no trouble recognizing faces. This double dissociation shows that the two systems can operate independently.

Faces Are Special

The fact that this disorder exists is evidence that identifying faces requires a special processing system, which in turn implies that facial recognition is evolutionarily important. The study of face-blindness has identified the fusiform face region and has shed light on the nature of neural interactions and higher order processing. Studies of individual neuron responses to faces have helped with these discoveries and in the process these studies have contributed to the theory of *grandmother cells.* Single-cell recordings in the inferotemporal cortex of macaques by Charles Gross (n.d.) in 1969 have identified that neurons can respond more strongly to some stimuli than others, such as the image of a macaque's paw. He also found cells that responded most strongly to faces. The selective activation behavior of these neurons resembles what would be expected of a grandmother cell. Gross's experiments were ignored until the 1980s due to disbelief that the recognition of specific categories of objects could rely on individual neurons.

In one study, a monkey was shown various images: faces of other monkeys, one of an experimenter's face, some that contained the most prominent features of a face (such as a circle for face shape, a grating for face symmetry), and some nonfacial stimuli. The neurons of the monkey's superior temporal sulcus responded only to a clear frontal photo of another monkey.

The next step to further research about prosopagnosia is currently being taken: raising awareness of the disorder so that those who have it know they do and can participate in family studies to begin identifying the genetic component of the disorder. Once this is accomplished, not only will it further our understanding of the disorder and its symptoms, but will contribute to the current understanding of neural developmental processes and higher order cognitive processing.

Face-blindness can be emotionally stressful and embarrassing for those who have it because others often attribute their "forgetfulness" to a lack of interest and even a lack of intelligence. The increased awareness of face-blindness as a neurological disorder will allow society to better accommodate and "forgive" those with the disorder.

Emma Boxer

See also: Grandmother Cell; Sacks, Oliver W.; Stroke; Visual Fields; Visual Perception (Visual Processing)

Further Reading

Behrmann, M., Avidan, G., Gao, F., & Black, S. (2007). Structural imaging reveals anatomical alterations in inferotemporal cortex in congenital prosopagnosia. *Cerebral Cortex, 17,* 2354–2363.

Duchaine, B.C., & Nakayama, K. (2005). Dissociations of face and object recognition in developmental prosopagnosia. *Journal of Cognitive Neuroscience, 17*(2), 249–261.

Farah, M.J., Wilson, K.D., Drain, H.M., & Tanaka, J.R. (1995). The inverted face inversion effect in prosopagnosia: Evidence for face-specific, mandatory perceptual mechanisms. *Vision Research, 35,* 2089–2093.

Kennerknecht, I., Grueter, T., Welling, B., Wentzek, S., Horst, J., & Edwards, S. (2006). First report of prevalence of non-syndromic hereditary prosopagnosia (HPA). *American Journal of Medical Genetics Part A, 140A*(15), 1617–1622.

Sacks, Oliver. (2010) *The mind's eye.* New York, NY: Alfred A. Knopf; London: Picador.

Psychology and Psychiatry

Psychology

The word *psychology* is derived from the Greek word *psyche,* meaning "soul" or "self" and *ology* means the "study of." Thus, psychology is the study of the human mind and behavior. Psychologists study the effects of mental functions on behavior, while also exploring the physiological and neurobiological processes that play a role in cognitive functions. There are several specialty fields within psychology including *abnormal psychology* (the study of abnormal behavior and psychopathology), *biological psychology* (the study of how biological processes influence the mind and behavior, utilizing tools such as magnetic resonance imaging and positron emission tomography scans to look at brain injury or abnormalities), and *cognitive psychology* (the study of attention, memory, problem solving, and language acquisition).

Wilhelm Wundt (1832–1920), a German psychologist, established the first scientific laboratory to study psychology in 1879. He was interested in describing structures that compose the mind, believing that psychology was the science of conscious experience and that trained observers could accurately describe thoughts, feelings, and emotions through internal reflection. Wundt separated psychology from philosophy through structured analysis of the brain, and his laboratory became a focus for those with an interest in psychology around the world.

William James (1842–1910) is considered the father of American psychology and was one of the first professors of psychology in the United States. His studies focused on a flow of consciousness and holistic concerns including the meaning of self and how the mind affects behavior.

Psychiatry

Psychiatry is a medical specialty devoted to the study and treatment of mental disorders, which include *affective, behavioral, cognitive, and perceptual abnormalities.* The term was first coined by the German physician Johann Christian Reil (1759–1813) in 1808 and literally means "medical treatment of the soul." The field of psychiatry encompasses a wide spectrum of human mental and behavioral experience—mood disorders, eating disorders, anxiety disorders, personality disorders, phobias, addiction, and many more. It is different from psychology in that its primary focus is illness or abnormality, as opposed to normal psychological functioning.

Psychiatry is dedicated to the investigation of abnormalities in brain function that manifest as diseases, which clinically may present as mild to severe. Modern psychiatry aims to determine how aberrations in normal function, through genetics or the environment, lead to the development of mental illness. Philippe Pinel (1745–1826) is considered to be the founding father of modern psychiatry. He worked as the director of hospitals in Paris for the mentally ill and his essay, *Memoir on Madness,* called for more diligent psychological study of individuals over time and more humanitarian asylum practices.

Development of Modern Psychiatry and Psychology

Ancient Greek philosophy, medieval Christianity, and post-Renaissance philosophers of the past several centuries have influenced contemporary psychology and psychiatry. Early civilizations associated madness with magic or divine forces. Greek and Roman societies hypothesized that psychiatric symptoms result from an imbalance of essential humors. Hippocrates (460–377 BC) introduced the theory that both physical and mental health required a harmonious balance of four humors: black bile, yellow bile, blood, and phlegm. Nearly five centuries later, Galen (130–201) expanded Hippocrates's ideas to include a typology of personality. The melancholic personality, or black bile, tended toward the depressed, while the choleric, or yellow bile, tended toward anger. In addition, the sanguine (from blood) tended toward the courageous, and the phlegmatic (from phlegm) tended toward calm. Each of these personality types was thought to result from an excess of its respective humor.

The European Renaissance brought a great change of cultural and intellectual values. Philosophers began to reexamine theories of the ancient Greeks and in doing so began to develop the field of modern psychology and psychiatry. Around the world, scientists, including Wundt, James, and Pinel, began to study human behavior, development, and happiness, and thus modern psychiatry and psychology began.

Schools of Thought

Throughout its history, psychology has had several major theoretical movements. These movements have shaped modern psychology and psychiatry and continue to have influence on research and clinical practice. Three important theories include *behaviorism, psychoanalytic theory,* and *humanistic theory.*

Behaviorism is based on the belief that behaviors can be measured, trained, and changed. Ivan Pavlov (1849–1936) studied classical conditioning. For example, a dog that naturally salivates at the sight of meat is conditioned to salivate at the sound of a bell when no food is present. The unconditioned stimulus (meat) is then paired with a conditioned stimulus (the sound of the bell). With time, the conditioned stimulus is able to elicit a response (salivation) even in the absence of the unconditioned stimulus. This simple example of classical conditioning can be applied to more complex human behaviors.

J.B. Watson (1878–1958), an American psychologist influenced by Pavlov, conducted experiments in classical conditioning that involved an 11-month-old boy named Albert B. In these experiments, Albert cried in response to loud noises (unconditioned stimulus). This unconditioned stimulus was then paired with the sight of a white rat (conditioned stimulus). Albert began to fear the white rat when it was no longer paired with the loud noise. Eventually, Albert avoided all objects that appeared similar to the white rat—an example of stimulus generalization. These types of experiments are no longer allowed as they result in fear conditioning.

Edward Thorndike (1874–1947) observed the behavior of cats and dogs when placed in a puzzle box to determine how the animal learned to escape. Based on this research, he developed the *law of effect,* which states that the effect of an action will determine the likelihood that it will be repeated. For instance, if the cat gets out of the box, then the action will be repeated. This contributed to B.F. Skinner's (1904–1990) theory of operant conditioning, which is based on the idea that consequences manipulate behavior. Skinner showed that positive reinforcement increases the frequency of a behavior, whereas punishment decreases the frequency of a behavior. Negative reinforcement describes the strengthening of a behavior through avoidance of a negative outcome or aversive stimulus.

Psychoanalytic theory continues to have a profound impact on theories of psychopathology and methods of treating mental illness. Sigmund Freud's (1856–1939) theory of psychoanalysis remains one of the most important in the field. This theory provides a comprehensive approach to understanding psychic development, emotion, and behavior in addition to psychiatric illness. Freud developed a psychic apparatus with three parts: *id, ego,* and *superego.* This structural theory defined the superego as the conscience, the id as the keeper of raw impulses (such as aggression), and the ego as the mediator between the expectations of the superego and the pressures for gratification of the id. Freud believed that the three related to each other in dynamic equilibrium. Freud also developed the psychosexual stages of development, which assume that a person must accomplish a series of tasks from infancy to adulthood in order to achieve psychological health. This theory implies that early experiences shape an adult's self-image and potential for success.

Carl Jung and Alfred Adler were followers of Freud who later developed their own theories of psychoanalysis. Carl Jung (1875–1961) is most known for his theories on the collective unconscious, which postulate that all humans go through life with a shared set of experiences and fundamental ways of dealing with situations, referred to as archetypes. Additionally, he established important theories on personality traits that influenced the development of the Myers-Briggs personality test. Alfred Adler (1870–1937) found his own school of psychology that focused on socially mediated phenomena including the role of birth order in personality development.

Humanistic psychology was a powerful counter to psychoanalysis and behaviorism, emphasizing free will, choice, and human consciousness. Abraham Maslow (1908–1970), an American psychologist, was one of the fathers of humanistic psychology. He is best known for his concept of the hierarchy of needs. He believed that human psychological needs are multidimensional and there is no single motivating force to explain all behavior. Maslow organized these needs hierarchically, with the most fundamental biologic needs (thirst, hunger, and warmth) at the bottom. Once these are met, the need for safety, psychological needs (love, belonging), and esteem needs can be met. At the top of the hierarchy, he theorized that humans encounter the need for self-actualization: an emotional and intellectual fulfillment of human potential.

Psychology and Psychiatry Today

Research in psychology and psychiatry continues to expand what is known about behavior, human development, personality, and the diagnosis and treatment of mental illness. The *Diagnostic and Statistical Manual Fifth Edition* (*DSM-V*) classifies mental illness or disorders according to symptoms, etiology, and progression over time (American Psychiatric Association, 2013). By categorizing mental disorders, the *DSM-V* provides a succinct communication tool for clinicians and researchers. Psychiatrists and psychologists use the *DSM-V* to diagnose and determine appropriate treatment plans.

Psychologists evaluate behavior and mental processes; they pursue a doctorate in psychology, and conduct research, teach, and treat patients. Clinical psychologists work in hospitals, mental health clinics, and schools to help those suffering from mental disorders or psychological distress. Psychologists conduct studies and experiments with human or animal participants that focus on cognition, neuroscience, personality, development, and social behavior.

Psychiatrists are medical doctors and mental health professionals that distinguish between physical and psychological causes of both mental and physical distress. Their training is mostly clinical and focuses on the evaluation and pharmacological treatment of severe mental illness. Psychiatrists utilize psychotherapy and medications, usually in combination, to treat mental illness. Psychiatric medications can help correct imbalances in brain chemistry that may lead to the development of psychiatric disorders.

There are several types of psychotherapy: *behavior therapy, cognitive-behavioral therapy, group therapy, individual therapy, couples therapy,* and many more. Behavior therapy stems from the theories of Pavlov, Skinner, Watson, and Thorndike and stresses the importance of working with objective, observable behavior that leads to habit formation. Behavior therapy does not necessarily help patients understand their emotions or motivations, but only their actions through reinforcement, relaxation training, and flooding—which is the continuous contact with an anxiety-prone situation. It is most helpful for disorders associated with abnormal behavioral patterns: alcohol and drug abuse, eating disorders, anxiety disorders, phobias, and obsessive-compulsive behavior.

Cognitive behavioral therapy is based on the assumption that schemas shape the way people react and adapt to situations. Each person has his or her own schemas that have been determined by their personal experience. Anxiety or depression develop when these schemas become overactive and predispose them to developing negative responses. Aaron Temkin Beck (1921–), a key clinical theorist in the development of cognitive behavioral therapy, developed the negative triad of depression: a negative view of oneself, a negative interpretation of experience, and a negative view of the future. The focus of cognitive behavioral therapy is to help patients restructure their negative cognitions so that they can perceive reality in a less distorted way and learn to react accordingly.

In addition to psychotherapy, psychopharmacology (drugs that are classified as antipsychotics and antidepressants) plays an important role in the treatment of mental illness. Antipsychotics are used to treat schizophrenia, psychotic mood disorders, and to control aggressive behavior. Antidepressants are primarily indicated for the acute and maintenance treatment of major depression. There are several classes of antidepressants that vary based on their mechanism of action, side effect profile, and dosing.

Conclusion

Psychology is the study of the human mind and behavior. Psychiatry is the study of abnormalities in brain function that lead to mental disorders. These dynamic fields continue to develop as research studies explore novel theories on human behavior and novel concepts concerning the treatment of mental illness. In a given year, 1 in 4 adults experience mental illness, while 1 in 17 live with a serious mental illness such as schizophrenia, major depression, or bipolar disorder (American Psychiatric Association, 2013). Psychologists and psychiatrists both play an important role in developing research projects and will continue to shape the fields of modern psychology and psychiatry.

Danielle Stutzman

See also: Addiction; Alcohol and Alcoholism; Attention Deficit Disorder/ Attention Deficit Hyperactivity Disorder; Behavior; Depression; Learning and

Memory; Magnetic Resonance Imaging (MRI); Schizophrenia; Wundt, Wilhelm Maximilian

Further Reading

American Psychiatric Association. (2013). *Diagnostic and statistical manual of mental disorders* (5th ed.). Arlington, VA: American Psychiatric Publishing.

Cohen, L. J. (2011). *The handy psychology answer book.* United States: Visible Ink Press.

Goldman, H. H. (2000). *Review of general psychiatry* (5th ed.). United States: Lange Medical Books/McGraw-Hill.

Tasman, A., Kay, J., Lieberman, J. A., First, M. B., & Maj, M. (2008). *Psychiatry* (3rd ed.). United States: Wiley.

Ptosis

When the upper or lower eyelid is drooping, the medical term used to describe this condition is *ptosis*. It is derived from a Greek word meaning "to fall" and the "p" in "ptosis" is silent. Thus, the word is pronounced / 'tōsəs/. Ptosis occurs when the muscles of the eyelid (the *levator palpebrae superioris* and the *superior tarsal*) are weakened or paralyzed and are unable to raise the eyelid. Over the course of the day, the weakened muscles become tired and the drooping becomes worse in the evening. Ptosis can affect one or both eyes. If ptosis is severe and untreated, it can produce other eye conditions such as *amblyopia* ("lazy eye") or *astigmatism* (blurry vision from a misshapen cornea).

Ptosis may occur at any age but it is predominantly seen in the elderly as the eye muscles weaken with age. However, if ptosis is diagnosed in a young child, it must be corrected quickly to avoid permanent damage to the sight. If an infant is born with ptosis, it is an inherited condition called *congenital ptosis* and its cause is currently unknown. Ptosis is generally caused by damage to the *superior cervical sympathetic ganglion* (part of the autonomic nervous system) or to the cranial nerve supplying the eyelid muscles, which is the *oculomotor nerve* (cranial nerve III). Damage to this nerve is usually a sign of an underlying disease or disorder such as a brain tumor, diabetes, drug abuse, myasthenia gravis, or stroke. Persons who abuse (high doses) opioid drugs (either illegal or prescription) may have a side effect of ptosis. The most common opioid drugs that can produce ptosis are heroin, hydrocodone (Vicodin), morphine, oxycodone (Oxycotin), or pregabalin (Lyrica).

Jennifer L. Hellier

See also: Addiction; Diabetes Mellitus; Oculomotor Nerve; Stroke

Further Reading

Finsterer, J. (2003). Ptosis: Causes, presentation, and management. *Aesthetic Plastic Surgery, 27*(3), 193–204.

Putamen

The primate brain, especially the human brain, has several deep structures that are located below the cortex. One such structure is the *basal nuclei* (previously known as the basal ganglia), which is a collection of neuronal cell bodies whose main function is to modulate motor movements for humans. The basal nuclei consist of three distinct structures: *caudate nucleus, putamen,* and *globus pallidus.* The word putamen is a Latin term meaning "falls off from pruning." This nucleus (a group of neuronal cell bodies) is round and is found between the caudate and the globus pallidus. The putamen is anatomically connected to the caudate, globus pallidus, and the substantia nigra, which means the "black substance." The putamen's main function is associated with voluntary movement, but it also has functions pertaining to learning and memory.

Anatomy and Function

Within the basal ganglia, the caudate is the most lateral (toward the side). Moving medially (toward the middle), the putamen is next followed by the globus pallidus. The caudate and putamen can be thought as one structure called the dorsal striatum (meaning "striped"). However, they are separated by a large fiber tract (group of myelinated axons) that is known as the internal capsule. The putamen and caudate have similar cell types and have integrated functions. The putamen receives input from the caudate and globus pallidus. It also receives dopamine (a neurotransmitter—which is a natural chemical used by neurons to "talk" to each other) from the substantia nigra. The output of the putamen is primarily inhibitory to the globus pallidus by two different pathways: direct and indirect. Both pathways use three neurotransmitters to produce the inhibition with the first two being the same for both pathways: GABA (gamma-aminobutyric acid) and dopamine. The direct pathway connects from the putamen to the globus pallidus internus and then to the substantia nigra. Its third neurotransmitter is substance P. When the putamen output ends in the globus pallidus externus, it makes up the indirect pathway. This pathway's third neurotransmitter is enkephalin. Together, these pathways help the putamen in modulating voluntary movement as well as modulating learning. Specifically, the putamen is necessary for category, implicit, and reinforcement learning functions. If there is damage to this nucleus, it results in abnormal movement of the body and limbs or difficulty in cognition. This is because it can no longer regulate or modulate these functions.

Diseases

The putamen's role in Parkinson's disease has been well studied. Specifically, as the neurons in the substantia nigra die, they can no longer release dopamine to the putamen. This means that both the direct and indirect inhibitory pathways are not completely functional, with the direct pathway having decreased activity and the indirect pathway having an increase. Together, it results in significantly more inhibition to the thalamus (a deep structure that modulates motor and sensory functions) causing abnormal tremors and motor movements.

Jennifer L. Hellier

See also: Basal Nuclei (Basal Ganglia); Caudate Nucleus; Globus Pallidus; Learning and Memory; Parkinson's Disease

Further Reading

Grahn, J., Parkinson, J. A., & Owen, A. M. (2009). The role of the basal ganglia in learning and memory: Neuropsychological studies. *Behavioral Brain Research, 199*(1), 53–60.

Purves, D., Augustine, G. J., Fitzpatrick, D., Katz, L. C., LaMantia, A., McNamara, J. O., & Williams, S. M. (Eds.). (2001). *Neuroscience* (2nd ed.). Sunderland, MA: Sinauer Associates.

R

Ramón y Cajal, Santiago (1852–1934)

Often referred to as Ramón y Cajal or just Cajal, *Santiago Ramón y Cajal* was a Spanish histologist, neuroscientist, and pathologist who investigated the morphology (shape) of brain cells by using a simple, light microscope. He is most famous for his remarkable detailed drawings of these microscopic structures, particularly of their delicate arborizations (fine-branching structures of dendrites and/or axons) and their connections in the central nervous system. With just a light microscope, his artistic drawings and anatomical analyses have proven correct in many brain regions. For his research and histological findings, Ramón y Cajal is considered to be the father of neuroscience. In fact, Ramón y Cajal's detailed drawings are still used today to teach neuroscience and neuroanatomy to students.

Ramón y Cajal was born in Navarre, Spain, and was the son of Justo Ramón, a physician and anatomy professor, and Antonia Cajal. Santiago was kicked out of many schools because of his rebellious behavior and disagreement with authority. In fact, he was imprisoned for demolishing a neighbor's gate with a homemade cannon at the age of 11. He was a natural artist and painter, but his father did not encourage Ramón y Cajal to develop these skills. Instead, his father made Ramón y Cajal an apprentice to a cobbler and a barber.

Eventually, Ramón y Cajal attended the University of Zaragoza School of Medicine, where his father taught. Ramón y Cajal graduated in 1873 and became a medical officer for the Spanish Army where he completed a tour in Cuba from 1874 to 1875. Ramón y Cajal returned to school and received his PhD in medicine in 1877. Ultimately, he became an anatomy professor at the University of Valencia in 1883 and then at the University of Barcelona in 1887. Ramón y Cajal's neuroscience research began while at the University of Barcelona where he learned of Camillo Golgi's (1843–1926) silver nitrate histological technique. Here he used his natural artistic skills with Golgi's stain and began his neuroanatomy research. Specifically, Ramón y Cajal studied and drew the central nervous systems of many animal species. During this time he identified dendritic spines as well as the axonal growth cone, which is the terminal end of an axon that seeks its synaptic target. Additionally, Ramón y Cajal was the pioneer in showing evidence for the neuron doctrine, which is the foundation of today's neuroscience. One fundamental concept of the neuron doctrine states that the central nervous system is made up individual cells and is not a continuous mass. Ramón y Cajal was able to draw these distinct cells and show how they connect to each other, meaning that the central nervous system is a contiguous system. For his findings and contribution to neuroscience, Ramón y Cajal received the Nobel Prize in Physiology or Medicine in 1906.

Jennifer L. Hellier

See also: Introduction: Neuroscience Overview; Neuron; Neuropil

Further Reading

Ramón y Cajal, Santiago. (1999) [1897]. *Advice for a young investigator* (Neely Swanson and Larry W. Swanson, Trans.). Cambridge, MA: MIT Press.

Rapid Eye Movement (REM)

When animals sleep, they enter different stages of sleep with one being *rapid eye movement (REM)*. REM is a quick, random movement of the eyes that occurs during sleep usually lasting 90 minutes to two hours. REM is one of five eye movement cycles that animals and humans go through when asleep. Each cycle lasts only for a short period of time, but each cycle gets longer as the sleep progresses. During REM sleep, the muscles become paralyzed and the brain cells (neurons) become quite active as if a person is awake. Thus, some scientists call REM paradoxical sleep.

The average adult has four to five cycles of REM sleep per night. However, the amount of time a person enters REM sleep depends upon her or his age. Younger persons experience more REM while older adults experience less REM sleep. It is hypothesized that REM is important for consolidating procedural and spatial memories. Thus, infants need a great amount of REM sleep, as it helps solidify procedural (like how to eat and crawl) and spatial (where their bodies are in space compared to other objects) memories of their external world. This assists in maturing an infant's neural connections and nervous system development.

People who go through the cycle of REM remember their dreams with vivid memories and clear pictures. REM is a very important stage of sleep. If a person is deprived of REM sleep the night before, the brain will try to recover the lost REM sleep, thus having the person enter REM sleep quicker and have many more cycles the next time they sleep. Consequently, REM sleep is considered part of man's evolutionary heritage. Furthermore, all mammals and birds go through the cycle of REM sleep.

History

In 1953, REM sleep was first identified and described by sleep researchers Nathaniel Kleitman (1895–1999) and Eugene Aserinsky (1921–1998). Together they are considered the fathers of modern sleep research. Kleitman and Aserinsky studied persons with sleep disorders and recorded the rapid eye movements during sleep, muscle tone, and low-voltage brain activity (discernible in a polysomnogram).

Anatomy and Physiology

Sleep has two main cycles non-REM and REM sleep. REM sleep is a cycle of sleep recognized by the rapid and random movement of the eyes. Animals and some humans tend to awake or are awake for a short time after an episode of REM. If a person wakes after a cycle of REM, they tend to remember their dreams. The activity of the brain's neurons during REM is similar to when awake, thus REM is often called paradoxical sleep.

Certain neurons in the brainstem (part of the central nervous system) that are located in the pontine tegmentum are especially active during REM sleep. It is suggested that these neurons are more likely responsible for REM. Additionally, the release of monoamine neurotransmitters (chemicals used to transmit neural impulses; norepinephrine, serotonin, and histamine) are turned off during REM. This causes REM atonia, almost a complete paralysis of the body, as the motor neuron is held back. It is suggested that this atonia ensures a person will not "act out" their dream and keeps them safe.

Disease

When a person lacks REM atonia, it results in a sleep behavior disorder where the sleeper acts out the movements of their dreams. This can cause them personal harm. Additional studies of sleep have shown that sleep deprivation early in life may cause behavioral problems, permanent sleep disruption, decreased brain mass, and an abnormal amount of neuronal cell death. Some of these problems may not be reversible. Thus, sleep is the best medicine and persons should try to get at least eight hours of sleep each night.

Patricia A. Bloomquist

See also: Sleep

Further Reading

Kiernan, J. A. (2005). *Barr's the human nervous system: An anatomical viewpoint.* Bethesda, MD: Lippincott Williams & Wilkins.

Purves, D., Augustine, G. J., Fitzpatrick, D., Hall, W. C., LaMantia, A.-S., McNamara, J. O., & Williams, S. M. (Eds.). (2004). *Neuroscience* (3rd ed.). Sunderland, MA: Sinauer Associates.

Reflex

From a surface level, *reflexes* do not appear very complicated. Most people have been to a doctor's office and had their knees hit with a rubber tool in hopes that the same leg will slightly kick. This action is called a *reflex.* Yet how does that slight force applied to the knee cause a kick without a conscious command from the brain? The topic of reflexes becomes even more complicated when examining cranial nerve, human infant, and post–spinal cord injury reflexes.

Simply defined, a reflex movement is an involuntary, rapid response to a given stimulus. The purpose of these quick, automatic movements is to avoid pain or injury. In the example of the knee-jerk reflex, a sensory nerve quickly transmits information about the force on the patellar ligament (a ligament attached to the knee cap) to the spinal cord. Nerves within the spinal cord relay a "contract now" motor signal to the quadriceps. The resulting "kick" is a way to relieve tension on the patellar tendon and prevent injury of the connected muscles or knee structure.

History

The study of reflexes reflects the evolving tensions between science and religion; between ongoing findings confirming or editing previous discoveries. Rene Descartes (1594–1660) was a pioneer in the study of reflexes. He reasoned that there was a central portion of the brain that housed the soul—the pineal gland—that served as the "conductor" of all physical activity. Knee-jerk, heartbeats, and movement rushed from the periphery toward the interface with the soul. His contemporary, Thomas Willis (1618–1678), was the first to use the term "reflex" but he argued that the sensory information and the soul met in a different region of the brain, the *corpus callosum.*

As the tension between religion and science began to slowly fade, anatomists began a more detailed study of the nervous system. Georg Prochaska (1749–1820) was the first to describe neuronal conduction as well as proposing a specific mechanism for limb reflexes. He identified the direct connection between sensory (peripheral) nerves and motor nerves in the spinal cord. Two notable scientists—anatomist

Santiago Ramon y Cajal (1852–1934) and physiologist Charles Sherrington (1857–1952)—further refined this work. Sherrington studied cat reflexes and described the concept of a "motor unit" as a group of muscle fibers innervated by a single motor neuron. This helped clarify the connection between a stimulus (such as increased patellar tension) and a coordinated response (the resulting quadriceps contracting) with relatively few neuron connections in the spinal cord.

Modern science continues to study reflexes. Sten Grillner (1941–) is associated with describing the concept of "central pattern generators" in voluntary muscle activity. Imagine for a moment the act of walking a few steps. Each step took place without consciously focusing on balance, heel strike, arm swing, or leg swing for each step. The act of walking is considered to be a complicated voluntary reflex that utilizes multiple parts of the brain/spinal cord simultaneously *without* consciously focusing on each step.

Anatomy and Physiology

It is useful to separate reflexes into monosynaptic (one neuronal synapse) and polysynaptic (multiple neuronal synapses) categories. The monosynaptic category is most commonly discussed through the lens of the knee-jerk reflex. Others in this category include the biceps, triceps, brachioradialis, and Achilles reflexes. To recap, a stretch sensation is detected by a sensory neuron in the muscle body. This signal is relayed to the spinal cord and a single synapse exists between the sensory fibers and the motor unit neurons. From this point, a signal to contract is relayed to a muscle in the hopes of reducing the stretch.

Several important concepts exist in this monosynaptic model. Firstly, how does the sensory neuron "detect" stretch? The answer can be found by examining the neuronal plasma membrane. Once there is an actual physical stretch, special chemical channels (or proteins) are opened in the neuronal cell membrane and the action potential signal of "stretch" is relayed to the spinal cord by traveling the length of the neuron's axon. Secondly, how does this reflex occur so quickly? This is because sensory and motor neurons are not all created equally. The fastest conducting neurons (Ia sensory and α-motor neurons) are utilized in these circuits in order to reduce the chance of injury from excessive muscle stretch. Lastly, how does the reflex reduce the muscle tone of opposing muscle groups, like the hamstrings in the leg? Each monosynaptic sensory signal not only activates specific motor neurons, but also simultaneously antagonizes/relaxes other motor neurons. This allows for a specific action based on a single sensory input.

With an understanding of the monosynaptic reflex concept, polysynaptic reflexes accomplish an end result, such as movement, just with more intermediate neuronal synapses. The previously mentioned central pattern generator (CPG) is one example. A conscious decision is made to walk, at which point the CPG is initiated. Parts of the complex reflex exist in the various areas of the brain that are involved in motion (the basal ganglia and cerebellum) as well as in the spinal cord. All work in symphony in order to coordinate the various movements involved in walking so a person can resume thinking of other matters.

Another example of a polysynaptic reflex is called the "flexor withdrawal." Imagine touching a hot stove or stepping on a sharp tack. Almost without thinking, the hand is quickly withdrawn or the foot is lifted up. Pain fibers (Ic) sense these types of noxious stimuli—though not as fast as stretch receptors—and synapse with interneurons in the spinal cord. These neurons amplify or mute pain before they synapse onto a motor fiber. Interestingly, the story gets a little more complicated than simply flexing to withdraw a hand or foot. The other limb simultaneously receives a signal from the contralateral (opposite side of) spinal cord neurons to extend certain muscle groups. This is important, for example, to maintain balance if one foot is lifted up into the air.

Any discussion of reflexes would be incomplete without mentioning those unique to human infants. Babies need certain "preprogrammed" responses to ensure survival early in life. Examples include those useful in eating such as the "suck" and "rooting" reflexes: an object placed in a baby's mouth immediately initiates sucking, an object lightly touching an infant's cheek causes the baby to turn toward that side, respectfully. Interestingly, these reflexes and many more begin to fade before the baby's first birthday. An important explanation arises from the changes that occur in the central nervous system during this time period. A baby continues to myelinate (an insulating covering of the axons) neurons—speeding conduction—and making more mature neuronal connections as learning takes place. These two factors lead to a slow dampening and eventual cessation of these reflexes.

Ultimately, the example of human infant reflexes drives home a final point: the conscious human brain is able to regulate reflexes. The antagonizing neurochemical signals (natural chemicals that block the action of a receptor) from the cortex can, for example, minimize or eliminate a knee-jerk reflex. Occasionally, patients will be so focused on the knee no reflex takes place. They might then be asked to interlock their hands and focus on pulling them apart while the rubber hammer lightly hits their knee. The shift in focus from the knee to the hands will allow the spinal cord reflex to occur in the absence of the cortex's inhibition.

A change in the corneal blink reflex with prolonged contact usage is another example of cortex affect on reflexes. The corneal reflex can be experienced when a hand or object comes close or actually touches the eye. Almost without control, both eyelids blink forcefully and rapidly (approximately within 10 milliseconds). This reflex involves the sensory trigeminal nerve (a cranial nerve that serves the head and face) with a quick relay to both facial nerve nuclei in the brainstem.

Interestingly, the reflex slowly diminishes with the constant touching of an eye during contact usage. A person will eventually be able to place and remove contacts without a blink. It is thought the conscious attention on this process reduces the reflex.

Reflexes in Disease/Injury

Knowledge of normal reflex patterns helps enlighten understanding reflex pattern in disease/injury states. Spinal cord injuries are extraordinarily unfortunate, but teach a great deal about reflex concepts. Once a spinal cord is injured, any function governed below that site is affected. The vertebrae overlying the region divide the spinal cord's anatomy into four general segments: cervical, thoracic, lumbar, and sacral. Imagine a spinal cord injury around the 12th thoracic to the fist lumbar section or T12–L1. At this level, the area around the waist and below would be impaired from both a sensation and motor standpoint.

Spinal shock—a term used to describe loss of motor function and sensation with eventual return of reflexes—begins instantly. The first 24 hours of injury would leave the lower limbs hyporeflexive (abnormal and decreased reflex activity) and hypotonic (flaccid). Reflexes such as the knee-jerk would return during days one to three, but then become hyperreflexive (abnormal and increased reflex activity) over the next few weeks. Finally, the muscles would become tighter during the weeks to years after the injury leading to a "hypertonic" state. This hypertonicity can be explained by unregulated neuron regeneration at and below the injury.

The return and progressive increase of the reflexes below the spinal cord injury reinforce concepts from normal reflexes. Polysynaptic reflexes return first due to the simple reason that more neurons contribute to these complex actions. The hyperreflexive state exists in the absence of central nervous system regulation in an analogous manner to human infant reflexes. Additionally, the attempt of spinal cord neurons to reestablish a connection leads to more connections below the injury leading to a stronger, more powerful circuit for the mono- and polysynaptic reflexes.

Injuries within the central nervous system (CNS) are identified and localized with an understanding of cranial nerve reflexes. Cranial nerve reflexes fall into the polysynaptic category due to interneurons that take sensory signals and transmit motor signals to bilateral sides. For instance, a bright penlight in one eye causes both pupils to constrict. If the light causes only the eye with the light to constrict, there is a problem with the motor neuron (oculomotor nerve) on the contralateral side. If there is no pupillary constriction when a penlight is shone, the problem likely exists with that ipsilateral (same side) optic nerve. This understanding can help identify problems with the nerves (such as inflammation or tumors) or with the brain itself (such as tumors or strokes).

In addition to injuries to the CNS, back injuries can be localized with an understanding of reflexes. Consider a person with significant lower back pain after lifting a heavy object. Is this a medical emergency? Upon close examination, it appears there is no Achilles reflex on the right side compared to the left. This subtle finding, taken with other evidence, might compel the doctor to order a magnetic resonance imaging (MRI) of the patient's lower back. It would be feared that the heavy lifting caused an intervertebral disk to bulge outward into the spinal canal and push against the right-sided S1 nerve root. Surgery to repair the herniated disk is often warranted in these situations.

Reflexes and Prosthetics

Limb prosthetics is a field currently encountering rapid growth and improvement. The demand continues to grow for more responsive, advanced devices. Integrating reflex response into these devices is currently in the early stages of position adjustment. For example, consider picking up a can of soup. If the person's grip is not strong enough, the can will begin to slip. A typical response would be to tighten the grip or potentially rapidly lower the arm in hopes of not letting it completely slip out. Current prosthetic devices are designed to give rapid muscular feedback in order to replicate the subconscious reaction to maintain the grip.

Future applications of reflex understanding to artificial devices are myriad. Could a device eventually be able to sense temperature and lead to a "flexor-extensor" reflex? Or might that same device be able to respond to signals arising from the contralateral side leading to a completion of the polysynaptic reflex?

Nicholas Breitnauer

See also: Areflexia; Axon; Blink Reflex; Central Nervous System (CNS); Hyperreflexia; Motor Neurons; Neurological Examination; Spinal Cord; Trauma

Further Reading

Alberstone, C. D., Benzel, E. C., Najm, I. M., & Steinmetz, M. P. (2009). *Anatomic diagnosis of neurologic diagnosis*. New York, NY: Thieme Medical Publishers, Inc.

Clarac, F. (2005). *The history of reflexes Part 1: From Descartes to Pavlov*. IBRO History of Neuroscience. Retrieved from http://ibro.info/wp-content/uploads/2012/12/The-History-of-Reflexes-Part-1.pdf

Clarac, F. (2005). *The history of reflexes Part 2: From Sherrington to 2004*. IBRO History of Neuroscience. Retrieved from http://ibro.info/wp-content/uploads/2012/12/The-History-of-Reflexes-Part-2.pdf

Costanzo, L. S. (2011). *Board review series: Physiology* (5th ed.). Philadelphia, PA: Lippincott Williams & Wilkins.

Restless Legs Syndrome

Restless legs syndrome (RLS), also known as *Willis-Ekbom disease,* is an increasingly common condition characterized by unpleasant sensations and an intense urge to move the legs. The symptoms associated with RLS range from mildly bothersome to unbearably painful and can change in severity from one day to another. Recognition of the disorder has become more frequent in recent years, with a current prevalence of 7–10 percent in the United States (Willis-Ekbom Disease Foundation, 2013). RLS affects people of all ages, but has a higher incidence in the elderly. Additionally, the condition presents in women two times more than men. Since the outcomes of RLS can chronically impact a patient's ability to sleep and perform daily activities, appropriate diagnosis and treatment may significantly improve their quality of life.

History

In 1685, the English physician Sir Thomas Willis (1621–1675) documented what is thought to be the first clinical account of RLS, with a patient who was experiencing difficulty sleeping due to uneasiness in the legs. His descriptions recalled that the patient felt tendon spasms causing restlessness to the point where he was no longer able to sleep and in a state of great torture. Years later in the 19th century, RLS reappeared in literature but with physicians then considering the disorder a sign of delirium. They termed it *anxietas tibiarum,* meaning anxiety of the legs. Finally, in 1945 the Swedish neurologist Karl A. Ekbom (1907–1977) used several personal observations to outline all of the characteristics of the condition in detail and coined the name "restless legs syndrome." Input from the two most prominent physicians involved in the discovery of RLS is the reason why it is also referred to as Willis-Ekbom disease.

Etiology

RLS is categorized into two different subtypes based on how it originates. Primary RLS is idiopathic, meaning there is no identifiable cause for the disorder. However, clinical observation suggests that primary RLS may have a strong genetic component. Over 40 percent of patients with RLS report a personal family history and twin studies have even demonstrated a high likelihood of hereditary contribution (Buchfuhrer et al., 2007). Also, genetic research has found that a significant percentage of people with RLS possess the same defects on certain chromosomes, which appear to be passed down in an autosomal dominant pattern. Primary RLS presents more commonly in the young and slowly develops over time. The other subtype is classified as secondary RLS, which occurs when there is a known nongenetic factor contributing to the disease. Contrastingly, this form presents with a faster onset and more often in older patients.

Although there is no well-defined mechanism explaining how RLS occurs, there have been many theories based on years of research. One of the most accepted models is that the condition stems from a dysfunction in the central nervous system, specifically with the naturally occurring neurotransmitter dopamine. Dopamine plays an important role in normal motor function and researchers speculate that decreased levels in the basal ganglia of the brain lead to problems with sensation and movement. This theory is supported by the fact that physiological dopamine levels follow cyclic variations that seem to mirror the rise and fall of daily RLS symptoms.

Several different medical conditions have been implicated in the etiology of secondary RLS. One of the more common causes of worsening symptoms is iron deficiency. Researchers hypothesize that this may be because of iron's function as a natural cofactor in the production of dopamine. In fact, magnetic resonance imaging (MRI) studies have even demonstrated lower brain iron concentrations in patients with RLS. Pregnancy is also frequently associated with the disease, possibly due to hormonal changes. Approximately 20 percent of pregnant women experience RLS, with peak symptoms occurring in the second to third trimesters and resolving after childbirth (Leschziner and Gringras, 2012). Other examples of medical conditions that may contribute to RLS are chronic kidney dysfunction, type 2 diabetes, or neurological issues. Studies have shown that people who have attention deficit disorder, Parkinson's disease, anxiety, or depression are all at a higher risk of developing symptoms. Deficiencies in many different vitamins, electrolytes, and hormones have also been linked to RLS. In addition, patient reports suggest that substances such as caffeine, alcohol, and tobacco or over-the-counter products such as antihistamines or antinausea medications may exacerbate symptoms. It is clear that there is a wide range of syndromes and compounds that may play a role in the etiology of RLS; however, the exact mechanisms by which they cause the disease are poorly understood.

Symptoms

The symptoms of RLS primarily reflect a dysfunction in both the motor and sensory regions of the brain. RLS presents with a spontaneous, uncontrollable urge to move the legs accompanied by uncomfortable sensations. Although occurring most often bilaterally between the ankles and knees, it can potentially present in other areas of the body such as the arms, trunk, or face. The sensory component of RLS can be difficult to describe but has been expressed by many patients as tingling, itching, creeping, crawling, and burning. Some patients even compare the condition to feeling as though there is an electric current, flowing water, or moving insects under their skin. In severe cases, RLS can manifest as very painful aches and throbs.

The motor component of the disorder involves involuntary movements, described as feeling like there is trapped energy in the legs. Patients can experience anything from subtle twitching and frequent pacing to full-extension muscle jerks. When they occur during the nighttime, these repetitive episodes are termed "periodic limb movements of sleep" and can significantly impact normal sleeping habits. Thus, RLS is a prominent cause of insomnia, making it difficult to both initiate and maintain sleep. Prolonged periods of sleep deprivation can lead to excessive daytime drowsiness and even serious organ dysfunction.

The rate of RLS symptoms and their severity can vary drastically from day to day. In general, symptoms are worse later in the day and during times of physical inactivity. Moreover, the extent of discomfort experienced from the disorder tends to worsen over time. Although it is a chronic condition, RLS patients may go through periods of remission where they function completely normal, especially if they are younger. This high fluctuation in symptoms can affect a patient's quality of life, potentially leading to severe mental and emotional problems.

Diagnosis and Management

Properly identifying RLS in patients can be difficult, because the symptoms of discomfort may be vague and consistent with several other conditions. In fact, it is not uncommon for cases to be misdiagnosed or go unrecognized. Diagnosis is based predominantly on clinical symptoms and elimination of other causes, as there are no laboratory markers (blood tests) to determine if a patient has RLS. To help with this issue, the National Institutes of Health outlines four cardinal criteria that must be met in order to truly diagnose a patient as having RLS. They are as follows: (1) a strong urge for leg (or upper body) movement accompanied by uncomfortable sensations; (2) symptoms that get worse with a lack of activity or while resting; (3) symptoms that get better, at least partially, with physical activity such as walking; and (4) symptoms that present more often in the evening or nighttime.

When a doctor assesses someone with suspected RLS they must perform a comprehensive exam. First, symptoms should be evaluated for severity and their impact on the patient's sleep. This can be assisted by having the patient complete a diary to document sensations and when they occur. Then, the provider should look for potential causes of secondary RLS by checking lab values from blood tests including iron levels and kidney function. Lastly, it is important to rule out all other possible causes for the symptoms such as *peripheral neuropathy* or *fibromyalgia* (a disorder in which a person has long-term, widespread pain that is due to abnormal pain processing). A proper neurologic exam can help differentiate these conditions, so they do not go untreated.

While there is no definite cure for RLS, many therapies have been tried in practice and demonstrate some success with relieving symptoms. As with most medical conditions, the safest option is to begin with a nonpharmaceutical remedy. All patients with RLS report that physical movement can help reduce symptoms. Therefore, it is important to encourage patients to engage in moderate physical exercise, such as walking, for at least a few days per week. Some patients report feeling relief from leg spasms after warm showers or baths. This may be due to the influence of increased temperature, which helps in relaxing the muscles. Likewise, massage therapy and muscle-stretching exercises have been shown to help with pain. Finally, implementing lifestyle changes may help RLS patients alleviate chronic sleep disruption. Performing appropriate sleeping habits, such as going to bed at a reasonable time and avoiding caffeine in the evening, can help improve nighttime symptoms.

The next step in treating patients with RLS is to consider if there are secondary causes that need to be addressed. Oral iron supplements should be given to people who are deficient, with close monitoring until levels are back to normal range. Other deficient substances that can be effectively normalized through oral supplementation are folate (a water-soluble B vitamin), vitamin B12, and magnesium. Studies have demonstrated that appropriate detection and reversal of these abnormalities can safely and effectively improve symptoms. Additionally, avoiding medications and substances that have been identified as contributory factors for a patient is a simple solution to reduce exacerbations.

When nondrug options are inadequately managing a patient's symptoms and after secondary causes have been addressed, they become appropriate candidates for medication therapy. The first-line options for RLS treatment are agents that stimulate the dopamine receptor. This is related back to the theory that low dopamine levels are a major factor in symptom severity. Examples of approved RLS medications by the U.S. Food and Drug Administration (FDA) that increase dopamine stimulation are Ropinirole, Pramipexole, and Rotigotine. Trials have shown that these medications perform superior to placebo (a substance that has no effect on alleviating symptoms) in improving RLS symptom severity, sleep, and quality of life. However, it is important to note that dopamine-enhancing agents can also cause serious neurologic side effects involving movement and sensation that may worsen RLS. Therefore, patients must be monitored closely and kept on low doses. Other treatment options include agents that affect nerve transmission such as antiepileptic medications, specifically gabapentin. Sedatives can be very useful in people with symptoms that are causing substantial difficulty sleeping. Benzodiazepines such as clonazepam and diazepam are commonly used in the treatment of insomnia and are a generally safe method to help initiate and maintain sleep. Finally, in patients with severe RLS, opiate drugs like codeine can be considered for pain reduction and improved tolerability of symptoms.

Future

While the therapies used in practice may provide patients with considerable relief, there is currently no cure for RLS. Therefore, organizations such as the National Institutes of Health are putting continuous efforts toward researching new medication options for the prevention and treatment of the disorder. A focus of research has also been to identify the poorly understood mechanism of RLS, to better target future management strategies. Improvements in the recognition and diagnosis of RLS have been associated with an increased prevalence in recent years. Since RLS is a chronic condition that significantly impacts patients' quality of life both physically and emotionally, the need for effective therapies is becoming evermore important.

Vidya Pugazhenthi

See also: Attention Deficit Disorder/Attention Deficit Hyperactivity Disorder; Central Nervous System (CNS); Depression; Diabetes Mellitus; Dopamine and Its Receptors; National Institutes of Health (NIH); Parkinson's Disease; *Sleep*

Further Reading

Aurora, R. N., Kristo, D. A., Bista, S. R., Rowley, J. A., Zak, R. S., Casey, K. R., . . . Rosenberg, R. S. (2012). The treatment of restless legs syndrome and periodic limb movement disorder in adults—an update for 2012: Practice parameters with an evidence-based systematic review and meta-analyses. *Sleep, 35*(8), 1039–1062.

Buchfuhrer, M. J., Hening, W. A., Kushida, C. A., Battenfield, A. E., & Dzienkowski, K. M. (2007). *Restless legs syndrome: Coping with your sleepless nights.* New York: Demos/ AAN Press.

Leschziner, G., & Gringras, P. (2012). Restless legs syndrome. *British Medical Journal, 344,* e3056.

Medline Plus. (2013). *Restless Legs.* Retrieved from http://www.nlm.nih.gov/medlineplus /restlesslegs.html

Willis-Ekbom Disease Foundation. (2013). *About WED/RLS.* Retrieved from http://www .rls.org

Retina

The *retina*, Latin for *net,* is a light-sensitive tissue that is found in the inside surface of the back of the eye. The eye captures light and creates an image of the visual world onto the retina. The retina's function can be compared to film in a camera. As the light hits the retina, it starts a chain reaction of chemical and electrical signals that trigger nerve impulses to be sent to various visual centers of the brain. These brain centers then interpret the signals as visual images.

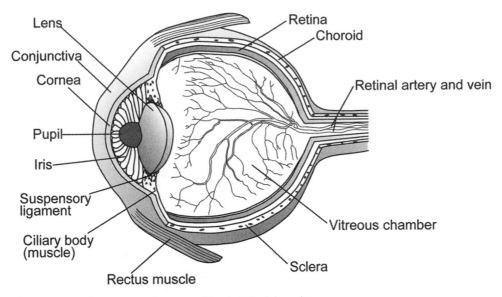

The anatomical elements of the eye. (Sandy Windelspecht)

History

The Greek physician Claudius Galen (AD 129–ca. 216) was the first person to document an examination of vision. Galen believed that the optic nerves were hollow and allowed psychic pneuma or "spirit" to flow from the brain to the eyes. This pneuma flowed out of the eyes to unite with the incoming light, and this was the process for vision. In Galen's opinion, the retina was formed by the optic nerve as it entered the eye and spread out. He also believed that the lens was the organ of vision. This theory remained static until the 17th century when a more accurate understanding of the gross anatomy of the eye and the function of each of its components was found.

Johannes Kepler (1571–1630) of Germany and René Descartes (1596–1650) of France, two prominent physicists of their time, discovered that the retina, not the lens, was responsible for the detection of light. Their work applied the physical behavior of light rays and used the geometry of optics to understand how animals process vision through their eyes. Kepler hypothesized that the lens at the front of the eye was necessary for focusing images. As the image of an object passed through the lens, he proposed that the image would then be projected in focus onto the retina. Several years later, Descartes confirmed Kepler's hypothesis by using eyes from an ox. Descartes carefully detached the eyes from their sockets and then removed the cells from the posterior portion of the eyes. This made the eye transparent so that he could easily look through it. Descartes looked at the back of the eye and saw the inverted image of the scenery outside. Later, in the 1830s, several German scientists used a crude microscope to closely examine the retina. Two different photoreceptor cells were discovered in the retina: the rod and cone cells. These retinal cells were named because of their shape as viewed under the microscope. Also during the 1800s, the visual pigments of the retina were discovered. Scientists dissected the retinas from the eyes of frogs and found that when these retinas were exposed to daylight they changed color. These scientists found that the retina is photosensitive and that the color they observed was due to the presence of a visual pigment. It was not until the 20th century, when new technologies and new conceptual ideas were understood, that more accurate information on the retina was made.

Anatomy

The retina is found on the inner surface of the back two-thirds to three-quarters of the eye. The wall of the eye consists of three different layers. The retina is the innermost layer. It lines the entire back portion of the eye with the exception of the area of the optic nerve. The total area of the retina is approximately 1,100 square millimeters. The average retina is 250 micrometers thick at the back of the eye, around the optic nerve. The retina then thickens to 400 micrometers around the macula's fovea—the center of the retina is the macula and the center of the macula is the fovea—and then begins to thin to 150 micrometers in the fovea. The retina thins even more as it gets closer to the edge of the eye and further thins to 80 micrometers at the edge. Retinal nerves attach to the optic nerve, which in turn exits the eye. The optic nerve is around the macula.

The cells that make up the retina consist of three basic types: photoreceptor cells, neuronal cells, and glial cells. Photoreceptor cells are known as cones and rods. Cones work best in bright conditions and provide color vision. Rods function in dim light and provide black-and-white vision. Each retina contains around 120 million rods and 6 million cones. There are three types of cones; each one perceives different wavelengths or colors of light and each one contains a different colored visual pigment. These pigments are called the red, blue, or green visual pigment. The center of the retina contains mostly cones while rods dominate the outer portions of the retina. The highest density of cones is at the center of the fovea. There are no rods at the center of the fovea.

Neural or nerve cells include bipolar cells, ganglion cells, horizontal cells, and amacrine cells. Bipolar cells connect the photoreceptors to the ganglion cells. Ganglion cells have dendrites that connect with bipolar cells. Horizontal cells connect bipolar cells with each other. And finally, amacrine cells connect bipolar and ganglion cells with each other. Glial cells are scattered between and within the axons of the ganglion cells in the retina and optic nerve. These supporting cells of the retina include Müller cells, astrocytes, and microglial cells.

The retina comprises 10 different cell layers. The inner surface of the retina is next to the vitreous of the eye, which is the glass-like portion of the eye. The outermost layer of the retina, the retinal pigment epithelium, is attached to the choroid (the brown-like vascular coat of the eye). Starting from the inner surface, the first layer is the inner limiting membrane. This basement membrane consists of Müller cells, which serve as support cells for the neurons of the retina. The second layer is the nerve fiber layer, which contain axons of the ganglion cell nuclei. The third layer is the ganglion cell layer. It comprises the nuclei of retina ganglion cells and axons of the optic nerve. This layer also contains displaced amacrine cells. The fourth layer is the inner plexiform layer and contains the synapse (the junction between two neurons where the neuronal impulse travels) between the dendrites of the retinal ganglion cells and cells of the inner nuclear layer. This layer also contains amacrine cells. The fifth layer is the inner nuclear layer. This layer is made up of three types of cells: bipolar cells, horizontal cells, and amacrine cells. The sixth layer is the outer plexiform layer, also known as the external plexiform layer. It consists of the synapses between the dendrites of horizontal cells from the inner nuclear layer and the rods and cones of the outer nuclear layer. In the macular region, this is known as the Fiber layer of Henle. The seventh layer is the outer nuclear layer and contains the cell bodies of rods and cones. The eighth layer is the external limiting membrane. This layer separates the inner segment of the rods and cones from their nucleus. The ninth layer is the photoreceptor layer also known as the layer of rods and cones or Jacob's membrane. As its name implies, it comprises both rods and cones. The 10th and outermost layer is the pigmented layer or retinal pigment epithelium. This layer is filled with densely packed pigmented hexagonal cells.

Physiology

The main function of the retina is to convert light into neural signals. This involves four basic processes: photoreception, transmission to bipolar cells, transmission to ganglion cells, and transmission along the optic nerve. Damage to any of these cells or processes can cause different visual problems including blindness.

In photoreception, light passes through the inner layers of the retina to reach the rods and cones. The photoreceptors contain a photopigment, which captures individual photons of light and turns them into neural signals. Cones work best in bright conditions and provide color vision. Rods function in dim light and provide black-and-white vision.

The next step is the transmission to bipolar cells through synapses. The rods and cones transfer the light and relay the signal to their cell bodies and out to their axons. These axons then contact the dendrites of both bipolar cells and horizontal cells. Horizontal cells are parallel interneurons and help with signal processing. Since there are 150 million photoreceptors and only 1 million optic nerve fibers, there must be convergence of signals.

The third step is the transmission to the ganglion cells. The bipolar cells pass the signal from photoreceptors to their axons. In the inner plexiform layer, bipolar axons contact ganglion cell dendrites and amacrine cells.

The final step involves transmission along the optic nerve. The ganglion cells send their axons through the nerve fiber layer and meet at the center of the retina. This forms the optic nerve. The ganglion cell axons leave the eye at the optic nerve. They then travel along with the signal all the way to the lateral geniculate nucleus in the brainstem. At the optic nerve, there are no photoreceptors, bipolar cells, or ganglion cells. Instead, the human optic nerve is made up of over 1 million ganglion cell axons.

Disease

A healthy retina collects light information and converts it into an electrical signal. This signal is then transmitted to the brain, which enables mammals to see. There are many genetic and acquired diseases or disorders that affect the retina. Retinitis pigmentosa is a group of genetic diseases that affect the retina and cause the loss of night vision and peripheral vision. This disorder is caused by the loss of rods and cones and may eventually lead to blindness. Similar to retinitis pigmentosa is cone-rod dystrophy (CORD), which is a number of diseases where vision loss is caused by the breakdown of the cones and/or rods. It involves vision loss, sensitivity to bright lights, and poor color vision.

Macular degeneration is a major disorder of the retina and describes a group of diseases characterized by the loss of vision in the center of the visual field caused by macula cell death. It is mainly age related and usually comes in two forms: wet and dry. In the dry form, cellular debris builds up between the retina and the choroid, which may cause the retina to become detached. Retinal detachment involves the retina peeling away from the choroid. In the more severe wet form, blood vessels form behind the retina, which may also cause the retina to become detached. Retinal detachment may also be caused by trauma, such as a blow to the eye or head. When a retina begins to detach, the patient's visual field may have one or more signs such as "floaters," bright flashes of light, or a black curtain over a portion of the field of vision. Retinal detachment can be repaired if it is done quickly before the retina is devoid of oxygen. If the retina does lose too much oxygen, its cells will die causing blindness. An ophthalmologist can repair retinal detachments or tears with a laser.

Retinopathy is a disorder caused by damage to the blood vessels that supply the retina. High blood pressure or hypertension can cause damage, which leads to hypertensive retinopathy. Diabetes mellitus can also cause damage that leads to diabetic retinopathy. Retinoblastoma is a cancer of the retina. It most commonly affects young children, but can occur rarely in adults.

Lipemia retinalis is a white appearance of the retina and occurs by fat (lipid) deposits. This disorder, called lipoprotein lipase deficiency, is caused by the inability to produce enzymes that break down fatty acids.

Color blindness is a common disorder of the retina and is caused by loss or abnormality of the certain type of cone cells. If just one type of cone is damaged or missing, the ability to distinguish between red and green is not possible. This is the most common type of color blindness. The most severe form of color blindness is *achromatopsia.* This condition is rare and causes no color to be seen. Persons with achromatopsia see everything as different shades of gray, and may also have a lazy eye, be sensitive to light, and have poor vision. In general, most types of color blindness are a genetic anomaly and are inherited by a mutation on the X chromosome. Therefore, more men will be color blind than women since men only have one X chromosome. For a woman to be color blind, she would need to have a mutation in both X chromosomes.

Mario J. Perez

See also: Color Blindness; Optic Nerve; Visual Perception (Visual Processing); Visual System

Further Reading

Kolb, H., Nelson, R., Fernandez, E., & Jones, B. (Eds.). (2011). *Webvision: The organization of the retina and visual system.* Retrieved from http://webvision.med.utah.edu/book/

Machemer, R., & Michelson, G. (2012). *The atlas of ophthalmology: Online multimedia database.* Retrieved from http://www.atlasophthalmology.com/atlas/frontpage.jsf

Retrovirus

General Virology

Retroviruses belong to a viral family called Retroviridae. Members of the family share several basic traits; they are all single-stranded RNA viruses, they have an envelope consisting of host cell membrane, and they share similar methods of replication. Several retroviruses infect humans, one of the best known is HIV (human immunodeficiency virus). Human DNA contains many stretches that may have come from retroviruses, but the significance of these endogenous retroviruses is not known. The observation that retroviruses can add DNA to the human genome, though, has led to research and trials using retroviruses for gene therapy.

Replication

The first step in viral infection is attachment. During this step, the virus attaches to the host cell using viral glycoproteins (specialized proteins containing sugar molecules) that recognize specific receptors on host-cell plasma membrane. Each virus infects a specific cell type; this is referred to as viral tropism. Viral tropism is a result of the attachment step; the cell must display receptors the virus can recognize.

Although viral attachment is mediated by binding to host-cell receptors, these receptors have other functions for the host that are merely exploited by the virus. The HIV virus, for example, is a retrovirus that is T-cell tropic, because one type of T-cell expresses the CD4 molecule that serves as a receptor for the virus. From the host-cell perspective, the CD4 molecule takes part in T-cell recognition of foreign molecules. Viral binding to CD4, however, allows the virus to enter the T-cell.

After the virus binds the host cell, the viral envelope fuses with the host-cell plasma membrane, and the virus enters the cell. The virus then uncoats, releasing the viral RNA and specialized enzymes necessary for viral replication. In human cells the flow of information is that DNA is transcribed into RNA, which is then translated into a protein. Human cells do not have an enzyme capable of making DNA from RNA. The virus must carry an enzyme to reverse transcribe RNA into DNA (hence the prefix *retro*) so the host cell can make copies of the virus. This enzyme is called reverse transcriptase.

Once viral reverse transcriptase transcribes the viral RNA into DNA, the DNA is referred to as a provirus. The provirus is carried to the nucleus where it can be integrated into the host genome using a viral enzyme, integrase. Most retroviruses require the host cell to divide in order to gain access to the nucleus and integrate. The location of viral integration is random and has potential to cause mutation in any gene. An established provirus is integrated into the host genome and will be replicated with the cell and passed on as part of the genome.

The provirus will be transcribed into RNA by the host cell and viral proteins will be translated on host ribosomes into proteins. The viral proteins are different than host-cell proteins in that they are synthesized in a long continuous string rather than as individual proteins. The virus needs an additional enzyme called protease to cleave the long protein into shorter proteins for virion assembly. Without protease to process the proteins, no infectious virions are formed.

The viruses are assembled in the cytoplasm (the "guts" of the cell) and bud out through the host-cell membrane. The host-cell membrane forms the viral envelope. After budding from the cell the viral particles are infectious. Viral glycoproteins project out through envelope, allowing the virus to recognize the next host cell. Thus, the infection cycle begins.

Classification

The Retrovirus family consists of single-stranded enveloped RNA viruses that are further divided into two subfamilies and a number of genera. The subfamily ortho-retrovirinae contains six genera, two of which contain retroviruses that infect humans, while the subfamily spumaretrovirinae does not contain any viruses known to be associated with human disease.

The Retrovirus family, subfamily orthoretrovirinae contains four genera of viruses that do not infect humans and two genera that infect humans. The retroviruses that do not infect humans infect a number of animals and cause various types of cancers.

The two genera that infect humans include the viruses HTLV-1 and HTLV-2 (human T-cell lymphoma viruses) and HIV. HTLV-1 causes adult T-cell leukemia. Other patients infected with HTLV-1 develop HTLV-1-associated myelopathy also known as tropical spastic paraparesis, an incurable viral infection of the spinal cord that causes weakness in the leg. HTLV-2 is associated with milder neurological disorders. HIV is part of the genus *Lentivirus,* originating from the Latin *lentus,* meaning "slow," which refers to the viruses' long incubation period. The disease caused by HIV infection is called acquired immunodeficiency syndrome (AIDS) and is characterized by immune dysfunction caused by a decline in T-cells. Similar Lentiviruses infect monkeys and cats, causing a milder disease that cannot be transmitted to humans.

Retroviruses in the subfamily spumaretrovirinae have not yet been proven to be associated with any human disease. The genus *Spumavirus* contains six species of foamy viruses that infect various animals including monkeys, cows, horses, and cats. At least one species, however, has been found in humans. Since these viruses can infect human cells and have not yet been associated with any disease, they may be candidate vectors for gene therapy, discussed in the following.

Human Endogenous Retroviruses

The retroviruses discussed previously are exogenous, or outside, of the host germ-line (egg and sperm) DNA and are passed from person to person. Analysis of human DNA reveals several retrovirus-like sequences called endogenous retroviruses. These sequences resemble genes found in known retroviruses such as HIV and HTLV, yet infectious viral particles are not produced. These integrated gene sequences are passed from parent to child, rather than from person to person. The significance of endogenous retroviruses is not known, but several roles have been hypothesized. Although viral particles are not produced from endogenous retroviral genes, viral proteins are transcribed and translated. Researchers speculate these viral proteins may have a role in cancer and autoimmune diseases, where the body's immune system attacks itself.

Human endogenous retroviruses may play a role in cancer, but the exact nature of this role is unknown and may vary with different cancers. When a retrovirus integrates into the host genome, the viral genes may control expression of host genes. These genes may then be abnormally expressed and cause malignant transformation of the cell. A variety of tumor cells have been shown to express increased amounts of various endogenous retroviral proteins, suggesting a possible role for these viruses in malignant transformation.

Endogenous retroviral elements may also play a role in autoimmunity. Over the past two decades many researchers have noted that patients with autoimmune diseases ranging from lupus to rheumatoid arthritis have antibodies to retroviruses, yet do not have HIV or HTLV. These patients do, however, have endogenous retroviral elements. Perhaps the body's reaction to these viral proteins causes the body to mistakenly recognize a self-protein as foreign. Or perhaps the retroviral protein directly activates the cells of the body's immune system to attack self-tissue. Alternatively the retrovirus may cause cells in the patient's body to express a unique foreign protein that the body recognizes and destroys, causing destruction of self-tissue. The challenge researchers face in making correlations between endogenous retroviruses and autoimmunity is that endogenous retroviral genes are expressed in normal tissues too.

Autoimmunity and cancer are undesirable effects to the host. Scientists are studying why these genes are kept in the human genome over many generations. It has been hypothesized that genes may offer an advantage to the host. For example, since endogenous retroviral DNA is translated into protein, these proteins may help the host gain resistance to other exogenous human retroviruses that may be more virulent.

Oncogenic Retroviruses

Retroviruses can cause tumors; these retroviruses are called oncogenic retroviruses. Infectious agents cause 10–15 percent of human cancers. Examples of oncogenic retroviruses include HIV and HTLV. Oncogenic viruses may cause cancer in a number of different ways. Some viruses carry genes that transform cells. In this case, a gene carried by the virus causes cell proliferation, and rapid tumor development. Other viruses are slow-transforming viruses that cause mutations as the virus integrates into the host genome. In this case, the virus destroys genes that regulate cellular growth. Still other viruses cause cancers because they affect the host's immune system, rendering the host incapable of recognizing a small tumor that would normally be destroyed, or unable to control another virus that can cause cancer.

Retroviruses as Vectors for Gene Therapy

Retroviruses make an ideal vector to transport a gene into a host cell because retroviruses can integrate into the host cell and this genetic material will be passed on when the cell divides. Unfortunately, the new gene will not be passed on to future generations unless the retrovirus integrates into sperm or egg cells. Caution must be used when using retroviral vectors, however, because the retrovirus could integrate into the host genome and cause mutation or cancer. Other hurdles yet to be cleared include the fact that target cells must be actively dividing in order for the retrovirus to infect the cell. This requirement for cell division means that cell types that don't divide often, such as neurons, are difficult to target using a retroviral vector.

Gene therapy of the disease severe combined immunodeficiency (SCID) provides an example of successful gene therapy as well as and illustration of some of the pitfalls. One type of SCID, ADA-SCID, results from a deficiency of the enzyme adenosine deaminase (ADA). Patients with this form of SCID are unable to produce functional lymphocytes. Treatments include lifelong enzyme replacement, or bone marrow transplant, if a genetically matched donor is available. Researchers engineered retroviruses containing the missing *ADA* gene. The viruses were allowed to infect lymphocytes collected from patients receiving ADA replacement therapy. Cells with the gene added back through gene therapy were found in patients, but patients still required ADA supplementation. Gene therapy trials are currently underway worldwide with the goal of finding a safe and effective method to replace the *ADA* gene.

Another form of SCID called X-SCID is caused by a mutation of a different gene, but also causes a decrease in lymphocytes. Twenty patients were treated by retroviral introduction of the missing gene into bone marrow stem cells. As a result of this trial, five of the patients developed T-cell leukemia. This leukemia was a result of the retroviral integration site. Although three of the five patients in the trial were cured of their leukemia, two died. As a result of these two deaths, gene therapy for X-SCID has been halted in the United States until better methods can be designed to ensure retroviral vector integration sites do not cause leukemia.

Neuroscientists are exploring several ways that gene therapy could be used to treat neurological diseases. Gene therapy has been used to treat animal models of epilepsy. One group (Wykes et al., 2012) used a rat model that is similar to one type of medication resistant human epilepsy. Researchers used a retroviral vector to introduce additional potassium ion channel genes into rat brains. These potassium channels caused potassium ions to flow out of brain cells, making it more difficult for a large number of neurons to fire at the same time and cause a seizure. This therapy prevented epilepsy, and when given to a rat with epilepsy, decreased seizures. Similarly, the same group has introduced genes for additional chloride channels into rodent brains. These chloride channels are light sensitive, so when a laser shines on the neurons, the chloride channels open, preventing neurons from firing and seizures. In the future this type of technology could allow an implantable laser that prevents seizures, similar to current implanted defibrillators that regulate patients' hearts.

Gene therapy may be applied to several neurological diseases in the future. Viral vectors could be used to deliver the genes coding for a missing protein, or for a growth factor to help resolve the disease. Viruses have the advantage of being able to deliver a gene to a specific cell type, and in the case of retroviruses, the gene will be integrated into the target cell and passed on as the cell divides.

Summary

Retroviruses have a significant impact on human health due to the diseases they cause and the role their infections may also play in human cancers. Nonetheless, scientists are learning new ways to use the retroviruses' engineering and mechanisms to treat other diseases by gene therapy. These treatments may prove to be beneficial in the future. For a more in-depth exploration of retroviruses and gene therapy, visit www.genetherapynet.com.

Lisa A. Rabe

See also: Acquired Immunodeficiency Syndrome (AIDS); Epilepsy; Poliomyelitis

Further Reading

Fischer, A., Havein-Bey-Abina, S., & Cavazzana-Calvo, M. (2010). 20 years of gene therapy for SCID. *Nature Immunology, 11*(6), 457–460.

Gene Therapy Net. (2012). Retrieved from www.genetherapynet.com

Wykes, R. C., Heeroma, J. H., Mantoan, L., Zheng, K., MacDonald, D. C., Deisseroth, K., . . . Kullmann, D. M. (2012). Optogenetic gene therapy in a rodent model of focal neocortical epilepsy. *Science Translational Medicine.* Rapid Publication on November 12, 2012. Published ahead of print. doi:10.1126/scitranslmed.3004190.

Rett Syndrome

Rett syndrome is a neurological disorder that primarily affects females and detrimentally affects postnatal development (growth after birth). Most commonly this syndrome presents as *inhibited motor function, degeneration of the heart,* and *decreased growth.* Another common and painful symptom of the syndrome is *gastrointestinal problems.* Rett syndrome is a developmental disorder and a child's inability to express themselves through the pain can lead to a misdiagnosis. Oftentimes a child is misdiagnosed as having *autism* or *Tourette syndrome.*

Every year, 1 in every 10,000–15,000 girls internationally is affected by Rett syndrome (NINDS, 2013). Research indicates that Rett syndrome affects all races and ethnicities. Although there is genetic testing available, it is often inconsequential because Rett syndrome is caused by a spontaneous gene mutation.

History

In 1954, Rett syndrome was first discovered by Andreas Rett (1924–1997), an Austrian pediatrician. He first observed two young girls in his waiting room who were compulsively wringing their hands, as if they were washing them. Rett went on to travel across Europe in search of patients with similar behaviors. In 1966, Rett published his findings for the first time in a German medical journal, and again in 1977 in English to bring about more awareness about the syndrome. Finally in 1999, Ruthie Amir (n.d.), a research fellow at Baylor University, discovered that the mutation of the *MECP2* gene caused Rett syndrome. This proved that Rett syndrome is an *X-linked disorder.* This means that the mutation occurs on the X chromosome and it also requires two X chromosomes for it to be expressed. This explains why Rett syndrome is almost only seen in young females.

Types and Symptoms

Rett syndrome as mentioned previously is caused by the mutation of the *MEPC2* gene on the X chromosome. The main function of the *MEPC2* gene is to provide instructions on the production of *methyl-cytosine binding protein 2.* This protein is responsible for proper brain development as well as a signal to turn on certain genomic expressions. The severity of the effects of the syndrome is dependent on the extent of the mutation. Since only one X chromosome is active in any given cell, some of the brain cells can have normal functioning. Therefore, if a higher percentage of the cells have the normal copy of the *MECP2* gene then the effects will be minimal. However, if the opposite is true, the effects can be extensive.

Since Rett syndrome is a developmental syndrome, there are many stages that a child will go through as they progress through the syndrome. *Stage 1* begins sometime between the age of 6 and 18 months. During this time, children show a decreased interest in toys and even human interaction. This stage can sometimes be overlooked by parents and health care professionals or incorrectly diagnosed as autism. *Stage 2* takes place between the ages of one to four years and is highly destructive. During this time, children lose learned behaviors and language. They also begin to wring their hands and other such habitual mannerisms. Dangerous symptoms such as *sleep apnea* and *hyperventilation* become common. *Stage 3,* or plateau stage, is the longest lasting stage. At this stage, children struggle with *motor function, seizures,* and *continued irritability.* This stage is also where most behavioral improvement can occur. Girls at this stage are more susceptible to learning coping methods to improve their lives. The *final stage* is the late motor deterioration stage. During this stage many girls begin to suffer from *decreased mobility, scoliosis,* and *decreased muscle tone.* Fortunately, communication and learned hand mobility are not affected. Also the repetitive hand movements and eye gaze become more steady and easier to manage.

Treatments

Currently there is no cure for Rett syndrome and all treatment is symptomatic. Most of the medication is used to treat the sleep disorders, seizures, and mobility functions of the patients. There is also physical therapy to help strengthen muscle tone and increase function in these limbs.

Research is focused on the function of the *MECP2* gene so that possible drugs can be discovered that produce the same effects as the gene to make an animal model. The International Rett Syndrome Foundation is on the frontlines of this research.

Future

As with any debilitating syndrome the quality of life for the individuals affected is low. However, there is hope as more research is being done and treatment methods become better. The life expectancy of someone with Rett syndrome is 40 to 50 years. Although there are individuals that live up to 60 years, they are in the minority. Currently, research is not performed on any patients that are past the age of 40. As research expands, hopefully life expectancy will increase and a more potent solution to this problem will be found.

Cynthia M. Joseph

See also: Autism; Seizures; Tourette Syndrome

Further Reading

Mayo Clinic Staff. (2012). *Diseases and conditions: Rett syndrome.* Retrieved from http://www.mayoclinic.org/diseases-conditions/rett-syndrome/basics/definition/con-20028086

National Institute of Neurological Disorders and Stroke (NINDS). (2013). *Rett syndrome fact sheet.* Retrieved from http://www.ninds.nih.gov/disorders/rett/detail_rett.htm

Reward and Punishment

In mammals, behavior is affected by consequences, which are both *rewards* (or reinforcements) and *punishments*. For example, hunting is a behavior that will result with a reinforcement of eating and satiation. However, attacking a porcupine will result with a punishment of quills in the attacker's skin. In neuroscience, this is called *operant conditioning* or instrumental conditioning. Specifically, operant conditioning is a learning experience whereby the animal's behavior is changed by what has happened in the past or consequences from outside experiences. Furthermore, the consequences can change the frequency, form, and strength of the behavior. It is important to note that operant conditioning is different from *classical conditioning,* which was performed by Ivan Petrovich Pavlov (1849–1936). Operant conditioning changes behavior by using reinforcements and punishments, while classical conditioning concentrates on conditioning reflex behaviors that will not maintain without consequences.

History

In 1937, American psychologist and behaviorist Burrhus Frederic "B.F." Skinner (1904–1990) first coined the term operant conditioning. He developed this term from his research studies on observable behavior and its observed consequences. Skinner invented the operant conditioning chamber (or the Skinner box) where pigeons or rats where isolated from all outside stimuli. In the box, the animal was free to make a choice of one or two repeatable responses, such as press a lever and receive food. Skinner would count the number of times the lever was pressed to determine a response rate of reinforcement schedules, which are the well-defined rules that control the reinforcement of an animal. The rules are either the time or the number of responses to be made available of the reinforcement.

Operant Conditioning

To shape behavior, scientists have found that certain consequences are needed: *reinforcement, punishment,* and *extinction.* Specifically, reinforcement is a consequence that will cause the behavior to occur more often. Punishment is a consequence that will cause the behavior to occur less often. Finally, extinction is a lack of consequence following a behavior. This means that if neither reinforcement nor a punishment is given after a behavior, then that behavior will occur less often. It is important to note that certain factors can alter the effectiveness of reinforcing or punishing consequences, such as satiation/deprivation, immediacy, contingency, and size.

There are five operant conditioning procedures: *positive (addition)* and *negative (subtraction) reinforcement; positive* and *negative punishment;* and *extinction.* In operant conditioning, the term "positive" means an addition following the behavior, while the term "negative" means a subtraction following the behavior. For a *positive reinforcement* (or reinforcement) example, pigeons in the Skinner box would receive a food pellet after pressing the lever. The reward (or positive reinforcement) was the food pellet. For a *negative reinforcement* (or escape) example, rats in the Skinner box would press a lever to stop an annoying and loud sound outside of the box. The reward (or negative reinforcement) is the removal of the noise, which increases the behavior of pressing the lever.

Positive punishment (or punishment) is contrary to what one would think, as it is the addition following a behavior. Specifically, it is the goal of positive punishment to decrease a behavior. For example, a cat owner does not want their kitten on the kitchen counter. Thus, a positive punishment would be squirting the cat with water each time it jumps onto the kitchen counter. Since cats do not like water, the kitten will try to avoid that behavior of jumping onto the kitchen counter. This is the same idea of spanking a child to stop a behavior.

Negative punishment (or penalty) is the subtraction or removal of a stimulus after a behavior. For example, a parent wants their child to stop hitting other children. Thus, a negative punishment would be for a parent to take away a favorite toy after their child hits another child. The removal of the favorite toy will decrease the bad behavior of hitting.

Finally, *extinction* occurs when reinforcement is no longer given for a certain behavior. For example, a rat in the Skinner box no longer receives food when a lever is pressed. Without receiving food, the animal will press the lever less often and will eventually stop pressing the lever. Thus, the behavior of pressing a lever is then considered extinguished.

Patricia A. Bloomquist

See also: Behavior; Behavioral Experiments; Behavioral Tests; Pavlov, Ivan

Further Reading

Dolan, R. J., & Dayan, P. (2013). Goals and habits in the brain. *Neuron, 80*(2), 312–325.

Jones, J. D., & Comer, S. D. (2013). A review of human drug self-administration procedures. *Behavioral Pharmacology, 24*(5–6), 384–395.

Skinner, B. F. (1988). The operant side of behavior therapy. *Journal of Behavior Therapy and Experimental Psychiatry, 19*(3), 171–179.

Romberg Test

The ability to balance oneself is dependent on the cooperation of a minimum of two out of three subjective factors: an individual's vision, their proprioception (the unconscious ability of the body to sense movement and orientation in space), and the proper functioning of the vestibular apparatus of the inner ear. Analyzing these three factors is the basis for the *Romberg test*. When giving a patient a complete neurological exam, doctors will often employ the Romberg test as one of many tools designed to screen for problems with balance particularly to determine disorders of proprioception and the vestibular apparatus. There are some variations to the test in practice, but in its purist form the subjects stands with their feet together, arms either folded across the chest or down at their side, and their eyes closed for 30 seconds. The clinician, while standing with his or her arms in front of and behind the subject to prevent falls, observes the subject for swaying and loss of balance. Mild rotational swaying may be perceptible and is considered a normal occurrence. For a true negative test, there should be no marked swaying or loss of balance, nor should the subject have to move their feet for stability. The results of the test are described as either a negative or a positive Romberg's sign.

History

It is interesting to note that the Romberg test has its roots in the treatment of syphilis (a sexually transmitted disease). The first written documentation of syphilis was in Italy in the 15th century. Syphilis is a bacterial infection caused by *Treponema-pallidum* and is readily cured by antibiotics; however, penicillin was not available until the 20th century. Without treatment of any kind, syphilis can be a devastating disease. In the later stages of the disease there is often a phenomenon called *tabes dorsalis*. Tabes dorsalis damages sensory nervous tissue around the dorsal columns of the spinal cord, which governs proprioception and sensory aspect of balance. The phenomenon leads to, among other symptoms, a loss of proprioception. Given the high incidence of syphilis prior to the discovery of penicillin and the lack of treatment options, patients with tabes dorsalis would have been abundant when Moritz Heinrich Romberg (1795–1873) began working as a physician and neurologist in the early to mid-19th century. Romberg did not know that tabes dorsalis was caused by syphilis. He posited that it was either due to excessive drinking or to sexual activity; but he did notice that patients suffering from it lost postural control when they could not see. He initially described this phenomenon in ca. 1840. In 1853, in the second edition of his textbook entitled *Lehrbuch der Nervenkrankheiten des Menschen* (*Textbook of Nervous Diseases in Humans*), he formally described the clinical assessment known as Romberg's sign (Lanska, 2003).

Another German physician, Bernardus Brach (n.d.), also described the assessment around this time. Thus, for a time, neurologists called it the Brach-Romberg sign. Another English neurologist, Marshall Hall (1790–1857), had actually documented his observations of the phenomenon several years before Romberg. However he did not parlay this knowledge into a clinical test as Romberg did, which is why Romberg earned the eponym.

Romberg was part of a zeitgeist in which neuroscience was flourishing and he was influenced by several significant individuals. There was his friend and teacher, Johann Peter Frank (1745–1821), who convinced Romberg to specialize in neurology; and also some English neurologists whose works Romberg translated into German. These included Andrew Marshall (1742–1813) who had published the *Morbid Anatomy of the Brain in Mania and Hydrophobia; with the Pathology of These Two Diseases*, and Sir Charles Bell (1774–1842) who published *Nervous System of the Human Body* (Schiffter, 2010). The idea that nerve pathways could either be sensory or motor was developing during this time, and indeed Romberg's own textbook was divided into two sections: "Neuroses of Sensibility" and "Neuroses of Motility." It is important to note that in this context, neuroses mean noninflammatory diseases of the nervous system, rather than the psychological "neuroses" which indicate less severe forms of mental illness. Romberg's test, which assesses sensory imbalance and ataxia and is often used to distinguish them from motor imbalance and ataxia stemming from cerebellar disorder, could not have been conceived without this idea. Based on the information gleaned from this time, later neurologists developed more precise and sensitive clinical tests for pathologies affecting balance.

The Test

In clinical practice, the Romberg test does not always give very precise results and today is used most often to monitor the progression of a patient diagnosed with a particular disease or as a general indication that the patient has difficulty with balance. The Romberg test is still sometimes used to distinguish between sensory and cerebellar ataxia, but truly more sophisticated measures are needed for this purpose. Often a patient with cerebellar ataxia will have difficulty balancing even with open eyes; however, this is not always true. The test was not designed to assess vestibular function, though it has come to be used for that purpose. There is still a lack of consistency regarding when to use the test and how to interpret the results; however, a positive Romberg's sign certainly indicates a need for further testing.

One of the most common uses of the test today is by law enforcement officials to confirm positive results from standardized roadside sobriety tests. The Romberg test removes visual stimuli that a person might use to maintain balance and can therefore detect problems with proprioception or the vestibular apparatus. The dorsal columns of the spinal cord carry sensory signals, which provide for proprioception are affected by tabes dorsalis, which is why the test was useful with sufferers of syphilis. Today there is little need for assessment of tabes dorsalis, but several other conditions affect these nerves as well including multiple sclerosis and amyotrophic lateral sclerosis (ALS). Vestibular disorders, such as Meniere's disease, can sometimes be detected with this test as well. There is less sensitivity with these disorders, however, and the test does not indicate whether there is a dysfunction with the inner ear itself or with the vestibulocochlear cranial nerve. Vitamin B deficiencies can cause problems with proprioception and therefore the test is often used as part of an assessment for this condition (Lemone and Burke, 2004).

Erin Slocum

See also: Ataxia; Multiple Sclerosis; Vestibular System

Further Reading

Lanska, D. (2003). The Romberg sign and early instruments for measuring postural sway. *Seminars in Neurology, 22*(4), 409–418.

Lanska, D., & Goetz, C. (2000). Romberg's sign development, adoption, and adaptation in the 19th century. *Neurology, 55*(8), 1201–1206.

Lemone, P., & Burke, K. (2004). Mental status and neurological techniques. In *Medical surgical nursing: Critical thinking in client care* (3rd ed., Vol. 2., pp. 917–979). Upper Saddle River, NJ: Pearson Education, Inc.

Schiffter, R. (2010). Moritz Heinrich Romberg (1795–1873). *Journal of Neurology, 257*, 1409–1410.

S

Saccades

The word *saccade* originally referred to the quick jerk of the reins to slow or change the direction of a horse. This concept applies directly to the eyes. A saccade is a small, rapid adjustment of the eye in order to bring an object into better focus. These movements are so rapid and small, they are hardly ever noticed. Typically, another person needs to watch in order to observe saccades.

Generally, these movements are necessary due to the small area of detailed vision in the eye named the "fovea." This area contains the largest concentration of high-resolution retinal cells (brain cells found on the photosensitive lining of the eye) and allows for detailed vision. A saccade relies on complicated neurological connection between the frontal cortex (of the brain), superior colliculus (in the brainstem), and three pairs of ocular muscles (these directly control eye movement). Ultimately, this quick motion helps build a rich, dynamic interpretation of the visual world.

History

Louis Emile Javal (1839–1907) is credited with the first documentation and discussion of ocular saccades. His choice to pursue a career in ophthalmology (medical study/surgery of eye disorders) began with experience within his family. Both his father and sister suffered from strabismus (where the eyes are not in alignment). During the course of his career, he developed devastating glaucoma (increase pressure in the eyes) that eventually led to his complete blindness.

During the course of his career, he became concerned with measuring the surface and movement of eyes. His was able to clarify the presence of saccades by placing a mirror directed to one eye while reading. Rapid, small adjustments were observed and it was reasoned that this perfectly normal movement allowed for more detailed sight.

The study of saccadic movement continues to modern times. Some believe these rapid movements are "ballistic," meaning it is impossible to change the direction/speed of the movement after it is initiated by the cortex and/or superior colliculus. Additionally, researchers studying animals other than humans have identified saccades as commonplace but often for different reasons than image focusing.

Anatomy and Physiology

A typical scenario of saccade initiation would be a new stimulus in the visual field. Imagine a balloon became loosened on a windy day. This mobile, bright object would enter the visual field and information from the retina (neurons responsible for vision in the back of eyes) would be transmitted to different parts of the brain. Once this new piece of information was recognized, both the frontal eye field and superior colliculus would coordinate eye movement toward the object.

Prior to the fovea centering on an object, peripheral retinal cells become activated. These neurons are especially sensitive to movement and make up "peripheral vision." In this part of the retina, a higher concentration of rod cells exists. Interestingly, the information gathered from these cells is only black and white. New information (such as the balloon) in the visual field is then sent to the frontal eye field.

The frontal eye field is a region in the frontal cortex named "Brodmann area 8." Korbinian Brodmann (1868–1918) was a neurologist who carefully labeled 52 total areas of the human brain. Each area possessed a unique compilation of neurons and connections to various parts of the brain. This frontal eye field is one area directly linked to axons arising from the retina.

It is believed that in this region of the cortex, attention is given to new information. This information—requiring further processing—is relayed to other portions of the visual pathways. One important connection from the frontal eye field is to a region in the midbrain responsible for initiating saccades. This area is known as the "superior colliculus."

A detailed map of the visual world exists in this part of the brain. Information from the retina is linked to specific portions of the superior colliculus, with the front portion dedicated to the fovea. This part of the brain exists in the rostral (toward the top of the head) and posterior (toward the back) part of the midbrain. Neuron bodies in this region directly control the muscles that move the eye.

Within the detailed visual map of the superior colliculus, the direction and speed of a saccade are dictated. In the case of the balloon, imagine this image is toward the left side of the visual field. The superior colliculus neurons are able to discern where the fovea is currently pointed and where the new stimulus exists. Based on the distance, a saccade is initiated at speeds usually around 400 degrees/second, but can go as fast as 700 degrees/second. The total right to left visual field, for reference, is typically 160 degrees.

The signal to initiate a saccade is a highly coordinated movement of ocular muscles. A leftward saccade is managed by the "paramedian pontine reticular formation" (PPRF). Here, the signal to activate leftward movement of the left eye is controlled by the abducens nerve and lateral rectus muscle. Simultaneously, the right eye is moved left through the "median longitudinal fasciculus." Both the oculomotor nerve and the medial rectus muscle facilitate this movement.

Once the saccade has completed, the image should now be directly placed on the fovea. This portion of the retina contains a higher proportion of cone cells (neurons dedicated to color and high-definition vision) than rod cells. This information is transmitted to the occipital cortex in the back part of the brain and the image is interpreted.

Interestingly, saccades also occur in the dark. This unique feature highlights the various functions of the superior colliculus. Not only does this part of the brain respond to signals from the frontal eye field, but it also receives somatic (peripheral sensory) stimulation. Touching of an arm could also be enough to trigger a saccade toward the stimulus.

Lastly, saccades can fall into multiple categories. This entry largely focuses on "visually guided" saccades. Specifically, the balloon example is a "reflexive" saccade in response to new information in the visual field. Other saccades include "scanning" (exploring visual field), "memory guided" (cortex driven, remembering where a point of focus existed), and "predictive saccade" (predicting the spatial location of a moving object).

Disease/Drugs

An exaggerated, biphasic (fast and slow) saccade is known as "nystagmus." There are instances where this type of movement is normal, such as with the rotation of the head, following a repetitively moving object with your eyes, and so forth. Brain lesions or the presence of drugs and/or alcohol can bring on this type of saccade.

Active substance usage or abuse can be detected with the aid of observing for nystagmus. Alcohol, for instance, specifically contributes to horizontal or lateral gaze nystagmus. An intoxicated person following the finger or pen light from left to right will reveal quick lateral saccades with a slow correction opposite of the fast movement. Phencyclidine (PCP) is an illegal drug known to induce vertical nystagmus.

Lesion or tumors within the brain, brainstem, or cerebellum can also be associated with nystagmus. Downbeat nystagmus is associated with lesions of the brainstem at the level of the foramen magnum (the large outlet for the spinal cord at the base of the skull). A person afflicted with this malady will experience a fast downbeat with a slow-upbeat saccade when focusing on an object in the center of the visual field.

Neurologic insults such as a stroke can be localized due to the lack of saccades. A stroke is either "hemorrhagic" (bleeding) or "ischemic" (absence of blood flow due to a blockage in the artery). One example is the deviation of gaze toward the location of a stroke in Brodmann area 8. If the left hemisphere of this area were to undergo a hemorrhagic stroke, the eyes would deviate leftward and be unable to make saccadic motion.

Finally, persons with Parkinson's disease have difficulty in maintaining ocular movements. They often will show abnormal smooth pursuit and saccadic movements that are associated with their motor deficits. These issues are more related to the disease process where substantia nigra neurons die and the target surviving neurons in the basal nuclei are no longer receiving dopamine (a neurotransmitter that is necessary for neuronal impulses) for activation. This in turn, causes the smooth motor movements to no longer occur.

Nicholas Breitnauer

See also: Abducens Nerve; Cerebellum; Frontal Lobe; Nystagmus; Oculomotor Nerve; Parkinson's Disease; Stroke; Superior Colliculus; Trochlear Nerve

Further Reading

Alberstone, C. D., Benzel, E. C., Najm, I. M., & Steinmetz, M. P. (2009). *Anatomic diagnosis of neurologic diagnosis.* New York, NY: Thieme Medical Publishers, Inc.

American Optometric Association. (2014). *Nystagmus.* Retrieved from http://www.aoa.org/patients-and-public/eye-and-vision-problems/glossary-of-eye-and-vision-conditions/nystagmus

Gorges, M., Müller, H. P., Lulé, D., Ludolph, A. C., Pinkhardt, E. H., & Kassubek, J. (2013). Functional connectivity within the default mode network is associated with saccadic accuracy in Parkinson's disease: a resting-state FMRI and videooculographic study. *Brain Connectivity, 3*(3), 265–272.

Purves, D., Augustine, G. J., Fitzpatrick, D., Hall, W. C., LaMantia, A.-S., McNamara, J. O., & Williams, S. M. (Eds.). (2001). Neural control and saccadic eye movements. In *Neuroscience* (2nd ed.). Sunderland, MA: Sinauer Associates. Retrieved from http://www.ncbi.nlm.nih.gov/books/NBK10992/

Wisconsin University. (2006). *Unit Nº. 2, brainstem: Superior colliculus.* Retrieved from http://www.neuroanatomy.wisc.edu/virtualbrain/BrainStem/23Colliculus.html

Sacks, Oliver W. (1933–)

Oliver Sacks, MD, is a British American neurologist and best-selling author. He currently lives in New York City where he sees patients and is a professor of neurology at New York University (NYU) School of Medicine. He is recognized for his 12 books that explore various neuroscience subjects, including *The Man Who*

Mistook His Wife for a Hat (1985), about various neurological disorders; *Musicophilia: Tales of Music and the Brain* (2007), which was made into a PBS Nova series called *Musical Minds; The Mind's Eye* (2010), about vision; and *Hallucinations* (2012). Many of his books are largely collections of his patients' neurological case histories and are known for being accessible and interesting to the lay public and neuroscientists alike. Sacks has won many awards for his books including the Lewis Thomas Prize by Rockefeller University, which recognizes the scientist as a poet.

Oliver Wolf Sacks was born in London, England, on July 9, 1933, to physician parents. He received his medical degree at Oxford University in 1958 and completed his residencies and fellowship at Mt. Zion Hospital in San Francisco and at University of California Los Angeles. He moved to New York City in 1965 pursuing a career in research. After a year, Sacks realized that he did not like lab work and accepted a position at Beth Abraham Hospital in 1966 as a consulting neurologist until 2007. Sacks worked as a consulting neurologist at several hospitals during this period and began teaching neurology in 1975 at Albert Einstein College of Medicine. He was a professor of neurology at NYU from 1992 to 2007, Columbia University from 2007 to 2012, and has returned to NYU where he still is as of this entry.

Sacks is known for his groundbreaking work in 1966 at Beth Abraham Hospital in the Bronx where he "awakened" a group of patients that had not moved or talked in decades. He discovered that these frozen patients had all survived *encephalitis lethargica* and their frozen state was due to the resulting brain damage. He experimentally treated them with L-DOPA, a drug that had recently been discovered as a treatment for Parkinson's disease. Sacks recounts this experience in his book, *Awakenings,* (1973) which was made into the 1990 movie *Awakenings* starring Robin Williams and Robert De Niro.

Sacks appears frequently on several news programs and his essays and articles have been published in magazines, newspapers, medical journals, and reprinted in several "Best of" anthologies. He has many hobbies and interests including chemistry and the periodic table of elements, botany, stereoscopic vision, and swimming. Sacks has a visual disorder called *prosopagnosia,* which impairs him from recognizing people by their faces. He discusses this disorder and his experience of recently losing vision in one of his eyes in his book, *The Mind's Eye.* Sacks's work has been supported by the Guggenheim Foundation and the Alfred P. Sloan Foundation. He is an honorary fellow of the American Academy of Arts and Letters and the American Academy of Arts and Sciences, and holds honorary degrees from many universities, including Oxford, Georgetown, Bard, Gallaudet, Tufts, and the Catholic University of Peru.

Emma Boxer

See also: Grandmother Cell; Levodopa; Neurologist; Prosopagnosia

Further Reading

Sacks, O. (2010). *The mind's eye.* New York, NY: Alfred A. Knopf.
Sacks, O. (2014). *Oliver Sacks, M.D.* Retrieved from http://www.oliversacks.com

Schizophrenia

Schizophrenia is a debilitating mental illness that affects approximately 1 percent of the population. The average age of onset is 18 for men and 25 for women; onset before age 10 or after age 60 is rare. The illness is characterized by a wide variety of symptoms, including hallucinations and delusions, depression and avolition (inability to be motivated), and cognitive deficits. Drugs and (occasionally) psychotherapy are used to treat schizophrenia. Current treatments effectively manage hallucinations and delusions in the majority of patients, but are ineffective at improving other symptoms. There is no cure for the illness, and symptoms usually persist across a lifetime, although they may vary in severity. Schizophrenia patients have a decreased quality of life because physicians are unable to effectively medicate many of their symptoms.

History

Although symptoms that resemble schizophrenia have been recorded in the texts of ancient civilizations, they were first classified as a unique illness by the psychiatrist Emil Kraeplin in the late 1800s. Kraeplin named the illness *Dementia praecox* or "premature dementia/precocious madness." Kraeplin chose the name due to its early onset compared to other dementias, its status as a "cognitive" illness as opposed to a "mood" illness such as bipolar disorder, and his belief that the disorder was progressive, organic, and incurable. In 1911, the psychiatrist Eugen Blueler first proposed the name *schizophrenia,* based on the Greek phrase for "split mind." The phrase referred to the disorganized, fragmented thinking of persons with the disorder. In contrast to Kraeplin, Bleuler did not believe the illness to be the incurable product of organic deterioration, and thus did not classify it as a "dementia." Nonetheless, early attempts to treat the symptoms of schizophrenia were unsuccessful and most diagnosed patients were institutionalized. In the 1950s, it was discovered that chlorpromazine, a drug that affects the dopamine receptor to treat both inflammation and nausea, was effective at treating hallucinations and delusions associated with schizophrenia. This discovery triggered the massive release

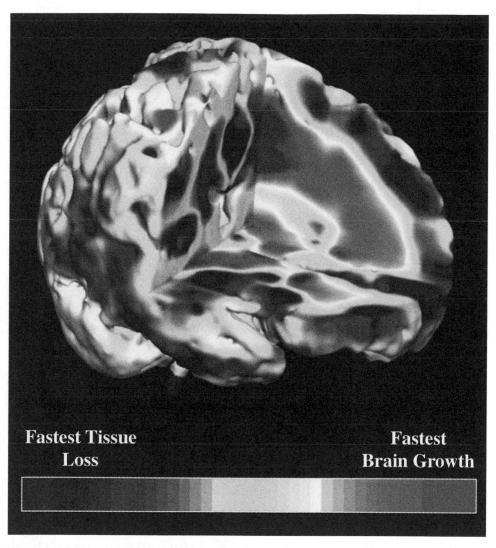

Fastest Tissue Loss

Fastest Brain Growth

Brain of MRI scan data for child onset schizophrenia showing areas of brain growth and loss of tissue. (National Institutes of Health)

of patients from hospitals and institutions in later decades. However, patients' quality of life remained poor because these treatments often caused severe movement disabilities and did not improve other symptoms (e.g., depression and cognitive deficits). A second wave of drugs in the 1970s was developed that did not have movement side effects; however, the range of symptoms they could treat remained the same. In the early 2000s, a third wave of drugs was developed to help treat depression (and related symptoms) in some patients.

Symptoms

Positive symptoms include hallucinations, delusions, disorganized speech, and bizarre behavior. Hallucinations can affect all of the senses: auditory (hearing), visual (vision), olfactory (smell), somatosensory (touch), or gustatory (taste), although auditory hallucinations are the most common. These inner "voices" may be accusatory and shaming, resulting in low self-esteem. Delusions include grandiose thinking and paranoia. Disorganized speech may involve rapidly changing ideas and illogical statements, and informal conversations may be difficult.

Negative symptoms include alogia (mental disabilities in generating speech), anhedonia (inability to experience pleasure), asociality (inability or unwillingness to develop interpersonal relationships), avolition (lack of motivation for everyday tasks, seeking employment, etc.), and depression. Currently, these symptoms are not well treated with medication and are associated with poor quality of life. Severe negative symptoms are a significant risk factor for suicide.

Cognitive symptoms include reduced mental processing speed, poor working memory (i.e., the ability to remember something for a short period of time, like a phone number, to use it soon afterward), inability to focus for long periods of time, susceptibility to distraction, and poor executive function (interpreting information and using it to make decisions). The average intelligence quotient (IQ) of a patient is around one standard deviation lower than the general population, although some patients may have high IQ scores.

Subtypes

Schizophrenia is divided into five subtypes, according to the *Diagnostic and Statistical Manual of Mental Disorders* (*DSM-IV*).

The *catatonic subtype* features dramatically reduced or abnormalities in voluntary movement. Patients of this subtype may sit or stand in one position for several hours. In addition, repetitive, purposeless movement may occur.

The *disorganized subtype* predominantly consists of disorganized thinking and communication. Patient speech and writing may be incomprehensible. Patients of this subtype may have difficulty with everyday tasks, such as bathing and brushing their teeth. Negative symptoms feature strongly in this subtype.

The *paranoid subtype* has prominent positive symptoms (hallucinations or delusions). Patients of this subtype may not show observable features of the illness and may be able to function relatively well in society.

The *residual subtype* no longer displays overt symptoms of the disorder, either due to medication or natural remission of the illness. Subtle abnormalities, such as unusual thoughts, may persist in patients of this subtype.

The *undifferentiated subtype* displays symptoms of schizophrenia, but specific features of the illness are not sufficiently prominent to enable classification in one of the other subtypes.

Risk Factors

Schizophrenia is a highly heritable disorder. An identical twin of a patient with schizophrenia has a 47 percent chance of developing the illness, a fraternal twin has a 12 percent chance, and a nontwin sibling has an 8 percent chance. If one parent has schizophrenia, a child has a 12 percent chance of developing it; if both parents have schizophrenia, a child has a 40 percent chance of developing it.

A number of genes have been associated with schizophrenia, particularly genes involved in brain development, cell metabolism, and the immune system. However, the variability is large and mutations in any single gene are unlikely (by themselves) to significantly increase the probability of developing the illness. Understanding how genes change the basic neurobiology of the brain to confer risk for schizophrenia is a major area of current research.

There are many environmental risk factors that increase the likelihood of developing schizophrenia. The disorder is associated with maternal infections and malnutrition during pregnancy. Mothers who develop influenza while in the second trimester are more likely to give birth to a child who will develop the illness. This association may be caused by an inflammatory response in the developing brain during the infection. Children who are born in the winter months (December–April) are also more likely to develop schizophrenia, perhaps from the increase in flu infections during this period. This is why it is important for pregnant women to receive a flu vaccination during their pregnancy. Malnutrition during pregnancy is also associated with schizophrenia in offspring, due to abnormal brain development in the womb. Another risk factor is childhood stressors; children from high-stress or neglectful environments are more likely to develop the illness. Rates of schizophrenia are also greater in high population density and urban environments.

The "first episode" of psychosis (when a patient first notices positive symptoms) is often triggered by stressful life events, such as a death in the immediate family or being expelled from school. High emotional stress in the mother during pregnancy also increases the risk that her children will develop schizophrenia. Research is actively studying how chemicals released during stress can influence brain development and function.

A combination of environmental and genetic factors is likely necessary to trigger the onset of schizophrenia. The effect of gene/environment interactions and their roles in increasing risk of schizophrenia are an emerging area of research.

Diagnosis

Schizophrenia is typically diagnosed by an interview with a doctor, generally following the first episode of psychosis. *DSM-IV* diagnostic criteria include presentation of positive and/or negative symptoms for a significant portion of time, social/occupational dysfunction (e.g., poor performance at work), exclusion of mood disorders (e.g., bipolar disorder), exclusion of the direct effects of a substance (e.g., drug abuse), and exclusion of a pervasive developmental disorder (e.g., autism).

Treatment

There is no cure for schizophrenia and medications only lessen some of the symptoms. As previously stated, positive symptoms are well treated in the majority of patients; however, cognitive and negative symptoms are not. Developing new drugs for the treatment of both cognitive and negative symptoms is a significant area of research.

Drugs that reduce the positive symptoms of schizophrenia are called antipsychotic medications. These medications primarily act on dopamine and/or serotonin receptors to reduce their activity resulting in reducing positive symptoms in most patients. Aripipazole is a relatively new medication that may be used to reduce negative symptoms in some patients. Nonetheless, antipsychotic medications often have debilitating side effects, including drowsiness, lethargy, movement abnormalities (tremor, rigidity), hypotension (low blood pressure), weight gain, impotence, and seizures. A confounding problem occurs when patients who initially present with only positive symptoms may also develop negative symptoms after beginning antipsychotic treatment.

Up to 25 percent of patients do not respond to antipsychotic drugs. Various types of psychotherapy may be prescribed in these cases to increase the effect of medication, although effectiveness can be inconsistent and occasionally worsen symptoms. A promising new method of psychotherapy is cognitive behavioral therapy (CBT). The goal of CBT is to teach the patient to cope with positive symptoms in a constructive manner. For example, inner voices (auditory hallucinations) often involve shaming language that is damaging to a patient's self-esteem. With the doctor's help, the patient learns to "interact" and "fight back" against these voices. The patient is also encouraged to think about delusional thoughts, and come to his own conclusions as to why these thoughts are illogical. Unlike most forms of psychotherapy, CBT is designed to help the patient cope with his symptoms, rather than stop them from appearing (which is often ineffective).

Finally, social support from family and friends is important. Patients may need help staying on track with medications, coping with symptoms, and with day-to-day activities. Social support also helps prevent relapses during remission.

Biological Causes

Although schizophrenia was once considered a purely "psychological" illness, the discovery of antipsychotic medication started a push toward understanding how biological changes in the brain may cause the illness. Brain imaging such as magnetic resonance imaging (MRI) was a key step in this process in that it allowed scientists to noninvasively study the brain of a living person. Although thousands of brain-imaging studies have observed changes in brain structure and function in schizophrenia, *how* these changes lead to symptoms remains unclear.

The first widely replicated structural brain finding in schizophrenia was increased size of fluid-filled spaces in the brain (ventricles). More recent studies observed a loss of gray matter (cell bodies) in many brain regions, including areas involved in memory, sensory processing, executive function (thinking), decision making, and self-awareness. It is unknown if changes in gray matter start before or after symptoms appear and "cause" schizophrenia. However, brain imaging has shown that losses in gray matter are present during the first episode of psychosis and may occur early in the disorder.

Functional MRI (fMRI) measures brain function in specific regions. Using fMRI, researchers have found altered brain function in patients with schizophrenia. For example, compared to healthy controls, patients are less likely to use areas involved in cognitive processing during mentally challenging tasks. During rest, patients also show increased activity in brain areas used for self-reflection and memory. An emerging area of research is determining how these changes relate to symptom severity and if they can be affected by drug treatment.

Outcomes

Although most patients are no longer institutionalized, long-term outcomes are poor. Average life expectancy is approximately 15 years less than that of the general population. The majority of patients lives in poverty and/or is unemployed, depending on family, friends, or government assistance programs for financial support. Many schizophrenia patients are homeless; indeed, up to half of all homeless people have the illness. Patients are 10 times more likely to commit suicide than the normal population. Schizophrenia is highly associated with drugs of abuse; over 80 percent of patients are chronic smokers, and heavy cannabis (marijuana) and alcohol use are common.

Future

Since the discovery of clozapine in 1971, relatively few new drugs have been developed that are significant improvements to existing medication. The high cost of research and limited knowledge of the disorder's brain effects has slowed drug discovery for schizophrenia. A major goal of current research is understanding changes in the brain that cause symptoms of schizophrenia. fMRI may prove useful in this process.

Other emerging therapies for schizophrenia include transcranial magnetic stimulation (magnetic pulses that stimulate the brain), cognitive behavioral therapy, and cognitive training/enhancement (basic mental exercises to improve brain function). Furthermore, preliminary studies show that physical exercise may be beneficial for patients. Strategies for preventing the disorder include close monitoring, early intervention in teens with a family history of schizophrenia, and adequate nutrition for pregnant women. Given the high financial costs (estimated in 2002, $63 billion annually in the United States) and that approximately 50 million people are affected worldwide, developing new treatments and ultimately a cure of schizophrenia is a high priority for research.

Jason Smucny

See also: Acetylcholine and Its Receptors

Further Reading

Green, M.F. (2003). *Schizophrenia revealed: From neurons to social interactions.* New York, NY: W.W. Norton.

Kingdon, D.J., & Turkington, D. (2008). *Cognitive therapy of schizophrenia (guides to individualized-based treatment).* New York, NY: Guilford Press.

Sadock, B.J., & Sadock, V.J. (Eds.). (2007). Schizophrenia. In *Kaplan and Sadock's synopsis of psychiatry: Behavioral sciences clinical psychiatry* (pp. 467–497). Philadelphia, PA: Lippincott Williams and Wilkins.

Schizophrenia. (2012). *Medline Plus.* Retrieved from http://www.nlm.nih.gov/medline plus/schizophrenia.html

Weinberger, D.R., & Harrison, P. (Eds.). (2011). *Schizophrenia* (3rd ed.). New Jersey: Wiley-Blackwell.

Schwannomas

A *schwannoma* (also referred to as a vestibular schwannoma, acoustic neuroma, and neurilemmoma) is a type of tumor that is usually benign and affects the outer covering of nerves, which is referred to as the nerve sheath. More specifically, these sarcomas arise from what are known as Schwann cells (hence, the name schwannoma), which are glial cells that are exclusively located in the peripheral nervous system. Schwann cells play a supporting role in functions such as nervous impulse conduction, neuron development and regeneration, and neuromuscular synaptic modulation. Due to the nature of the cell that the neoplasm is created from, the general symptoms include either a painful or painless mass that is slow growing. Additionally, when the affected area is palpated (touched or manipulated), an electric-like shock known as a Tinel shock is experienced by the patient.

The etiology of schwannomas is largely unknown; however, evidence does show that people with a genetic disorder called neurofibromatosis type 1 (NF1; formerly known as von Recklinghausen disease) are more likely to develop this neoplasm. Vestibular schwannomas are also genetic disorders but these are linked to neurofibromatosis type 2 (NF2). Another factor that increases the chance of having these timorous Schwann cells is a rare genetic disorder called schwannomastosis, which has recently been identified as another neurofibromatosis (NF). These tumors, on average, affect one out of every 40,000 people. Standard treatment involves complete surgical resection followed by radiation therapy to reduce the risk of any recurrence. However, there exists a great deal of complexity with surgical resection, as these tumors tend to exist within very important nervous pathways. If the mass is present in an area that carries a great amount of risk for the patient (meaning, that it will be difficult for the surgeon to remove it), the course of action then turns to high-dose radiation therapy. The prognosis for schwannomas is dependent upon the location of the tumor, how much it has spread to other regions, the extent of resection, and the overall health and well-being of the patient. Since less than 1 percent of schwannomas are malignant, patients can typically expect an optimistic prognosis with a strong chance to survive following tumor removal. Furthermore, evidence suggests that, if the tumor is completely removed during surgery, then the possibility of a recurring tumor is almost zero.

Types of Tumors

As schwannomas are primarily benign tumors of Schwann cells, the symptoms reflect manifestations of the malfunctions of these cells relative to their locations in the peripheral nervous system. Although these tumors can grow anywhere in the peripheral nervous system, there is a prevalence of schwannomas on certain cranial nerves, specifically the vestibulocochlear nerve, which is the 8th of 12 cranial nerves (cranial nerve VIII). These tumors are also known as acoustic neuromas. Schwannomas are also prevalently found in major peripheral nerves such as the sciatic nerve, which travels from the lower back, through the buttocks, and down the posterior side of the legs to the feet.

Schwannomas can be histologically categorized into two groups: (1) Antoni type A, and (2) Antoni type B. Antoni type A schwannomas present with elongated bipolar cells with poorly defined borders that are arranged in a parallel fashion.

Antoni type A schwannomas resemble a palisade (fence-like) structure. Antoni type B schwannomas possess the histological characteristics of reticular-shaped cells with lymphocyte-like nuclei. The Antoni type A have a histology that is linked more with spinal schwannomas; whereas, Antoni type B have characteristics that are correlated with intracranial schwannomas. Some prominent forms of these neoplasms are acoustic (cranial nerve VIII), trigeminal (cranial nerve V), facial nerve (cranial nerve VII), and jugular foramen schwannomas.

Acoustic schwannomas (acoustic neuromas) are the most common form of this tumor making up 75–90 percent of all cerebellopontine angle (where the cerebellum and the pons meet) masses, and 7–8 percent of all primary intracranial tumors. This schwannoma arises along the vestibulocochlear nerve, primarily on the inferior division of the vestibular portion of the nerve and participates in both Antoni type A and B growth patterns. Additionally, instances where schwannomas present bilaterally serve as indices that the neoplasm is the result of NF2. Individuals who present with acoustic neuromas display symptoms such as hearing loss, balance issues, cerebellar and brainstem malfunctions, and in some cases hydrocephalus (excess cerebrospinal fluid in the brain) may occur. Radiographic evidence of this neoplasm includes widening and attrition of the internal acoustic meatus on X-ray computed tomography (CT) scans. Treatment of acoustic neuromas includes both stereotactic radiosurgery and microsurgery. With respect to microsurgery, a number of approaches the surgeon can take; however, the choice of action is dependent on factors such as risk of hearing loss and the overall complexity and finesse of the procedure. Prognosis for acoustic schwannomas is optimistic with a recurrence rate of 1–9 percent after resection.

Trigeminal schwannomas are the second most common form of schwannomas making up one-third of the tumors of Meckel's cave, although still being very rare as this type of tumor accounts for less than 0.2 percent of all intracranial tumors. This sarcoma occurs most frequently in the fourth decade of life and arises from Schwann cells of the trigeminal nerve. These schwannomas are found in three different locations in the body, relative to the ganglion (a distinct group of cell bodies). They can be preganglionic, ganglionic, and postganglionic schwannomas. Individuals presenting with a trigeminal schwannoma display symptoms of facial numbness, hyperesthesia (increased sensation to sensory stimuli), pain, and in some cases, memory loss and seizures may occur. Radiographic evidence for trigeminal schwannomas is similar to all other schwannomas, however, this type of tumor is more likely to have cystic components as well as greater variance in composition relative to acoustic neuromas. Prognosis of trigeminal schwannomas is dependent largely on location and size of the tumor. Factors such as limited surgical exposure, encasement of blood vessels, and adherence to the brainstem affects the extent of resection. However, with today's surgical techniques, roughly 70–80 percent of trigeminal resections are complete. Additionally, the chance of recurrence is highest the first three years posttreatment.

Facial nerve schwannomas (FNS; also known as a facial nerve neuroma/neurilemmoma) are the third most prevalent form of neurilemmomas. FNS make up less than 1 percent of all temporal bone tumors, and this schwannoma arises along the facial nerve. As with all other schwannomas, FNS obstructs the facial nerve by displacing it, which causes the neurons to splay apart. This subset of schwannomas is similar to acoustic neuromas in that it can grow into the cerebellopontine angle, thus having similar effects. Individuals with FNS present with symptoms such as facial nerve palsy (mimicking a similar progression as Bell's palsy), hearing loss (both sensory neural and conductive), and in less than 10 percent of cases, a palpable mass may be felt if the tumor is extracranial (outside of the cranium). Radiographic evidence for this tumor is congruent with all other schwannomas; although, an index that distinguishes trigeminal schwannomas from acoustic neuromas is the presence of a neural expansion along the facial nerve canal of the skull. Treatment for this type of tumor follows the standard treatment protocol for schwannomas: surgical resection and/or radiation therapy (the choice of which is dependent on location, size, and other typical risk factors). Prognosis for this neurilemmoma is similar to all other schwannomas in that it is dependent on the degree of complete removal.

Jugular foramen schwannomas (JFS) are the fourth most common subtype of schwannomas that involves cranial nerves IX, X, and XI (also known as the glossopharyngeal, vagus, and spinal accessory nerves, respectively). JFSs are typified by involvement of the jugular foramen (a Latin word for "natural opening"). This sarcoma arises predominantly on the glossopharyngeal nerve sometime during the third to sixth decade of life. This is generally when the individual no longer expresses NF2. JFSs have a higher occurrence in women relative to men. Symptoms for JFS vary widely as they involve multiple cranial nerves; the most prevalent symptoms are hearing loss, tinnitus (ringing in the ear), dysphagia (difficulty swallowing), ataxia (decreased muscle coordination), and hoarseness. Radiographic evidence includes a well-demarcated dumbbell-shaped mass at the affected jugular foramen. Treatment is typical for schwannomas with surgical resection being favored along with radiation therapy, although in some cases high-dose radiation therapy is favored over surgery. Prognosis is akin to all other schwannomas although surgery is highly complex due to the brainstem being adjacent and connected to the jugular foramen.

Future

Current research for schwannomas is exciting and abundant with focuses on laminectomy, radiosurgery, radiation therapy, and even some adjuvant chemotherapy.

In one study, Dr. Xing Su (2012) and his team have gathered data that suggests laminectomy is a safe and effective way to treat schwannomas of the spinal cord, opening yet another therapeutic option for patients with these sarcomas. Another study has demonstrated that the use of certain calculations can significantly reduce setup error for radiosurgical instruments, thus making radiosurgical procedures safer and more effective. The amount of research concerning this, and other types of tumors, is substantial and progressive, aiming to deliver a more optimistic outcome to all individuals affected.

Eric W. Prince

See also: Bell's Palsy (Bell Palsy); Glioma; Meningioma; Schwann Cells—Building with Clay Activity

Further Reading

Bakar, B. (2008). The jugular foramen schwannomas: Review of the large surgical series. *Journal of Korean Neurosurgical Society, 44*(5), 285–294. Retrieved from http://www.ncbi.nlm.nih.gov/pmc/articles/PMC2612565/

Genetic and Rare Diseases Information Center (GARD). (n.d.). *Schwannoma.* Retrieved from http://rarediseases.info.nih.gov/GARD/Condition/4767/Schwannoma.aspx

Newton, H.B. (2011). *Sporadic schwannomas and neurofibromas.* Retrieved from http://www.medmerits.com/index.php/article/sporadic_schwannomas_and_neurofibromas/P10

Su, X., Shi, W., Huang, Q., Shen, J., & Chen, J. (2012). Hemi-semi laminectomy approach for the microsurgical treatment of spinal schwannomas. *Chinese Medical Sciences Journal, 27*(2), 96–100.

Tivorsak, T., & Westesson, P.L. (2006). *Neuroradiology case of the week: Case 140.* University of Rochester Medical Center—Radiology. Retrieved from http://www.urmc.rochester.edu/smd/rad/neurocases/Neurocase140.htm

Secondary Messengers

Within all cells and particularly in brain cells (neurons), biochemical reactions are necessary for keeping the cell healthy and for interacting with other cells. This activity usually occurs by *secondary messengers (or second messengers),* or naturally occurring chemicals that start signaling pathways within the cell. Thus, second messengers are an element of signal transduction. Second messengers are molecules that relay signals received at receptors (specialized proteins) on the cell surface to aim at the molecules inside the cell. This binding of a ligand (chemical) to a single receptor at the cell surface changes the biochemical activities within the cell. Second messengers also supply and broaden the strength of the signal. Today, there are three known major classes of second messengers: *cyclic nucleotides (cyclic AMP* and *cyclic GMP), inositol trisphosphate (IP)*, and *diacyl-glycerol (DAG)*.

History

In the 1940s, American pharmacist and biochemist Earl Wilbur Sutherland Jr. (1915–1974) was the first person to identify the second messenger cyclic AMP and its function in glycogen metabolism within the liver. For this discovery, he won the 1971 Nobel Prize in Physiology or Medicine. Sutherland found that epinephrine (adrenaline, a natural hormone) would stimulate the liver to change glycogen to glucose in liver cells but it could not do it alone. Thus, Sutherland looked for another molecule to start the process and discovered cyclic AMP. Several years later, American cell physiologists Martin Rodbell (1925–1998) and Alfred G. Gilman (1941–) worked to find the signaling protein that would start the activities of cyclic AMP and discovered G proteins. For their discovery and for expanding on Sutherland's findings, they won the 1994 Nobel Prize in Physiology or Medicine.

Anatomy and Physiology

Within the central nervous system and other hormone-sensitive systems, the systemic hormone (a regulatory, natural, and/or manmade chemical) does not directly enter the target cell but instead binds to a receptor located within the cell membrane. This receptor is usually a G protein. When the G protein becomes bound with the hormone or other chemical, it causes a conformational change in the shape of the G protein and begins complex, intracellular, signaling pathways. This activity spreads to the target enzymes or intracellular receptor and the mediator is a second messenger. Thus, a hormone will indirectly affect the creation of another molecule within the cell.

The second messenger cyclic adenosine monophosphate (cyclic AMP or cAMP) is derived from adenosine triphosphate (ATP, the energy of a cell) and used for intracellular signal transduction in many different organisms, along the cyclic AMP–dependent pathway. Additionally, the second messenger cyclic guanosine monophosphate (cyclic GMP or cGMP) has been shown to activate intracellular protein kinases (enzymes that assist in transferring a phosphate group from ATP to another molecule) to the binding of membrane impermeable peptide hormones to the external cell surface. This is called *phosphorylation*. Finally, diacyl-glycerol (DAG) is a lipid that acts as a second messenger by stimulating PKC (protein kinase C), which may also lead to phosphorylation of other molecules.

Disorders

The cognitive deficits in age-related illnesses (like dementia) and attention deficit hyperactivity disorder (ADHD) are of interest of scientists who study the brain. Recent studies have shown that cyclic AMP affects the function of thinking in the prefrontal cortex through ion channels (specialized proteins within the cell membrane) called hyperpolarization-activated cyclic nucleotide-gated channels (HCN). When cyclic AMP affects a HCN channel, it causes the channel to open. This in turn closes the brain cell to transmit or communicate, and ultimately interfering with the function of the prefrontal cortex. This abnormal activity may be due to the second messenger and other signal transductions. However, more research is needed to better understand the causes and effects of such disorders.

Patricia A. Bloomquist

See also: Attention Deficit Disorder/Attention Deficit Hyperactivity Disorder; Auditory System; Dementia; G Proteins; Olfactory System (Smell); Visual System

Further Reading

Antoni, F. A. (2012). Interactions between intracellular free Ca2+ and cyclic AMP in neuroendocrine cells. *Cell Calcium, 51*(3–4), 260–266.

Lodish, H., Berk, A., Zipursky, S. L., Matsudaira, P., Baltimore, D., & Darnell, J. (2000). *Molecular cell biology* (4th ed.). New York, NY: W. H. Freeman.

Willard, S. S., & Koochekpour, S. (2013). Glutamate, glutamate receptors, and downstream signaling pathways. *International Journal of Biological Sciences, 9*(9), 948–959.

Seizures

A *seizure* is a sudden, erratic increase of abnormal electrical activity in the brain that temporarily affects actions and/or cognition and perception. Seizures can last for a few seconds as in absence seizures (formerly called "petit mal" seizures) and up to a few minutes as seen in complex-partial seizures. Symptoms can be as mild as a momentary blank facial expression caused by impaired consciousnesses in absence seizures, or as severe as the violent convulsions of tonic-clonic seizures (formerly called "grand mal" seizures). In some cases, seizures can be life threatening. A condition in which seizures last longer than five minutes or when one seizure immediately follows another is called status epilepticus. This can cause significant brain damage and death if not promptly treated. A seizure is not a disorder itself, but rather a symptom indicating underlying central nervous system (CNS) disturbance. Individual symptoms and prognosis vary depending on the type of seizure and causative agent.

While most seizures occur as part of an epileptic disorder, sometimes they can be isolated events. Seemingly unrelated conditions like a high fever (febrile seizures) can lead to seizures, particularly in young children. A stroke can cause single-incident seizures in adults as well. Approximately 5 percent of the population has experienced a single-incident seizure, whereas only 1–2 percent of the population has epileptic seizures. The risk of developing recurrent epileptic seizures can increase after an individual has a single-incident seizure. There are many different types of epilepsy, and they can come from genetic, structural-metabolic, or unknown sources.

Types of Seizures

I. Generalized seizures

    A. Tonic-clonic (in any combination, formerly called "grand mal" seizures)

    B. Absence (formerly called "petit mal" seizures)

        1. Typical

        2. Atypical

        3. Absence with special features

            a. Myoclonic absence

            b. Eyelid myoclonia

    C. Myoclonic

        1. Myoclonic

        2. Myoclonic atonic

        3. Myoclonic tonic

    D. Clonic

    E. Tonic

    F. Atonic

II. Focal seizures (formerly partial seizures)

III. Unclassified

    Classification of partial seizures (Outdated)

    A. Simple

        1. Motor symptoms

2. Sensory symptoms
3. Psychic symptoms
4. Autonomic signs

B. Complex

1. Delayed consciousness impairment
2. Impaired consciousness at onset

C. Secondarily generalized seizures

Source: Berg, A. T., Berkovic, S. F., Brodie, M. J., Buchhalter, J., Cross, J. H., van Emde Boas, W., Engel, J., French, J., Glauser, T. A., Mathern, G. W., Moshe, S. L, Nordli, D., Plouin, P., Scheffer, I. E. (2010). Revised terminology and concepts for organization of seizures and epilepsies: Report of the ILAE Commission on Classification and Terminology 2005–2009. *Epilepsia, 51*(4), 676–685. doi:10.1111/j.1528–1167.2010.02522.x.

History

The Greek root for the word *epilepsy* means to seize or attack. Ancient physicians described the symptoms as though a demon had seized or attacked the victim. The earliest record of epileptic seizures comes from Babylon in the 11th century, BC. Ancient Greeks and early Christians also documented seizures with attributing such violent convulsions to demonic possessions, witchcraft, or contagious diseases. Thus, the remedies described in medical literature from before Christ's birth through the Middle Ages were barbaric by today's standard. Medicinal treatments varied from herbal elements such as mistletoe and peony root to remedies of human and animal origin like camel's hair or organs, blood, and bones of other humans. Ancient physicians would sometimes attempt to release the demon by making a hole in the afflicted person's skull. Others would try to pin the evil spirit by driving an iron nail into the first vertebra of the victim's neck. During the Middle Ages, progress was made as physicians considered the idea that seizures were a natural (and not demonic) disease caused by an imbalance of the Hippocratic humours (black bile, yellow bile, phlegm, and blood). Ironically, the Renaissance period brought a regression in this area and medical scholars once again attributed seizures to demons and witchcraft.

It was not until the Age of Enlightenment that physicians began to disregard the idea that seizures were caused by witchcraft, supernatural powers, or demonic possession. The advancements of anatomy and pathology, as well as the development of new sciences such as chemistry, pharmacy, and physiology, promoted this change in ideology. In 1836, English physician and physiologist Marshall Hall (1790–1857) described epilepsy as an "irritable" reflex arc at the level of the spinal cord. His hypothesis was refined in 1858 by Charles-Édouard Brown-Séquard (1817–1894), a physician who suggested that the irritated reflex involved the medulla oblongata (part of the brainstem that controls breathing and heart rate). Near the end of the 19th century, English neurologist John Hughlings Jackson (1835–1911) rejected these ideas of exaggerated reflex activity as the mechanism of epileptic seizures. Hughlings Jackson demonstrated that epilepsy began in the cerebrum, and not from altered functions at lower levels of the nervous system. Modern science has confirmed Hughlings Jackson's hypothesis and has identified several regions in the brain that are most susceptible to seizures and epilepsy.

Subtypes and Symptoms

The wide variation not only in seizures, but also in etiology has led to the opinion that "epilepsy" is more accurately termed "the epilepsies." The International League against Epilepsy (ILAE) is currently responsible for the governing of terminology and classification relating to the different types of seizures and epilepsies (see Types of Seizures sidebar).

Depending on the subtype of epilepsy, seizure symptoms can vary from visible muscle contractions to sensory and psychic symptoms only perceived by the person experiencing the seizure. Focal seizures were formerly called partial seizures, and though this terminology is now outdated it is useful in describing the symptoms. Motor symptoms in simple partial seizures cause visible muscle twitches. Sequential involvement of muscle groups is called a "march" and is identified as Jacksonian seizures. Sensory symptoms are usually not noticeable to a bystander, but can cause considerable distress to the patient. These include both somatosensory and special sensory disturbances. Tingling, visual, auditory (sound), olfactory (smell), and gustatory (taste) hallucinations may ensue. The sensory aspect of the partial seizures preceding the generalized tonic-clonic seizure is called an "aura." People with this type of epilepsy often come to recognize an aura as an indicator before the start of a seizure. Psychic symptoms include senses of déjà vu and jamais vu (failure to recognize familiar scenes, people, or words). When the autonomic nervous system is involved changes in blood pressure and heart rate have been observed along with diaphoresis and pupil dilation.

Absence seizures are a subtype of epilepsy and are typically only seen in children. Victims of this type of epilepsy will either outgrow the seizures or the seizures will progressively worsen. Symptoms present as almost unnoticeable blank stares or unresponsiveness, but can also include some autonomic and mild clonic symptoms. Increased disturbances in muscle tone and more gradual onset are atypical traits of this type of seizure.

Atonic seizures are characterized by momentary loss of muscle-tone, whereas myoclonic seizures are brief involuntary muscle contractions. Tonic seizures are rigid contraction of muscles particularly those of the limbs. Major muscle groups repeatedly contract and relax during clonic seizures. The notorious tonic-clonic seizures involve nearly immediate loss of consciousness followed by both tonic and clonic symptoms.

Complex-partial seizures originating in or involving the mesial temporal limbic structures are the most common type of seizures, and the most common cause is temporal lobe epilepsy (TLE). These seizures will frequently evolve into secondarily generalized seizures. Most patients with TLE have had some prior brain injury such as trauma to the head from riding a bicycle or a car accident, febrile convulsions, or status epilepticus. TLE is usually a permanent condition with variable seizure frequencies within a population of afflicted individuals.

Risk Factors

Seizures can be clinically diagnosed as either unprovoked or provoked. Unprovoked seizures are also known as "primary" seizures and have a genetic cause. Predictably, the greatest risk factor for this type of epilepsy is having a parent with the disorder. The link is particularly strong in cases in which the mother is affected, with up to 9 percent of their children also presenting symptoms (Fisher, 2012). Generalized epilepsy is more heritable, but injury or illness can trigger partial seizures. TLE typically follows a specific insult to the CNS, but the intervening period between the initial event and the diagnosis of epilepsy can be months to years.

Provoked seizures are classified as having a structural-metabolic cause. They are most likely to follow a high fever, alcohol withdrawal, an injury or illness affecting the CNS, or a systemic metabolic condition such as extreme hypoglycemia. Stroke, brain tumors, and trauma can also damage the CNS and cause seizures. As previously discussed, an individual's risk of having another seizure greatly increases following a first episode. Thus, preventing the first episode like wearing a bicycle helmet or drinking moderately (less than three alcoholic drinks at a sitting) is crucial for avoiding provoked seizures.

Diagnosis, Treatment, and Outcomes

A complete history and physical examination, including detailed descriptions of symptoms, is the first step in diagnosing seizures and the subtype of epilepsy. Other conditions can sometimes share overt symptoms with epilepsy, which can lead to misdiagnosis. For example, the psychic and sensory symptoms of partial seizures can sometimes lead to a misdiagnosis of schizophrenia and atonic seizures have been mistaken for narcolepsy. Not only does a misdiagnosis delay effective treatment, but it can also lead to treatments that are actually contraindicated. Therefore, additional testing is necessary. Laboratory blood work can uncover causative metabolic disorders, and computed tomography (CT) or magnetic resonance imaging (MRI) scans can identify abnormalities in brain structures. Electroencephalogram (EEG) is particularly useful as it can record changes in electrical activity, which is the defining feature of seizures. Whether the seizures are generalized or partial will also be apparent on an EEG.

Modern research has indicated that some of the ancient treatments may have actually been beneficial. Peony root, though toxic in large doses, does seem to inhibit the surge of electrical activity associated with seizures (Aiko, 1991). The practice of drilling holes into the skull was an ancient treatment for many other conditions, including depression. This may have been anecdotally successful when the cause of the symptoms was a tumor because the hole could have relieved pressure on the affected area of the brain. These practices, however, do not play a role in the modern treatment of epilepsy. Some people prefer alternative herbal medicine in place of or in conjunction with standard treatment; however, these can have negative drug interactions or other side effects that worsen symptoms.

During the course of a tonic-clonic seizure, the primary goal of the treatment is to prevent injury. Ties should be loosened and the head should be cushioned; other than that there is very little to be done but wait. Nothing should be placed in the patient's mouth, nor should any attempt be made to restrain him or her. Status epilepticus requires emergency medical services, like an ambulance, as this condition is life threatening. Beyond immediate care for a person experiencing a seizure, treatment primarily involves preventing and ameliorating symptoms. Usually, a combination of medication and avoidance of triggers can manage epilepsy. Over 20 drugs have been approved to treat epilepsy, but the appropriate medication varies based on the specific type of diagnoses. Some medications may be given concurrently, but monotherapy is preferred as there are fewer side effects and drug interactions.

Ideally, the underlying cause of the seizures can be identified and treated. However, this is not always possible or practical. Surgery can be an option for patients who do not respond to pharmaceutical therapy. For the secondarily generalized seizures, cutting the corpus callosum prevents the electrical discharges from spreading between the hemispheres.

In many cases, complex-partial seizures in TLE cannot be treated with conventional anticonvulsant drugs, and surgical removal of the hippocampus and closely associated limbic structures is required to eliminate seizures. Studies have shown that when the surgical intervention was successful in stopping seizures the epileptic tissue had a common pathology of mesial temporal sclerosis (tissue scarring). Predictably, these surgeries have significant side effects but until recently were the only option for patients who did not respond to medication. A new treatment has begun gaining popularity in which a device can be implanted under the skin on the chest in proximity to the vagus nerve. Much like a pacemaker regulates the heart, this device sends an electrical signal at regular intervals to the brain. This signal prevents a large build-up of electrical charge that could trigger a seizure.

Roughly half of all children with epilepsy will outgrow it, and 80 percent of adults will experience a five-year remission. About 70 percent of patients are able to manage their condition with medication, and the greatest predictor of patient outcomes is their compliance with taking medication. Some patients are unable to control their symptoms with monotherapy, but find good control with two or more medications. About 1 in 10 patients have "intractable epilepsy" that is refractory to medication and is not suitable for surgery. In these cases, vagus nerve stimulation typically reduces their seizure frequency by 50 percent within a year.

Future

The older terminology and classification for seizures are still often used; however, the changes recently implemented by the ILAE will be used by most scholarly sources in the future.

More directly impacting patient outcomes, geneticists are working to identify the specific gene or genes responsible for genetic epilepsy. Once identified, testing will begin to explore the possibility of gene therapy to cure the epilepsy. Currently, research is underway to test the efficacy of implanted electrodes in the brain. These electrodes would theoretically detect impending seizures and apply electrical stimulation to avert them. The limitations of human testing necessitate the use of appropriate animal models for this and other groundbreaking discoveries.

Erin Slocum and
Jennifer L. Hellier

See also: Epilepsy; Hippocampus; Limbic System

Further Reading

Aiko, S., Tsukasa, S., Eiichi, S., Noriyuki, Y., Kazumi, Y., & Tadashi, T. (1991). Inhibitory effect of peony root extract on pentylenetetrazol-induced EEG power spectrum changes and extracellular calcium concentration changes in rat cerebral cortex. *Journal of Ethnopharmacology, 33*(1–2), 159–167.

Eadie, M. J. (1994). The understanding of epilepsy across three millennia. *Clinical & Experimental Neurology, 31,* 1–12.

Fisher, R. S., & Saul, M. (2012). *Genetic causes of epilepsy.* Stanford School of Medicine. Retrieved from http://neurology.stanford.edu/epilepsy/patientcare/videos/e_09.html

International League against Epilepsy. (2012). Resource Center. Retrieved from http://www.ilae.org/Visitors/Centre/ctf/documents/ILAEHandoutV10_000.pdf

Sensory Receptors

Living organisms have the ability to sense stimuli from the environment around them and respond in an appropriate manner. The sensory system deals with information being delivered to the nervous system by neurons that have receptors for various stimuli. A *receptor* is defined as either a specialized protein that detects chemical signals or as a specialized cell that detects environmental stimuli and generates a response. A stimulus is defined as a change in one or more conditions in the environment, both internal as well as external. A stimulus can be one of a variety of changes in the environment such as temperature, pressure, pain, or visible light, to name a few.

Sensory receptors are important because they provide the necessary information about the environment, and allow for the appropriate response to follow. They are involved in an animal's, and particularly a human's, sense of taste (gustation), smell (olfaction), sight (vision), touch, and hearing (audition). Sensory receptors are also involved with an animal's ability to breath and move. Sensory receptors have different-sized receptive fields—the area or region where an external or internal stimulus will activate the neuron. In general, large receptive fields cover a large area but tend to have less perception while small receptive fields cover a small area and have strong perception. For example, in touch sensation, small receptor fields in the fingers allow for discriminative touch giving the ability to sense detailed structures.

Types of Sensory Receptors

To date, sensory receptors have been categorized into five groups: *mechanoreceptors, chemoreceptors, thermoreceptors, photoreceptors,* and *nociceptors.* Some of these different receptor types are found throughout the body or in almost every sensory system.

Mechanoreceptors

Mechanoreceptors are receptors that respond to a physical stimulus such as mechanical pressure or distortion. These receptors are important for discerning

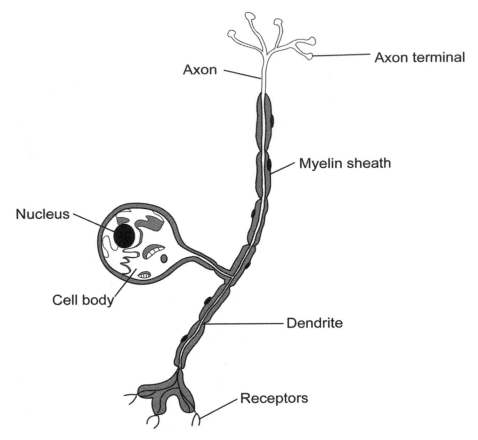

A sensory neuron. This neuron structure details a sensory neuron, which carries impulses and messages to the spinal cord and brain. These sensory neurons, which have cell bodies, are located in the CNS and close to the body so they are protected from damage. The axon moves these messages away from the nucleus and cell body, and the dendrites work in reverse to bring the impulses into the cell body. The myelin sheath works as an insulator to protect the neuronal signal from degrading over distances. (Sandy Windelspecht)

between different sensations such as light touch, touch, positional change (balance), and pressure. Perhaps the most notable stimuli that mechanoreceptors respond to are *sound waves* (used for hearing) and *proprioception* (the sense of position in space).

The mechanoreceptors that respond to sound waves are the hair cells within the cochlea, which are found in the inner ear. These sound waves bend the stereocilia (also called a hair bundle) on the top of the hair cells, which are "trapped" or protrude into a fluid-filled tube. The sound wave pushes the fluid that bends the stereocilia causing a mechanical change in their position. This activates the hair cell, which in turn transmits the signal from the cochlea in the ear to the brain where the information is processed. Thus the process of hearing results from a sound wave to a mechanical movement of a cell's apical hair bundle to a chemical signal so that a person is able to understand its meaning.

Similar to the change of position for a hair cell, proprioceptors sense the body's position in relation to space. These receptors are found in the bellies of skeletal muscles, joints, and tendons. They are referred to as *muscle spindles* and *Golgi tendon organs*. These receptors sense stretch in the muscle or tendon and the information is used to determine where the body is positioned in space. For example, when a person is typing, their finger joints change positions from one key to another and alter their position in space or in reference to the person. This in turn changes the stretch of the muscles and tendons within the fingers, like extending the right pointer finger to press the "&" key and relaxing and bending the left pointer finger to press the "f" key. These same signals of changing joint angles occur in all motor movements, such as the angles of the knees, ankles, and hips while walking, jumping, or running.

Other mechanoreceptors include (1) *Pacinian corpuscle* for the sense of pressure; (2) *Meissner's corpuscle* for the sense of touch; (3) *Merkel cell* for the sense of light touch; and (4) *semicircular canals* for the sense of balance or positional change.

Chemoreceptors

Chemoreceptors are receptors that respond to chemical stimuli in the environment. The two prominent classes of chemoreceptors are those involved in *olfactory* and *gustatory systems.* The olfactory system deals with the sense of smell and the gustatory system deals with the sense of taste.

Olfactory receptors are found in the membranes of olfactory sensory neurons located in the olfactory epithelium, which lines the insides of the nose. Olfactory sensory neurons have a long apical dendrite that ends with a bulb. The bulb has several long hair-like cilia that span several micrometers within the mucous layer of the olfactory epithelium that meet the external air. Volatile odor molecules in the environment enter the nose when breathed in and bind to receptors specific for that odor molecule. The information transmitted from the binding of the odorant molecule is sent to the olfactory bulbs (located at the base of the brain just below the frontal lobes) via the olfactory nerve (cranial nerve I) and then processed and perceived as a particular smell.

In the gustatory system, taste cells located in taste buds of the tongue operate in the same way as olfactory sensory neurons except these respond to aqueous chemical stimuli. For example, if an individual is eating an apple, the fruit is broken apart by the teeth and mixes with saliva. This turns the food particles into an aqueous solution so that the taste cells can bind to the specific chemical structures of the food, such as sugar for a sweet taste. The signal is brought to the brain for processing via three cranial nerves that supply sensory information for the tongue and soft palate: the facial nerve (cranial nerve VII), the glossopharyngeal nerve (cranial nerve IX), and the vagus nerve (cranial nerve X).

Other chemoreceptors include the *carotid bodies* to sense oxygen in blood and nociceptors to sense pain from trauma. More information about nociceptors is given in the following.

Thermoreceptors

Thermoreceptors are specialized sensory receptors that determine temperatures that are generally not painful (not too hot and not too cold). Thermoreceptors do not have a specific form, like a hair cell or olfactory sensory neuron, but are considered to be free nerve endings or free nonspecialized endings. These receptors are found throughout the skin, cornea (the covering of the eye), and the bladder. There are two fiber types used to sense temperature. For warmth, *unmyelinated C-fibers* will increase their firing rate when they are warmed between 32 and 48°C (or 90 and 118°F). However for some persons, temperatures over 40°C (104°F) are considered painful. For cool or cold temperatures, both unmyelinated C-fibers and *lightly myelinated A delta fibers* are activated. Specifically, the C-fibers reduce their firing when cooled while A delta fibers increase their firing rate when cooled between 10 and 30°C (or 50 and 86°F).

Nociceptors can act as thermoreceptors to determine pain from temperature, such as when a person burns their hand. Additionally, nociceptors are activated as thermoreceptors when temperatures are too cold that it becomes painful.

Photoreceptors

Photoreceptors are specialized sensory receptors that convert visible white light into the sense of vision. Specifically, these receptors absorb photons of light and transduce that absorption into a membrane potential, which activates the neuron. Photoreceptors are found in neurons located in the retina, which is the photosensitive lining of the back of the eye. There are two main types of photoreceptors: *cones* and *rods*.

Cone cells are shorter, wider, and have a tapering end compared to rod cells, thus receiving its name "cone." Cone cells are densely packed in the *fovea centralis* (or fovea, which is located in the center of the macula region of the retina) and reduce in number toward the outer edges of the retina. Cone cells need bright light to be activated and can absorb all *short, medium,* and *long wavelengths of visible light.* The different wavelengths represent different colors within the visible light spectrum, with short wavelengths being bluish in color, medium wavelengths being greenish in color, and long wavelengths being reddish in color. In humans, there are three types of cone cells: S-cones (absorb short wavelengths), M-cones (absorb medium wavelengths), and L-cones (absorb long wavelengths). Each cone cell type will absorb all visible light wavelengths but will absorb a specific wavelength more readily than the other two wavelengths. For example, an S-cone will absorb short wavelengths in bright light but will need significantly brighter light to also absorb medium and long wavelengths. This means that as each cone cell type is activated in bright light, the human brain uses these different wavelengths to see and perceive all possible colors within visible light.

Rod cells are longer and thinner compared to cone cells; thus giving its name "rod." Rod cells are more packed along the outer edges of the retina and absent in the fovea. With their location at the edge of the retina, rod cells are also used during peripheral vision. Rod cells are activated with dim lighting, meaning they can absorb a single photon of light to be activated. This makes rod cells to be more sensitive to light compared to cone cells. Thus, rod cells are the main photoreceptor neurons used for night vision. Because rod cells are activated in dim visible light, they have no role in color vision.

Nociceptors

Pain receptors or nociceptors (from Latin meaning "hurt") are specialized sensory receptors that determine when a stimulus is painful. These receptor types are generally called free nerve endings or free nonspecialized endings. Nociceptors send their signal to the brain and spinal cord so that the body can appropriately respond, such as to let go of a hot handle. Nociceptors are found in all locations of the body, both internally (such as the gut, heart, joints, and muscles) and externally (like the cornea, mucosa, and skin—also known as cutaneous nociceptors). This is because pain is an important signal that should not be ignored. Similar to thermoreceptors, nociceptors use two different fiber types: lightly myelinated or unmyelinated C-fibers (for slow conducting signals) and myelinated A delta fibers (for fast conducting signals).

Nociceptors respond to many types of noxious stimuli: *chemical, mechanical, polymodal, silent,* and *thermal*. A chemical nociceptor is one that is activated by chemicals or environmental irritants such as spices that are typically used for cooking. For example, capsaicin is a common spice found in peppers that can be noxious to the eyes, nose, and mouth.

A mechanical nociceptor responds to extreme pressure or mechanical deformation. For example, when sounds that are extremely loud like a fire truck siren, it causes the hair cells in the cochlea to move in such a way that it deforms the cell, which activates the A delta fibers and causes pain.

In general, a neuron will respond to only one type of stimulus. However, since pain is an important signal, there are polymodal nociceptors that respond to several types of noxious stimuli. Meaning they can respond to both chemical and mechanical stimuli, to both thermal and mechanical stimuli, or to all three types of noxious stimuli.

Silent nociceptors are those that are activated only when a specific threshold of stimulus is received or when injury has been induced. These types of sensory receptors will be stimulated after inflammation of the surrounding tissue occurs. For example, a silent nociceptor will only be activated after the skin has been cut and the area becomes inflamed.

Finally, a thermal nociceptor will respond to extreme temperatures such as hot temperatures over 42 C (or over 108 F). Extreme cold temperatures are painful and may feel "hot." However, scientists are still unsure of the exact pathway used to transmit cold pain to the brain and spinal cord.

Jennifer L. Hellier and
Roberto Lopez

See also: Auditory System; Discriminative Touch; Neuron; Olfactory System (Smell); Taste System; Thermal Sense (Temperature Sensation); Touch; Visual System

Further Reading

Abraira, V. E., & Ginty, D. D. (2013). The sensory neurons of touch. *Neuron, 79*(4), 618–639.

Fetsch, C. R., DeAngelis, G. C., & Angelaki, D. E. (2013). Bridging the gap between theories of sensory cue integration and the physiology of multisensory neurons. *Nature Reviews: Neuroscience, 14*(6), 429–442.

Kandel, E. R., Schwartz, J. H., Jessell, T. M., Siegelbaum, S. A., & Hudspeth, A. J. (Eds.). (2012). *Principles of neural science* (5th ed.). New York, NY: McGraw-Hill.

Kinnamon, S. C. (2013). Neurosensory transmission without a synapse: New perspectives on taste signaling. *BMC Biology, 11*, 42.

Purves, D., Augustine, G. J., Fitzpatrick, D., Hall, W. C., LaMantia, A.-S., McNamara, J. O., & Williams, S. M. (Eds.). (2004). *Neuroscience* (3rd ed.). Sunderland, MA: Sinauer Associates.

Serotonin and Its Receptors

Serotonin is a naturally occurring chemical that is used in the body and central nervous systems of animals. Within the body, serotonin is found in the blood (platelets) and gastrointestinal tract. Within the central nervous system it acts as a neurotransmitter, which is used for neuronal signaling. This signaling is how neurons "talk" to each other. For mammals and particularly humans, it is the neurotransmitter that has been associated with appetite, mood elevation producing feelings of happiness and well-being, and sleep. Serotonin is derived from the amino acid tryptophan and has the chemical name of *5-hydroxytryptamine*. It is universally denoted as 5-HT.

History

Serotonin was first identified in 1935 by Italian pharmacologist and chemist Vittorio Erspamer (1909–1999). At the time, Erspamer did not know what chemical he extracted from enterochromaffin cells (neuroendocrine cells found in the lining of the digestive tract). He placed the extract on intestines causing them to contract. In 1937, Erspamer was able to show that this extract was an unknown amine and named it "enteramine." It took a decade for Maurice M. Rapport (1919–2011) and colleagues to find serotonin in blood serum. They discovered that it caused blood vessels to constrict. Based on its action (giving vascular tone) and location (serum), Rapport and colleagues named it "serotonin." A few years later in 1952, it was shown that enteramine and serotonin were the same compound, but the name serotonin remained. In 1953, Betty Twarog (1927–2013) and Irvine H. Page (1901–1991) identified serotonin in the brain. Scientists worked on understanding serotonin's function in the central nervous system over the next 10 years, which led to the discovery of antidepressants. These drugs, called serotonin reuptake inhibitors, act on serotonin by blocking its ability to be recycled into the presynaptic neuron (see "Clinical Uses" in the following).

Anatomy and Physiology

In the body, serotonin is critical for blood clotting. When a blood vessel is damaged, active bleeding occurs. To stop the bleeding and to return to homeostasis, blood platelets are recruited to the site. Here, serotonin is released from the platelets to begin the clotting sequence with serotonin acting as a vasoconstrictor. This causes the damaged blood vessel to constrict (become smaller) and slow down its active bleeding. In the nervous system, serotonin is a ligand or agonist because it is a chemical that binds to specific sites on the serotonin receptor. The binding of ligands will cause receptors to fold and reshape until a channel or pore is exposed. Once this conformational change occurs, a physiological response in the neuron can ensue.

In the brain, serotonin is largely produced in neurons that are located in the brainstem's reticular formation, particularly in the *raphe nuclei* (a group of neuronal cell bodies). These seven or eight nuclei project their axons throughout the brain and spinal cord, making a complex neurotransmitter system that reaches almost every part of the central nervous system. The neurons in the lower raphe nuclei project to the cerebellum and the spinal cord while the neurons in the upper raphe nuclei project to the cerebral cortex and deep structures.

Serotonin receptors, therefore, are also spread throughout the central and peripheral nervous systems. These receptors are mainly G protein–coupled receptors. To date, only one known serotonin receptor family (the 5-HT$_3$) has been shown to be a ligand-gated ion channel. Ligand-gated channels tend to affect the neuron quickly with a short affect (a few seconds), where G protein–coupled receptors can modulate the neuron resulting in a long-term change within the neuron (over a few hours). Depending on where the receptor is located, it can have either an excitatory or inhibitory function.

In general, serotonin receptors modulate a neuron's ability to release other neurotransmitters, such as acetylcholine, dopamine, glutamate, and GABA (γ-aminobutyric acid), or hormones like cortisol, oxytocin, and vasopressin. To date, there are seven known serotonin receptor families with each having several subtypes. Of the six G protein–coupled receptors, three increase a cell's level of cyclic adenosine monophosphate (cAMP; 5-HT$_4$, 5-HT$_6$, 5-HT$_7$), two decrease the level of cAMP (5-HT$_1$ and 5-HT$_5$), and one increases a cell's levels of IP3 (inositol trisphosphate) and DAG (diacylglycerol; 5-HT$_2$). IP3, DAG, and cAMP are all second messenger molecules that are used in signal transduction and/or lipid signaling within the cell.

Clinical Uses

Because serotonin and its receptors affect appetite, mood levels, and sleep, drugs have been designed to be agonists or antagonists of 5-HT receptors as well as to affect the time serotonin remains in the synaptic cleft (see the following text). Specifically, drugs have been developed as antidepressants (to reduce depression), antipsychotics (to reduce psychoses), anxiolytics (to decrease anxiety), antiemetics (to decrease vomiting), and antimigraines (to inhibit migraine headaches).

Many drugs have also been designed to inhibit the reuptake of serotonin within the synaptic cleft, the space between two neurons (a presynaptic and postsynaptic neuron) where chemical signaling occurs. When a neurotransmitter is released into the synaptic cleft from the presynaptic neuron, the concentration of the neurotransmitter increases quickly in the small space. The neurotransmitter will then bind to its receptor on the postsynaptic neuron. However, the neurotransmitter also diffuses, recycles (reuptake), or breaks down in the synaptic cleft resulting in a fast decrease in concentration. This is so that the synapse "resets" for the next chemical wave. By creating drugs to block the reuptake or break down of serotonin, it results in serotonin increasing its length of time within the synaptic cleft and possibly rebinding to the serotonin receptor on the postsynaptic neuron. Increasing this binding time has been associated with improving depression and mood elevation in depressed patients. This is how monoamine oxidase inhibitors (MAOIs) or selective serotonin reuptake inhibitors (SSRIs) work. There are side effects with both MAOIs and SSRIs; however, SSRIs have fewer side effects.

Jennifer L. Hellier

See also: Behavioral Health; Depression; Dopamine and Its Receptors; G Proteins; Glutamate and Its Receptors

Further Reading

Berger, M., Gray, J. A., & Roth, B. L. (2009). The expanded biology of serotonin. *Annual Review of Medicine, 60,* 355–366.

Mayo Clinic Staff. (2013). *Depression (Major depression). Selective serotonin reuptake inhibitors (SSRIs).* Retrieved from http://www.mayoclinic.com/health/ssris/MH00066

Mohammad-Zadeh, L. F., Moses, L., & Gwaltney-Brant, S. M. (2008). Serotonin: A review. *Journal of Veterinary Pharmacology and Therapeutics, 31*(3), 187–199. doi:10.1111/j.1365–2885.2008.00944.x.

Nichols, D. E., & Nichols, C. D. (2008). Serotonin receptors. *Chemical Reviews, 108*(5), 1614–1641.

Shatz, Carla J. (c. 1948–)

Carla J. Shatz, PhD, is a neurobiologist who is well known for her discoveries regarding how the eye and the visual system develop in mammals. Her work has been instrumental in discerning the basic principles of early brain development. Specifically, she has shown the role of neural activity in understanding how and when neuron connections are formed. These findings have helped neuroscientists to better understand learning and memory as well as diseases like autism and schizophrenia.

Dr. Shatz graduated from Radcliffe College in 1969 with a bachelor of arts in chemistry. In 1971, she received a master's degree in physiology from the University College London while on a Marshall Scholarship. In 1976, she was the first person to receive a doctor of philosophy in neurobiology from Harvard Medical School, where she studied with Nobel laureates David Hubel and Torsten Wiesel. During this period, she was appointed as a Harvard Junior Fellow. From 1976 to 1978, Dr. Shatz obtained postdoctoral training with Dr. Pasko Rakic in the Department of Neuroscience at Harvard Medical School.

During Dr. Shatz's postdoctoral training, she discovered that long before vision is possible, the retina generates spontaneous wave activity that is critical for cellular pattern formation in the brain. Her efforts aimed to discover how brain circuits are tuned by experience during critical periods of development both before and after birth.

Since then, Dr. Shatz has elucidated several cellular and molecular mechanisms that transform early fetal and neonatal brain circuits into mature connections. By studying the visual system of mammals, the Shatz Lab discovered that adult wiring emerges from dynamic interactions between neurons, particularly during synaptic plasticity and the gene expressions involved in the process of circuit tuning. Through efforts to understand mechanistic underpinnings of circuit tuning, her work has examined functional screens for genes regulated by neural activity and studied these functions for vision, learning, and memory. Dr. Shatz's work has led to a better understanding of many neuro developmental disorders and resulting interactions between the nervous and immune systems.

From her groundbreaking discoveries in neuroscience, Dr. Shatz has become a member of the American Academy of Arts and Sciences, the National Academy of Sciences, and the Institute of Medicine. Her academic career has included Stanford University School of Medicine, University of California-Berkeley, and Harvard University Department of Neurobiology. Dr. Shatz is currently performing research and teaching at Stanford University where she is a professor of biology and neurobiology as well as directing the Bio-X program (http://biox.stanford.edu).

Dr. Shatz has received several awards for her research. She has received the Society for Neuroscience Young Investigator Award in 1985, the Silvio Conte Award from the National Foundation for Brain Research in 1993, the Charles A. Dana Award for Pioneering Achievement in Health and Education in 1995, the Alcon Award for Outstanding Contributions to Vision Research in 1997, the Bernard Sachs Award from the Child Neurology Society in 1999, the Weizmann Institute Women and Science Award in 2000, the Gill Prize in Neuroscience in 2006, the Sapp Family Provostial Professorship, Stanford University Inaugural Chair Holder in 2010, the Physiological Society Prize Lecture, Physiological Society Prize Lecture Oxford England in 2011, and the 2011 Ralph Gerard Prize in Neuroscience.

Karen Savoie

See also: Retina; Visual System

Further Reading

Bio-X Stanford University. (n.d.). Retrieved from http://biox.stanford.edu

Richardson, M. W. (2012). *Carla Shatz: Shattering the glass ceiling.* Retrieved from http://www.brainfacts.org/About-Neuroscience/Meet-the-Researcher/Articles/2012/Carla-Shatz.aspx

Shingles

Herpes zoster, a painful rash of blisters presenting along a well-defined region of the body such as the face or mid-section, is more commonly known as *shingles*. Fluid-filled vesicles forming a distinctive line that has come to be called a zoosteriform rash characterize this disease. Shingles is caused by the varicella zoster virus (VZV), which is also the cause of the once-common childhood illness chickenpox (varicella).

In people who have had varicella, the virus may lie dormant in sensory nerve ganglia for decades only to become activated when the individual experiences significant physiological or psychological stress. This reactivation of the virus is the disease known as herpes zoster. Immunocompromised individuals are certainly more at risk for developing herpes zoster, though most sufferers are immunocompetent. In fact, the current lifetime risk for developing the disease is 32 percent (Atkinson et al., 2012). Adults over 60 experience the greatest risk. Most people recover quickly within two to four weeks, and the antiviral drug acyclovir greatly speeds recovery.

History

In 1888, Austrian physician Janos von Bokay (1858–1937) established the link between varicella and herpes zoster by observing that children who had not been exposed to chickenpox—and therefore lacked natural immunity—developed chickenpox following exposure to herpes zoster lesions (Vincent, 2011). He had many examples of this phenomenon available to him due to the prevalence of multigenerational households at the time. Older adults would live with their grown children and grandchildren and when they would develop shingles their young, previously unexposed grandchildren could contract chickenpox. Ancient civilizations including the early Greeks documented symptomology consistent with herpes zoster, and it is believed that the virus may have first emerged 70 million years ago (Nogueira and Traynor, 2004). However, von Bokay's discovery was the first true step toward understanding the disease.

Some skeptics remained unconvinced that these two illnesses were caused by the same virus until well into the 20th century. The advent of the electron microscope gave scientists the power to observe that virions cultured from both diseases appeared to be similar. In 1952, the virus was definitively isolated from both diseases (Vincent, 2011). This was enough proof to finally satisfy the scientific community that these diseases shared a common infectious agent and in 1958 the names of the varicella virus and the zoster virus were merged to reflect this discovery. In 1968 the complete genome was mapped and the virus was given the official name of *human (alpha) herpes virus 3* (Vincent, 2011).

Herpes zoster is a recurrent infection of VZV following the primary infection that caused varicella. Though the virus is present in the vesicles, herpes zoster cannot be directly spread through contact. Contact with a ruptured vesicle could potentially cause a primary infection in an individual who lacks immunity, as seen by von Bokay, and that in turn carries the risk of the individual later developing herpes zoster.

Signs, Symptoms, and Treatment

The rash itself is extremely painful and is preceded by a prodromal (presymptomatic) period of two to four days of hypersensitive skin and occasionally other symptoms such as erythema, fever, chills, malaise, and gastrointestinal upset. Flat macules (distinct, discolorations of skin that are less than one centimeter in diameter) and papules (distinct, fluid-less, bumps of skin that are less than one centimeter in diameter) then develop, eventually leading to the fluid-filled vesicles. The affected area may be severely itchy and the patient is likely to experience *allodynia*— meaning that even very mild stimuli causes considerable pain. As with varicella, the vesicles ultimately crust over and the rash resolves in most cases. This phase usually lasts 7 to 10 days. Habif (2005) noted that in the majority of cases the rash presents in the thoracic area, though it is not uncommon to see it in the cervical, lumbar, trigeminal, and sacral areas (Ebersole et al., 2008).

Diagnosis is made primarily based upon the patient's signs and symptoms, especially the zosteriform rash. Herpes zoster is not the only cause of this type of rash, and other factors including the patient's medical history are necessary for diagnosis. The presence or absence of prior infection with VZV is important, as well as any history of other herpiform diseases as these can sometimes present in a similar manner. If there is a question as to whether or not the patient has herpes zoster, polymerase chain reaction can be performed on a sample of the fluid from one of the lesions. This will confirm the genetic identity of the virus, if present. Biopsies are obtained from the vesicles using a Tzanck smear that shows enlarged and abnormal cells (Leeuwen and Poelhuis-Leth, 2009).

Once diagnosed, the patient is treated systemically with an oral antiviral nucleoside analog, such as acyclovir, which blocks both virus deoxyribonucleic acid (DNA) polymerase and host-cell DNA replication (Albanese and Nutz, 2012). Acyclovir not only shortens the healing time but also reduces the incidence of postherpetic neuralgia, which is severe pain that is caused by nerve damage from the viral infection. Topical treatments such as Burow's solution (aluminum acetate) and calamine lotion (zinc oxide and iron oxide) help relieve the itching and stinging of the rash as well as help prevent bacterial infections of the lesions. Analgesics are often indicated. Gabapeptin is useful for treating neuropathic pain and some patients require opioids for adequate pain control (Ebersole et al., 2008).

Prevention is possible, and there are two types of vaccines available to this end. The varicella vaccine became available for those 12 or older in the United States in 1995; and a combination vaccine for measles, mumps, rubella, and varicella was approved for children 1 to 12 years of age in 2005. It effectively prevents the primary infection and therefore the secondary infection in 70–100 percent of those immunized, depending upon the age of the patient and whether or not they receive the second dose (Atkinson et al., 2012). This is a live-attenuated vaccine and is contraindicated in anyone with a weakened immune system. For people who have already been infected with VZV, the vaccine Zostavax prevents herpes zoster in 51 percent of those vaccinated and postherpetic neuralgia in 67 percent (Atkinson et al., 2012). There is a limited supply of the latter vaccine, and so it is available only to those over the age of 50 and only recommended for those over the age of 60.

The severity of the infection and risk of complications may be increased if multiple skin rashes are found, if the face is affected, or if the affected individual is an older adult (Ebersole, 2008). Most people recover completely within two to four weeks; however, there are some complications which may draw out the recovery period. The most common of these is postherpetic neuralgia affecting 40–60 percent of those with herpes zoster (Ebersole, 2008). This is an unfortunate condition in which the allodynia from the rash persists for months or years after the lesions have resolved. A condition called *herpes zoster opthalmicus* can cause permanent blindness if untreated and can occur when the virus is present in the ophthalmic division of the trigeminal nerve or following contact with the lesions and then with the eyes. As with any open wound, bacterial infections are always a risk. Scarring is not a normal sequela of herpes zoster, but a bacterial infection can lead to it. Keeping the lesions clean and covered with bandages usually prevents infection. Infections are treated based on the extent of the infection and the specific bacteria present. Most of severe of the possible complications is the potential for the virus to enter the central nervous system, lungs, and liver. This only occurs in immunocompromised patients and though possibly fatal is also quite rare.

The recent development of vaccines to prevent both the primary and secondary infections of VZV is likely to significantly reduce the prevalence of herpes zoster, though they may not completely eradicate it. While the Zostavax vaccine only prevents herpes zoster in 51 percent of those immunized, the varicella vaccine prevents varicella in 70–100 percent of those immunized (Atkinson et al., 2012). As the children immunized against VZV age, they will not be susceptible to herpes zoster as are today's older adults. Of immunocompetent children, only those whose parents either object to vaccination or do not pursue the second dose of the vaccine in the appropriate window will be at risk for this disease in the future. This is a great opportunity for public health officials to raise awareness about the importance of the varicella vaccine. There is an investigational product that is useful in treating immunocompromised patients called varicella zoster immune globulin (Atkinson et al., 2012). It provides artificial passive immunity to those who cannot receive the vaccine. As this product becomes more widely available, it will likely improve the outcomes for these patients.

Erin Slocum

See also: Retrovirus; Trigeminal Nerve

Further Reading

Albanese, J., & Nutz, P. (2012). *Mosby's nursing drug cards* (21st ed.). St. Louis, MO: Mosby, Inc.

Atkinson, W., Hamborsk, J., & Wolfe, S. (2012). Varicella. In *Epidemiology and prevention of vaccine-preventable diseases* (12th ed., pp. 301–306). Washington, DC: Public Health Foundation.

Ebersole, P., Hess, P., Touhy, T., Jett, K., & Luggen, A. (2008). Biological maintenance needs. In *Toward healthy aging human needs and nursing response* (7th ed., pp. 157–193). St. Louis, MO: Mosby, Inc.

Leaden, A., & Poelhuis-Leth, D. (2009). *Davis's comprehensive handbook of laboratory and diagnostic tests with nursing implications* (3rd ed.). Philadelphia, PA: F.A. Davis Company.

Nogueira, R., & Traynor, B. (2004). The neurology of varicella-zoster virus: A historical perspective. *Archives of Neurology, 61*(12), 1974–1977.

Vincent, W. (2011). Varicella-zoster infections—An overview. *Quest Diagnostics Infectious Disease Update, 18*(8), 97–108.

Short-Term Potentiation

Short-term potentiation, also known as posttetanic potentiation or PTP, is short-term synaptic plasticity found in excitably cells called neurons. PTP is caused by short bursts of excitatory postsynaptic potential (EPSP) or mini-EPSP (mEPSP) called tetanic stimulation. These short bursts do not result in any enhancement of the postsynaptic signal—which is called *potentiation*—and PTP usually only lasts for up to a few minutes long. Any potentiations shorter than this are considered *augmentations.* PTPs result when synapses are stimulated with repetitive pulses at high frequencies for a short amount of time. The results of a PTP can vary between depression and potentiation following stimulation and are thought to be the result of a buildup of calcium ions (Ca^{2+} ions) in the presynaptic neuron's axon terminal. In this way, it either strengthens or weakens a synapse. PTPs usually take a while to onset, but then only up to a few seconds to develop. PTP works closely with long-term potentiation (LTP), which is required for learning and memory functions of the brain.

Mechanism

In mammalian hippocampal slice experiments, researchers use a recording electrode to measure changes in the neuronal network's excitability and a stimulating electrode to produce the electrical stimulation of neurons. For both LTP and PTP, these stimulations are both types of *high-frequency stimulation* such that each pulse of the stimulation is very short (in milliseconds) as well as their interval (in milliseconds to seconds). A train of pulse stimulations (termed a *tetanic stimulation* or a *tetanus*) that last for one second delivered at a frequency of 100 hertz (Hz) and then repeated 20 seconds later will induce LTP and last for more than an hour or two. To induce PTP, however, the train of pulses is shorter with a shorter interval or frequency, usually between 10 and 50 hertz and with an interval in the milliseconds.

Since both LTP and PTP events are stimulated by an excitatory potential, the EPSP and mEPSP respectively, it seems like intuitively they would share a similar mechanism. Research completed by Schulz and Fitzgibbons (1997) proved otherwise in the mammalian hippocampus *in vitro*. They were able to show that even when occluding LTP expression, they were able to still see the expression of PTP and vice versa. However, in their experiments they were able to show that PTP prior to LTP stimulation would lower the threshold for LTP to develop. Thus, the proximity of the two mechanisms indicates that there may be some shared induction step (Schulz and Fitzgibbons, 1997). PTP does seem to be dependent on calcium ion levels near the synapse in the presynaptic neuron. It is thought that the calcium ion buildup occurs in the mitochondria during the stimulation of the synapse. These excess calcium ions then get packaged into vesicles and transported from the mitochondria down the axon to the axon terminal. Once there, an action potential signals the vesicles to release calcium ions into the synapse. The stimulation of the synapse triggers the release of the calcium ions, which are important in carrying the action potential to the postsynaptic neuron. Increasing the calcium concentrations in the synapse triggers calcium channels on the dendrite of the postsynaptic neuron to open allowing calcium ions to flow into the cell. This influx of calcium ions into the postsynaptic neuron depolarizes it propagating the action potential from the dendrite through the cell body and to the neuron's axon.

PTP has previously been thought to have contributed to temporal processing on a scale of tens to hundreds of milliseconds. PTP has been shown to be completely independent of postsynaptic membrane potential, N-methyl-D-aspartate (NMDA) receptors, or retrograde neuropeptide release. Tetanic stimulation can be used in medicine to determine if and where a depolarizing block in a neuromuscular junction was located. If the tetanic stimulation fades, then this is an indication that there is a depolarizing block in this neuromuscular junction. The usage of tetanic stimulation is debated, however. This is because it can be painful for the patient in some stimulation frequencies.

Riannon C. Atwater

See also: Calcium Channels; Excitation; Learning and Memory; Long-Term Potentiation; Membrane Potential: Depolarization and Hyperpolarization; Membrane Potential Experiment—Understand Membrane Properties; Neuroplasticity; NMDA and Its Receptors; Postsynaptic Potentials

Further Reading

Balakrishnan, V., Srinivasan, G., & von Gersdorff, H. (2010). Post-tetanic potentiation involves the presynaptic binding of calcium to calmodulin. *Journal of General Physiology, 136*(3), 243–245. Retrieved from http://www.ncbi.nlm.nih.gov/pmc/articles/PMC2931153/

Bao, J.X., Kandel, E.R., & Hawkins, R.D. (1997). Involvement of pre- and postsynaptic mechanisms in posttetanic potentiation at Aplysia synapses. *Science, 275*(5302), 969–973.

Marder, C.P., & Buonomano, D.V. (2003). Differential effects of short- and long-term potentiation on cell firing in the CA1 region of the hippocampus. *Journal of Neuroscience, 23*(1), 112–121. Retrieved from http://www.neurobio.ucla.edu/~dbuono/PDFs/MarderBuono03.pdf

Schulz, P.E., & Fitzgibbons, J.C. (1997). Differing mechanisms of expression for short- and long-term potentiation. *Journal of Neurophysiology, 78*(1), 321–334. Retrieved from http://www.ncbi.nlm.nih.gov/pubmed/9242283

Sinuses

Humans have many *sinuses,* natural openings or cavities found in bone or other tissue. Sinuses are usually named for the bones where the sinuses are found. The most commonly known sinuses are those found in the nasal cavities, as these can fill with mucous when a person is ill and may lead to infection. Other sinuses that are found in the head are the *dural venous sinuses,* which are part of the cardiovascular system particularly of the veins. This entry will focus on venous sinuses.

The dural venous sinuses—also known as dural sinuses, cerebral sinuses, or cranial sinuses—are located in the brain between the meningeal layers of the dura mater (a tough, thick covering—the meninges—that surrounds the brain for protection). Although these sinuses are part of the venous system, they do not have valves. The dural sinuses receive and drain the blood from internal and external veins of the brain, which helps maintain homeostasis. They also receive cerebrospinal fluid (CSF, a colorless fluid that surrounds and protects the brain) from the subarachnoid space (between the dura and the brain), and drains into the internal jugular vein located in the neck.

Anatomy and Physiology

The walls of the dural venous sinuses are made of dura mater that is lined with endothelium (a special layer of flattened cells found in blood vessels). This endothelium lining is contiguous from the sinuses and also lines the veins. Within the cardiovascular system, all vessels—veins and arteries—have a set of vessel layers (basement membrane, Tunica intima, Tunica media, and Tunica externa). However, the dural sinuses are not true vessels, so they lack some of these layers.

There are two groups of sinuses within the dura: the posterosuperior sinuses at the upper and back of the skull, and the anteroinferior sinuses at the base of the skull. The posterosuperior group comprises the superior sagittal, straight inferior sagittal, and the two transverse occipital sinuses. The anteroinferior sinuses are found in each hemisphere, thus comprising the cavernous, superior petrosal, intercavernous, and inferior petrosal sinuses. Some of the smaller sinuses will drain into the larger sinuses. Nonetheless, all blood and cerebrospinal fluid will eventually drain into the left and right internal jugular veins.

Injury

The sinuses can be damaged by trauma, for example, a skull fracture. This may cause a blood clot (thrombosis) within the dural sinuses. Sometimes such a thrombosis can cause a hemorrhagic infarction (blockage of a vein) that may lead to seizures (or epilepsy), neurological deficits, or death.

Patricia A. Bloomquist

See also: Cerebrospinal Fluid; Epilepsy; Meninges; Seizures; Stroke

Further Reading

Kiernan, J. A. (2005). *Barr's the human nervous system: An anatomical viewpoint.* Bethesda, MD: Lippincott Williams & Wilkins.

Purves, D., Augustine, G. J., Fitzpatrick, D., Hall, W. C., LaMantia, A.-S., McNamara, J. O., & Williams, S. M. (Eds.). (2004). *Neuroscience* (3rd ed.). Sunderland, MA: Sinauer Associates.

Skull

In vertebrates, particularly craniates, the brain is protected by a hard, bony structure called the *skull.* The skull is the most anterior part of the skeleton; it forms the shape of the face and facial structures like the ears, eyes, and nose. The skull is made up of the *cranium* (which surrounds the brain) and the *mandible* (the jaw bone). The cranium of the skull looks like one bone in adults, but is actually several flat bones that fuse together during the first year after birth. These fusions are called *sutures,* which are immoveable joints. The skull has many more functions than just housing the brain, it also is necessary for determining the distance between the eyes, fixing the position of the ears, allowing smells to enter the brain, and making the opening of the digestive system (mouth). Thus, it is essential for helping (1) the visual system in producing stereoscopic vision; (2) the auditory system for determining sound localization; (3) the olfactory system in receiving odors; and (4) the body in receiving nutrients.

Anatomy and Physiology

At birth, the human skull has 44 separate bones. These bones begin to fuse during the first year of age. The result is 22 distinct bones and two distinct regions: the *neurocranium* (that houses the brain) and the *viscerocranium* (the makes up the face). The neurocranium consists of the ethmoid, the frontal, the occipital, two parietal, the sphenoid, and two temporal bones. The lobes of the brain are named after the bones that overlie them. There are 14 bones of the viscerocranium, which are two conchae, two lacrimal, the mandible, two maxilla, two nasal, two palatine, the vomer, and two zygomatic bones.

There are several natural openings within the skull called *foramina* (plural; *foramen,* singular form). These holes allow the cranial nerves to enter or exit the skull so that the head, neck, and face can have sensory and motor functions. The largest opening is the *foramen magnum,* which allows the spinal cord to be contiguous with the brainstem.

Injury

The skull is extremely strong and generally very difficult to break. However, penetrating injuries can occur causing brain damage and/or death. The brain can also be injured by other means, such as falling off a bike or hitting the head in a car accident. When this occurs, the brain can bump against the inside of the skull and tear the *meninges,* the hard membranous coverings of the brain. Within the meninges, blood vessels travel and can be torn causing internal bleeding. Since the skull is rigid and inflexible, the active bleeding will increase the intracranial pressure and potentially have the brainstem and brain herniate through the foramen magnum. If this occurs, significant brain damage or death is inevitable. Thus, the intracranial pressure must be relieved by surgery. This is why head injuries and specifically concussions must be monitored and/or treated as soon as possible by a health care provider.

Jennifer L. Hellier

See also: Brain Anatomy; Concussion; Cranial Nerves; Hematoma (Hemorrhage); Meninges; Trauma

Further Reading

Thorogood, P. (1988). The developmental specification of the vertebral skull. *Development, 103*(Suppl.), 141–153.

Sleep

Sleep is the naturally recurring state described by the reduced or the absence of consciousness and the inactivity of nearly all voluntary muscles. Sleep is more easily reversible than hibernation (a dormant state) or coma (a state of extreme unconsciousness and unresponsiveness). Sleep is a heightened anabolic state, meaning it accentuates growth and rejuvenation of the immune, nervous, skeletal, and muscular systems. Although energy is conserved during sleep, metabolism does not decrease during sleep. In most animals, and particularly in mammals, sleep timing is controlled by an internal circadian clock called the *suprachiasmatic nucleus*, sleep-wake homeostasis, and willed behavior meaning animals can fight the urge to sleep.

Sleep Stages

In 1937, the stages of sleep were first described by Alfred Lee Loomis (1887–1975) and his coworkers. These scientists separated the different electroencephalography (EEG) features of sleep into five levels from wakefulness to deep sleep; however, rapid eye movement (REM) sleep was not discovered until 1953. It was the study performed by Nathaniel Kleitman (1895–1999), Eugene Aserinsky (1921–1998), and Jon Birtwell in which REM was identified and defined as a unique sleep stage.

Sleep progresses in a cyclical fashion through five stages. Four stages are referred to as non-REM (NREM) sleep and the fifth is known as REM sleep. One cycle typically lasts about 90–110 minutes in humans.

Presleep is a period of decreased perceptual awareness. In this stage, brain activity is characterized by alpha waves, which are normal brain frequencies (8–10 hertz or 8–10 cycles per second) that can be measured on EEG during wakefulness with eyes closed. In general, alpha waves are more rhythmic and have higher amplitudes compared to beta waves. Alpha waves also have a lower frequency compared to beta waves, which normally range from 12 to 30 hertz and are associated with waking consciousness. Beta waves are categorized into three groups based on the frequency of the waveforms: low beta waves range from 12.5 to 16 hertz, beta waves consisting of 16.5–20 hertz, and high beta waves which occur between 20.5 and 28 hertz. During beta wave activity, humans are highly alert and focused. Beta waves usually occur throughout the day when humans are engaged in any form of activity while being awake. Presleep occurs right as a person begins to fall asleep or when they start to get drowsy. During this stage, a person experiences their muscles as still being active and their eyes rolling slowly while opening and closing moderately.

Stage one is characterized by light sleep and lasts for only about 10 minutes. The brain waves gradually transition from alpha waves to theta waves, which range from 4 to 7 hertz and are associated with drowsiness and light sleep.

Synchrony

Brain cells that are responsible for nerve impulses are called neurons. Within the brain, neurons make up a local circuit that may consist of a few to hundreds of interconnected neurons. These smaller circuits will connect with other circuits making up the entire brain circuitry. Some circuits are responsible for sensory information while others are responsible for motor function. Nonetheless, neurons become activated from other neurons and the output signal can be modulated or processed to the next circuit. Synchrony is a phenomenon where neuronal output signals (or action potentials) occur at the exact same time. In general, neurons only synchronize when it is part of the processing. Abnormal synchrony in the brain causes seizure activity, which may result in damage to the brain.

The most common type of synchrony is an oscillation. In general, an oscillation occurs when a population of neurons release action potentials (or fire) at the same time and then go quiet. This activity repeats over and over resulting in an oscillation. A group of synchronized neurons produce a "burst" of activity and are said to be bursting. The speed of bursting or oscillations is called a frequency (the incidence over time), which is a measurement of hertz (Hz). When two separate circuits are oscillating at different frequencies they are desynchronized. If they both oscillate at the same frequency they are synchronized.

Neuroscientists have found that synchronized oscillations are important for many physiological processes such as sleep. Sleep spindles or sigma waves are oscillatory brain activity ranging from 12 hertz to 14 hertz that last for a short amount of time, less than 1 second. Scientists have suggested that the brain uses these sleep spindles to inhibit its complex processing; thus, allowing the sleeper to be in a tranquil state.

Jennifer L. Hellier

See also: Epilepsy; Oscillations; Seizures

Further Reading

Lachaux, J. P., Rodriguez, E., Martinerie, J., & Varela, F. J. (1999). Measuring phase synchrony in brain signals. *Human Brain Mapping, 8*(4), 194–208.

Stage two also contains theta waves but random short bursts of increased frequency called sleep spindles are the defining characteristic in this stage. Sleep spindles or sigma waves are oscillatory brain activity ranging from 12 to 14 hertz and last for less than one second. It is hypothesized that sleep spindles are how the brain inhibits its complex processing so that the sleeper can remain in a tranquil state. K-complexes are the largest amplitude and brain activity that is normally found in healthy persons, and sleep spindles generally occur with K-complexes. In general, K-complexes are more frequently observed in the first few cycles of sleep. It is hypothesized that K-complexes are necessary for sleep-based memory consolidation as well as to reduce arousal from external stimuli that are not signals of danger, like a sneeze, an air conditioner turning on, or a baby crying. Stage three and stage four are very similar and are typically grouped into one stage. They are considered to be deep sleep. Brain activity transitions from theta waves to delta waves, which are the lowest in frequency ranging between 0.5 and 4 hertz. Delta waves have the highest amplitude compared to alpha, beta, and theta brain waves. Both stages three and four are also known as slow wave sleep (SWS). This is caused by the brain's preoptic area, which is thought to be the main region to drive delta waves. The sleeper is less responsive to the environment and environmental stimuli no longer produce a reaction. When a person is extremely tired from a hard day, they tend to fall into a deep sleep easier. During this type of sleep, delta waves have been shown to trigger the release of a growth hormone that is necessary for the process of healing. This is one of the hypotheses for why animals sleep, to heal their bodies from the day's activities.

Stage five is when the sleeper enters REM sleep where most muscles are paralyzed. This is one of the most interesting stages as brain wave patterns are similar to those in relaxed wakefulness. REM sleep is turned on by acetylcholine secretion as well as neurons that secrete serotonin. Adults reach REM sleep roughly every 90 minutes. Thus a healthy adult would have about four to five sessions of REM sleep a night. REM sleep is shorter in the first few sleep cycles and longer in the last few cycles when the sleeper is near waking. REM sleep is hypothesized to play an important role in cognitive development of infants and children as they spend much more of their sleep in REM periods compared to adults.

REM Sleep

REM sleep accounts for 20–25 percent of total sleep in most human adults and is identified by rapid eye movements accompanied with a rapid low-voltage EEG that is similar to the bioelectric outputs of a person who is awake. Memorable dreaming occurs in this stage, which is thought to aid in memory formation as well as creativity for the sleeper. If a person is deprived of REM sleep, they will "rebound" during their next sleep cycle such that they will spend more time in REM than in any other sleep stage. It is this rebound effect that makes researchers think that REM sleep is essential for normal physiological needs required by animals, particularly in mammals and birds.

REM sleep has also been associated with depression. For example, a recent study deprived REM sleep in patients with depression caused by an imbalance of certain brain chemicals. The following day, these patients showed less signs of depression; however, as soon as the patients fell asleep they would rebound and lose the effect when they awoke.

Circadian Clock

The circadian clock is an inner timekeeping device that couples with the neurotransmitter, adenosine. Adenosine is necessary for blocking bodily activities that are needed for wakefulness. This means that adenosine helps animals prepare for sleep. Adenosine is produced while an animal is awake and builds up over the course of the day. When the levels of adenosine are high it induces sleepiness, which tends to correlate with the lack of light (or nighttime). As a person gets sleepier, melatonin begins to be released, resulting in a decrease of the person's core temperature. This cycle is known as the circadian rhythm of the body and it helps induce a structured sleep-wake cycle. The suprachiasmatic nucleus (SCN) is a tiny region in the brain's midline that is responsible for controlling circadian rhythm in animals. The SCN receives inputs from specialized photosensitive ganglion cells in the retina. If a light is turned on during the night, information is relayed throughout the SCN through a process called entrainment. If the SCN is destroyed then the length and timing of sleep may become erratic.

Sleep Apnea

Sleep apnea is a condition where a person suffers major pauses in breathing during sleep. This disrupts the normal progression of sleep and often can cause more severe health problems. Apneas (without breathing) occur when muscles around a person's airway relax during sleep and cause the airway to collapse and block the intake of oxygen. Oxygen levels in the blood drop and causes the person to come out of deep sleep in order to resume breathing. Diagnosing sleep apnea usually requires a sleep study performed in a sleep clinic. Patients typically do not remember any episodes of wakefulness due to sleep apnea. They just feel really tired even after getting several hours of sleep and they have no idea why.

Sleep apnea can affect anyone at any age. Risk factors of sleep apnea include but are not limited to being male, overweight, and old age. If left untreated, sleep apnea can cause a number of health problems. The most common side effects of sleep apnea are high blood pressure and stroke.

Common symptoms of sleep apnea are waking up with a very sore and/or dry throat, loud snoring, or morning headaches. The most common treatment at home for sleep apnea is to lose weight and exercise as well as sleeping on one's side. If home care treatments do not work, then doctors might recommend a continuous positive airway pressure (CPAP) machine, which includes wearing a mask over the nose and mouth while sleeping. The mask is hooked up to a machine that delivers a continuous flow of humidified air into the nose. This positive air pressure helps by opening the collapsed airway, thus returning normal and regular breathing.

If a CPAP does not alleviate the problem, then the next option for a patient with sleep apnea is surgery. This path of treatment is more geared for patients with a deviate septum, enlarged tonsils, and/or a small lower jaw. The most commonly performed surgeries to correct for sleep apnea are nasal surgery to correct nasal problems, uvulopalatopharyngoplasty (UPPP) which is a procedure to remove soft tissue on the back of the throat and palate (roof of the mouth) to increase the width of the airway, and mandibular maxillar advancement surgery to correct certain facial problems or throat obstructions.

Insomnia

Insomnia is generally described as difficulty falling asleep or staying asleep. Insomnia can have many different causes that are not limited to but include psychological stress (work deadlines), a poor sleep environment (television is turned on), or an inconsistent sleep schedule. Insomnia is often treated through behavioral changes like keeping a regular sleep schedule, avoiding strenuous activities right before bed, and reducing stimulants such as caffeine. Patients are encouraged to keep televisions and radios off at night as well as having heavy, darkening drapes that block out all sunlight. White noise appears to be a promising treatment for insomnia.

Causes of insomnia can include illness, depression, anxiety, or interferences in a normal sleep schedule such as jet lag or switching work schedules from day to night. Symptoms include sleepiness during the day, irritability, and problems with concentration and/or memory. The most common and effective treatment for insomnia is practicing good sleep habits and avoiding taking over-the-counter medication for insomnia. These medications may have undesired side effects as well as lose their effectiveness over time.

Good sleep habits or sleep hygiene consist of:

1. Going to sleep at the same time every night and waking up at the same time every morning. This includes weekend days—Saturdays and Sundays.
2. Not taking naps during the day as they can make the person less sleepy at night.
3. Avoiding caffeine in the afternoon or late at night as caffeine stimulates the brain and keeps a person from falling asleep.
4. Following a nighttime routine such as reading a book, listening to quieting music, and/or taking a warm bath to increase relaxation before going to sleep.
5. Setting a time limit. For example, if a person lies in bed for more than 20 minutes and cannot fall asleep, then they should get up and do something that is not overstimulating and may increase drowsiness. After the quieting activity, then try to sleep again.

Research

At the University of California-San Diego, a psychiatric sleep study was performed and enrolled more than 1 million adults. The results showed that people who live the longest report sleeping for six to seven hours every night. Another study performed in women that looked at sleep duration and its association with mortality risk showed similar results. In fact, other studies show that persons who sleep more than seven to eight hours per day have an increased risk of depression, which can cause a change in socioeconomic status.

Researchers at the University of Warwick and University College in London found that the lack of sleep can more than double the risk of death by cardiovascular disease (Ferrie et al., 2007). Too much sleep, however, can also result in doubling the risk of death but not primarily from cardiovascular disease. Finally, short sleep has been shown to be a risk factor for weight gain, hypertension, and type 2 diabetes. It is quite clear that REM sleep and sleep in general are active areas of research. Scientists are still trying to determine the function of sleep and REM sleep as well as why it is necessary for humans to sleep at all.

Renee Johnson

See also: Circadian Rhythm; Depression; Rapid Eye Movement (REM); Sleep Apnea (CPAP Treatment)

Further Reading

Ferrie, J. E., Shipley, M. J., Cappuccio, F. P., Brunner, E., Miller, M. A., Kumari, M., & Marmot, M. G. (2007). A prospective study of change in sleep duration: Associations with mortality in the Whitehall II cohort. *Sleep, 30*(12), 1659–1666.

National Institute of Neurological Disorders and Stroke (NINDS). (2007). *Brain basics: Understanding sleep.* Retrieved from http://www.ninds.nih.gov/disorders/brain_basics/understanding_sleep.htm

National Institute of Neurological Disorders and Stroke (NINDS). (2010). *NINDS sleep apnea information page.* Retrieved from http://www.ninds.nih.gov/disorders/sleep_apnea/sleep_apnea.htm

National Sleep Foundation. (2011). *Insomnia.* Retrieved from http://www.sleepfoundation.org/article/ask-the-expert/insomnia

Sleep Apnea (CPAP Treatment)

Sleep is essential for humans to properly function both mentally and physically. When a person does not receive the sleep they need, their immune system cannot fight illnesses and their brain cannot focus on complex ideas. *Sleep apnea* is a disorder where a person has difficulty breathing when asleep and does not receive the oxygen required, resulting in a change in blood chemistry. This causes the baroreceptors in the carotid artery to have the brain "wake" the person to breathe, which usually results in loud snoring and microarousals. The most common and best treatment for sleep apnea is to give the person a continuous positive airway by means of a machine. This machine is called a *continuous positive airway pressure* (CPAP), which applies and maintains a mild and continuous level of positive air into the mouth and nose of an abnormally breathing person. CPAP is often used most commonly for people who have breathing problems, such as sleep apnea, and for infants with underdeveloped lungs.

History

Australian physiologist Colin Sullivan (1945–) invented the CPAP machine to treat sleep apnea and sudden infant death syndrome (SIDS). The first of these machines were loud and bulky, but today they are much improved. Because of this invention many persons with sleep apnea can live more fulfilled lives.

Disease Types and Symptoms

Sleep apnea is a type of sleep disorder where breathing is shallow or infrequent during sleep. Each pause is called apnea, and can last up to 10 seconds to several minutes. In contrast, each shallow breathing episode is called a hypopnea. Physicians are able to diagnose sleep apnea by having the person complete an overnight sleep test, or *polysomnogram*. There are three types of sleep apnea: (1) *central* (CSA), (2) *obstructive* (OSA), and (3) *complex* (a combination of central and obstructive). In CSA, the person's breathing is interrupted because the part of the brain controlling breathing is compromised. In OSA, there is a true physical block to the airflow, such as the soft palate. Thus, the brain tells the respiratory centers to work harder to breathe, which usually results in snoring. In general, an individual with sleep apnea is rarely aware of having difficulty breathing while asleep. Sleep apnea is usually noticed by others observing the individual or by the effects on the body. The main side effect of sleep apnea is daytime sleepiness and fatigue. However, the individual has adjusted to this fatigue and thinks it is normal to feel tired all the time.

Treatment

Continuous positive airway pressure as a treatment or therapy for breathing disorders uses mild air pressure to keep the airway open. Infants with respiratory distress syndrome or bronchopulmonary dysplasia may be treated with CPAP to ease their breathing. Finally, in premature infants whose lungs have not fully developed, CPAP improves survival and decreases the need for steroid treatments for their lungs.

Patricia A. Bloomquist

See also: Baroreceptors; Sleep

Further Reading

National Heart, Lung, and Blood Institute. (2011). *What is CPAP?* Retrieved from http://www.nhlbi.nih.gov/health/health-topics/topics/cpap/

National Institute of Neurological Disorders and Stroke (NINDS). (2013). *NINDS sleep apnea information page.* Retrieved from http://www.ninds.nih.gov/disorders/sleep_apnea/sleep_apnea.htm

Society for Neuroscience

The *Society for Neuroscience* (www.sfn.org) is a professional group that supports scientists who are interested in furthering scientific research of the brain, nervous systems, and diseases of the nervous systems. Ralph W. Gerard created the Society for Neuroscience in 1969 so that neuroscientists and physicians throughout the world could share their scientific findings with each other. By integrating basic scientists and physicians from diverse cultures, members of the group are able to improve their knowledge as well as develop professional collaborations that may not have occurred otherwise. Members of the Society for Neuroscience range from undergraduate and graduate students to postdoctoral fellows and faculty from all stages of their career (such as middle school teachers to professors in college).

The Society for Neuroscience has an annual meeting that occurs generally in the fall of each year in North America. During the annual meeting, members present their data during poster sessions, platform presentations, symposia, and special lectures. The Society for Neuroscience also reaches out to thousands of communities in more than 80 countries through their annual Brain Awareness Week. This week is typically in the spring of every year, however, members present neuroscience education and outreach to their communities year round.

The Society for Neuroscience publishes the peer-reviewed journal: *The Journal of Neuroscience.* The goal of this journal is to include the most up-to-date and scientifically sound research in several neuroscience areas such as behavioral, systems (e.g., limbic, sensory, motor), cognitive (thinking), cellular, molecular, developmental, plasticity (changes induced by activity), and repair neuroscience as well as the neurobiology (the mechanisms) of neurological diseases. Another publication offered by the Society for Neuroscience is *BrainFacts.org*. This publication is for students of all ages and for the layperson that is interested in learning more about the central nervous system. *BrainFacts.org,* the book used during Brain

Awareness Week, is scientifically correct information that dispels several myths about the brain and nervous system.

Jennifer L. Hellier

See also: Introduction: Neuroscience Overview; Transgenic Mice

Further Reading

Society for Neuroscience. (2013). *Mission and strategic plan.* Retrieved from http://www .sfn.org/about/mission-and-strategic-plan

Sodium Channels

Sodium (Na^+) is a positively charged ion. In the central nervous system, it is essential for the development and continued propagation of an action potential (a neuronal signal or impulse). Sodium ions are highly concentrated in the extracellular fluid between neurons, which are specialized cells found only in the nervous system. However, when neurons send neural impulses between each other, specifically at the junction of where two neurons are located (the synaptic cleft), it causes a significant change in the receiving neuron (or postsynaptic neuron). Within the postsynaptic neuron, certain integral membrane proteins, called receptors or ion channels, will open allowing sodium ions to rush through. Because these ion channels conduct sodium through the plasma membrane they are generically called *sodium channels.* Sodium will flow down its concentration gradient and enter the postsynaptic neuron. This results in a change in the resting membrane potential (voltage difference across the membrane at rest, which is typically around −70 mV) of the postsynaptic neuron such that it is depolarized (becomes more positive and closer to 0 mV). If a cell depolarizes enough (to about −55 or −40 mV), it may result in the production of an action potential.

Types of Sodium Channels

Sodium channels are named by the way the protein is activated to allow sodium to flow. To date, there are two main classifications: *voltage-change receptors* and *ligand-gated receptors.* The voltage-change receptors are activated when the voltage of the membrane is altered. These receptors are also called voltage-dependent, voltage-sensitive, and voltage-gated sodium channels. They are universally designated as Na_v to denote the voltage requirement. Ligand-gated receptors are opened when a specific chemical (neurotransmitter) binds to specific sites on the receptor, such as acetylcholine. The binding of a ligand (which is also called an agonist) will induce a conformational change in the receptor, such that a closed pore or channel will open. Most ligand-gated sodium channels are nicotinic acetylcholine receptors found at the neuromuscular junction. The remainder of this entry will focus on voltage-change receptors as the ligand-gated sodium channels are discussed in the *Neuromuscular Junction* and *Acetylcholine and Its Receptor* entries of this encyclopedia.

Structure

For voltage-change sodium channels, there are two types of subunits: *alpha* and *beta*. This means there are different genes that encode for alpha subunit proteins and beta subunit proteins. To date there are nine known alpha subunits that are named $Na_v1.1$ through $Na_v1.9$, and four known beta subunits named SCN1B, SCN2B, SCN3B, and SCN4B. The alpha subunit is large enough that it can form its own channel, but usually it combines or interacts with one or two beta subunits. However, if a neuron only expresses alpha subunits, this protein will make its own channel that is functional, meaning it will conduct sodium ions in a voltage-gated way. In general, an alpha subunit will interact with a SCN1B or SCN3B subunit noncovalently, but will associate with a SCN2B or SCN4B subunit by a disulfide bond.

Alpha subunits consist of four repeat domains that are labeled I through IV. In each domain, there are six membrane-spanning segments that are labeled S1 through S6. This shows that the subunit is highly integrated within the membrane as it passes through the plasma membrane 24 times, forming a circle or pore. Segment S4 is highly conserved—meaning it has almost identical sequencing in all alpha subunits—and is the voltage sensor for the channel. When this sensor detects a change in transmembrane voltage, each segment S4 moves within the cell membrane to be closer to the extracellular side so that the pore is formed and will open. To ensure that only sodium ions can pass through the newly opened pore, the external portion of the pore (in the extracellular space) makes a narrow passageway that is large enough for sodium ions but not for other ions. This is performed by the "P-loops" that are found between each S5 and S6 segment on the extracellular side. With the rotation of the S4 segments, the P-loops come closer together forming the passageway into the pore. On the intracellular side of the pore, the S5 and S6 segments of each domain make up the internal portion of the pore. Finally, the pore can be blocked or "plugged" by the linking sections between the III and IV domains. This is a safety mechanism for the cell to inactivate the channel if its activity has been prolonged.

A way to imagine how a sodium channel opens and closes, one can think of a movable bridge, with the bridge being the pore or channel and the automobiles the sodium ions. Think of the bridge as being in the up position the majority of the time so that the boats below can travel along the river. Imagine one side of the bridge as the outside of the cell or extracellular, the other side of the bridge as the inside of the cell or intracellular, and the bridge itself as the sodium channel. When the bridge is up, the "extracellular cars" cannot get inside the cell. However, when the bridge is down, meaning the sodium channel changed its shape, the "extracellular cars" can now cross and enter the cell. The signal to move the bridge is a line of cars or the time of day, which represents the voltage change across the membrane.

Function

Voltage-change sodium channels are commonly called voltage-gated based on their gating activities or states. There are three main states a sodium channel can be in at one time: *activated* (open), *deactivated* (closed), and *inactivated* (closed). In the activated state, the sodium channel opens in a response to a change of transmembrane voltage, specifically at the site where the sodium channel is located. This is important because depolarization is a localized event that can propagate through the neuron's plasma membrane. If several synapses arrive at the same time to a single neuron, these localized depolarizations can summate and propagate together and possibly produce an action potential.

When the sodium channel is closed it can be in one of two different states. The deactivated state is the normal state of the channel. The sodium channel has activation gates (part of the protein channel) on the extracellular side that block the pore. It is when these gates move out of the way so that the pore can form during the movement of the S4 segments and the P-loops when the membrane potential begins to depolarize. This then causes the open state when sodium ions rush into the cell further depolarizing the cell. However, there is a maximum amount a cell will depolarize, resulting in the sodium channels inactivating themselves by plugging the pore with the intracellular linking section between the III and IV domains. These are called the inactivation gates, which are like a ball and chain where the ball will plug the intracellular portion of the pore. Thus, sodium can no longer enter the cell, which stops the depolarization. Sodium is removed from the cell to reset the "stage" by ion exchange pumps or by exiting through other channels. When the voltage returns near resting membrane potentials, the inactivation gates unplug the pore while the activation gates close the pore from the extracellular side. This is a process called deinactivation.

The function of beta subunits has recently been better understood. When the alpha subunit is coexpressed with a beta subunit, the result is modulation of the kinetic properties of the sodium channel. This means that the speed the sodium channel conducts sodium ions through it will alter, the length of inactivation periods will change, and/or the voltage change required to activate the channel will differ. Since there are several combinations of sodium channels with each having the same goal of depolarizing the neuron (by fluxing sodium ions), small changes in their kinetic properties define their specialized roles in different parts of the central nervous system.

Diseases and Disorders

There are so many different types of sodium alpha and beta subunits and the genes that encode for them, if a mutation occurs it can result in significant neurological diseases and/or disorders. In fact, studying these disease states, such as epilepsy, helped researchers better understand the role and function of voltage-change sodium channels. For instance, the *SCN1A* gene encodes for the Nav1.1 protein, which is typically found throughout the central nervous system and cardiac myocytes. Mutations in the *SCN1A* have been associated with inherited febrile epilepsy, West syndrome, intractable childhood epilepsy with generalized tonic-clonic seizures, familial hemiplegic migraine, familial autism, and Lennox-Gastaut syndrome, to name a few. The *SCN2A* gene encodes for the Nav1.2 protein, which is typically found through the central and peripheral nervous systems. Mutated Nav1.2 proteins, have been associated with inherited febrile seizures and epilepsy. Finally, the last sodium channel mutation that is known to be associated with epilepsy is within the Nav1.6 protein (*SCN8A* gene). These channels are found in the central and peripheral nervous systems, cardiac myocytes, and glia cells. Because several voltage-change sodium channels have such a large role in the pathophysiology of seizures and epilepsy, about 24 antiepileptic drugs have been designed to block these abnormal sodium channels (Zuliani et al., 2012). This is a therapeutic attempt to stabilize the inactivation period of these sodium channels that have shown some success in reducing the chances of additional seizures. It is important to note, however, that antiepileptic drugs do not cure the epilepsy. Instead it just lessens the chances for future seizures.

Jennifer L. Hellier

See also: Acetylcholine and Its Receptors; Autism; Epilepsy; Ion Channels; Lennox-Gastaut Syndrome; Migraine; Neuromuscular Junction; Seizures

Further Reading

Albuquerque, E. X., Pereira, E. F., Alkondon, M., & Rogers, S. W. (2009). Mammalian nicotinic acetylcholine receptors: From structure to function. *Physiological Reviews, 89*(1), 73–120.

Hillel, B. (2001). *Ion channels of excitable membranes* (3rd ed.). Sunderland, MA: Sinauer.

Kandel, E. R., Schwartz, J. H., Jessell, T. M., Siegelbaum, S. A., & Hudspeth, A. J. (Eds.). (2012). *Principles of neural science* (5th ed.). New York, NY: McGraw-Hill.

Yu, F. H., & Catterall, W. A. (2003). Overview of the voltage-gated sodium channel family. *Genome Biology, 4*(3), 207. Retrieved from http://www.ncbi.nlm.nih.gov/pmc/articles /PMC153452/

Zuliani, V., Fantini, M., & Rivara, M. (2012).Sodium channel blockers as therapeutic target for treating epilepsy: Recent updates. *Current Topics in Medicinal Chemistry, 12*(9), 962–970.

Somatosensory Cortex/Somatosensory System

In the mammalian central nervous system, the *somatosensory cortex* (or *somatosensory system*) is crucial to senses such as pain, touch, temperature, and spatial orientation (a sensation termed proprioception). The system consists of a network of neurons that work together to sense and then to process this information. The network of neurons will be described in three different divisions called *first-order neurons, second-order neurons,* and *third-order neurons.*

Location

The sensing portion of the system involves a somatic (body) receptor that is within the skin, bones, muscles, joints, eyes, and ears. These specialized receptors will pick up sensory information and begin a sensory impulse. This sensory receptor is on a neuron that is considered the first-order neuron or primary afferent neuron for sensory information. This neuron comes from the periphery and will travel the afferent pathway (toward the central nervous system.) For most of the sensory neurons, their cell body (or soma) is located in the dorsal root ganglion (a group of cell bodies outside of the central nervous system) just lateral of the spinal cord. For sensation to the head, neck, and face, these nuclei (a group of cell bodies inside of the central nervous system) are found in the brainstem and are named for the cranial nerve that carries the sensory and/or motor information to the central nervous system.

The secondary neuron is an interneuron. This secondary neuron will receive information from the first-order neuron's axon terminal, where neuronal information is transferred from one neuron to another. Some of these second-order neurons may send their axons to cross over to the other side of the spinal cord or brainstem before carrying the information to the thalamus, which is a deep relay structure within the brain. All second order-neurons will synapse in the thalamus, except for the sense of smell.

Lastly, the third-order neuron is located in the thalamus, which is made up of several different nuclei. The second-order neuron synapses on the third-order neuron. Here the sensory information is transferred and then carried to the correct sensory area of the cerebrum, such as the primary visual cortex for vision and the somatosensory cortex for pain, temperature, touch, and proprioception.

In the brain the somatosensory system involves the thalamus, reticular formation, and the postcentral gyrus, which is found posterior to the central sulcus in the parietal lobe of the cerebral cortex. Along the surface of the postcentral gyrus, the body is mapped from the midline to the temporal lobe. This means that a specific body region is located in a specific region of the postcentral gyrus. This map is called a *homunculus,* meaning "little man." The purpose of the thalamus is to act as the relay center from the spinal cord or brainstem to the homunculus. This is the same as the reticular formation, but the reticular formation acts as a relay for the spinal cord or brainstem to the thalamus. The homunculus is the main processing center of the somatosensory system. It processes the sensory impulses received from the thalamus. If a reaction is necessary, such as to move away from a heat source, this sensory information in the cerebral cortex will be transferred to the motor cortex to respond.

Pathways

The somatosensory system has specific ascending pathways that are dependent on the information carried and how they ascend. It is important to note that the terms "tract" (a group of fibers or axons) and "pathway" may be interchangeable, and that these tracts are named by where they are located in the central nervous system and/ or where they originate and then terminate. One of the pathways is the *anterolateral tract.* In these *spinothalamic pathways,* the first step is the first-order neuron. It carries the sensory impulse for touch, pressure, pain, and temperature. The neuron then enters the spinal cord and synapses in the posterior gray horns. The secondary neuron then decussates (crosses) the impulse by the ventral white commissure to the contralateral (opposite) side where it ascends to the thalamus. The thalamus then directs the signal to the correct area.

There are three types of pathways for the anterolateral tract. They are (1) *lateral spinothalamic tract,* (2) *anterior spinothalamic tract,* and (3) *spinoreticulothalamic tract.* The lateral spinothalamic tract is a pathway that carries pain and temperature. The cell body of the secondary neuron is located in the dorsal horn of the spinal cord. It will decussate via the ventral white commissure and then ascend within the lateral funiculus. Upon reaching the posterolateral nucleus of the thalamus, it will then project the impulse to the postcentral gyrus of the cerebrum. The anterior spinothalamic pathway is much like the lateral pathway except it carries crude touch sensory information. Additionally, instead of ascending through the lateral funiculus the anterior spinothalamic tract will ascend through the anterior funiculus. Finally, the spinoreticulothalamic tract is different as its cell bodies are located in the substantia gelatinosa, a more anterior and slightly medial region of the dorsal horn. These then decussate to the spinoreticular tract and ascend to the reticular formation in the brainstem. From there the impulse is sent to the thalamus. This is different from all the ascending pathways because it synapses into the reticular formation in the brainstem rather than going straight to the thalamus.

Another type of ascending pathway is the *posterior column* or *lemniscus pathway* of the spinal cord. This pathway carries highly localized information to the central nervous system. There are two important nuclei that these paths with terminate. One of these pathways, called the *fasciculus gracilis,* sends impulses that involve fine touch, proprioception, vibration, and pressure from the inferior half of the body (legs and trunk) to the central nervous system. The first-order neuron synapses to the nucleus gracilis where it will then decussate and ascend to the thalamus. The *fasciculus cuneatus* pathway sends those same impulses but from the arms and upper body to the central nervous system. However, the fasciculus cuneatus will go through the nucleus cuneatus before decussating and ascending to the thalamus.

Since these pathways involve multiple relay stations they can be vulnerable to injury. If there were damage to an area anywhere along these pathways, it can lead to the loss of sensation. However, these paths act as a type of anastomosis of the nerves and will provide backup routes for pain and temperature impulses, as these sensations are important for survival. For example, if the spinal cord is damaged on one side, the person would still be able to feel pain and possibly temperature. However, if the spinal cord is damaged completely through, the person may not be able to sense anything.

Aaron Jones

See also: Anterolateral Tract (Anterolateral System); Discriminative Touch; Homunculus; Motor Cortex; Sensory Receptors; Pain; Thalamus; Thermal Sense (Temperature Sensation); Touch

Further Reading

Dougherty, P., & Tsuchitani, C. (1997). Somatosensory systems. In *Neuroscience Online, an electronic textbook for the neurosciences* (Chap. 2). Open-access educational resource provided by the Department of Neurobiology and Anatomy at the University of Texas Medical School at Houston. Retrieved from http://neuroscience.uth.tmc.edu/s2/chapter02.html

Kandel, E. R., Schwartz, J. H., Jessell, T. M., Siegelbaum, S. A., & Hudspeth, A. J. (Eds.). (2012). *Principles of neural science* (5th ed.). New York, NY: McGraw-Hill.

Purves, D., Augustine, G. J., Fitzpatrick, D., Hall, W. C., LaMantia, A.-S., McNamara, J. O., & Williams, S. M. (Eds.). (2004). *Neuroscience* (3rd ed.). Sunderland, MA: Sinauer Associates.

Spasm

In medical terms, a *spasm* is an involuntary muscle contraction with a sudden burst of pain. It is usually recognized as a muscle cramp or a "Charley horse." Muscle cramps are usually harmless and end within a few minutes. As a result of an involuntary muscle activity, a spasm can also be a burst of activity, anxiety, emotion, energy, eustress (good stress), or stress. Abnormal nerve stimulations or abnormal muscle activities have been attributed to spasms. In rare cases, *spasmisms* may occur, which is a series of spasms or permanent spasms of a muscle or a group of muscles.

Spasms are classified based on what part of the body is affected. There are artery spasms, bladder spasms, coronary spasms (of the heart), esophageal spasms, facial spasms (tics), infantile spasms (seizures), and muscle spasms, just to name a few.

Causes, Signs, and Symptoms

The causes of spasms may include overloading the muscle, causing fatigue, being dehydrated, and having insufficient electrolytes within the body (which may be associated with dehydration). Electrolytes include sodium, potassium, calcium, magnesium, chloride, hydrogen phosphate, and hydrogen carbonate, which are generally added to Pedialyte and sports drinks like Gatorade. However, sports drinks generally have added sugars that are not necessary for rehydration and should be taken sparingly.

Similar to seizures, spasms are symptoms of *paroxysmal attacks* or *paroxysms* (a sudden attack or outburst). These short, frequent symptoms can be observed in many clinical conditions such as asthma, breath-holding spells, dystonias (abnormal tone of the muscles), encephalitis, epilepsy, general head trauma, malaria, multiple sclerosis, pertussis, stroke, and trigeminal neuralgia (pain of the trigeminal nerve). In any type of spasm, it may damage the muscles, tendons, or ligaments that are involved in the spasm. This occurs only when the force of the spasm is greater than the tensile strength of the underlying connective tissues.

Syncope, or simple fainting, can be characterized with spasms that look like epileptic seizures. However, syncope and epileptic seizures are not the same condition. Syncope occurs when there is decrease in cerebral perfusion by oxygenated blood, meaning the brain does not receive enough oxygen. This causes the person to faint and have muscle spasms. Syncope can occur at anytime (like in a hot room) without any serious side effects. In some cases, however, an underlying cause or neurological disorder may trigger syncope that may become serious or life threatening.

Other types of spasm include hypertonic spasm and colic. Hypertonic spasm is a malfunctioning of nerve feedback to the central nervous system. This causes the muscle to continually contract and not to relax. It is a serious type of spasm as it can become permanent and damage the muscles, tendons, and ligaments. It is often seen in patients with a neurological condition such as Huntington's disease, spinal cord injuries, and/or stroke. Colic is the pain of smooth muscle spasms in a particular organ. The sensation of colic makes a person to want to move around, but the pain can cause nausea or vomiting if severe.

Patricia A. Bloomquist

See also: Aneurysm; Epilepsy; Stroke

Further Reading

Pavone, P., Striano, P., Falsaperla, R., Pavone, L., & Ruggieri, M. (2013). Infantile spasms syndrome, West syndrome and related phenotypes: What we know in 2013. *Brain Development.* pii: S0387–7604(13)00298–2.

Zaya, M., Mehta, P. K., & Bairey-Merz, C. N. (2013). Provocative testing for coronary reactivity and spasm. *Journal of the American College of Cardiology.* pii: S0735–1097(13)05882–8.

Speech

Speech is a neurological process in which the brain executes a verbal response to various forms of stimuli. Stimuli may be auditory (temporal lobe), visual (occipital lobe), or sensory via touch (parietal lobe). Because there are numerous triggers for speech production, the process involves a complicated connection of circuits in the brain. As a result of the varying stimulations, the brain integrates the incoming information into *Wernicke's area,* the language center, to interpret the stimuli. The information then activates *Broca's area,* the inferior region of the frontal lobe that houses speech, to produce a verbal response. In order for the muscles of speech to function, however, *Broca's area* must communicate with the precentral gyrus region on the frontal lobe to initiate the literal lexical movements. Understanding these functions is essential for analyzing effective communication and speech disorders. A lesion or dysfunction of some sort to any of these areas may result in speech difficulty or inability altogether. The process of speech also reveals the complexity of the cranium in its ability to integrate many types of information and activate a chain of responses in a matter of milliseconds. Most importantly, speech is an essential factor in everyday life, and thus determines lifestyle and one's ability to interact with the outside world.

History and Development

The first primary discoverer of speech functions was Pierre Paul Broca (1824–1880), a French surgeon from the mid-19th century. His research escalated when one of his patients had severe speech difficulties, leading him to believe that such dysfunction was a result of frontal lobe damage. Soon after the patient's death in 1861, the autopsy revealed a lesion to the frontal lobe, confirming his theory. In following years, Broca's expanded findings were well received by various societies and research centers, as fellow scientists were anxious to localize speech functions to specific areas in the brain (Dronkers et al., 2007). In analyzing future patients, Broca became more convinced of his frontal lobe speculation. He found that those suffering from speech disorders had lesions in the area of the inferior frontal gyrus of the frontal lobe, primarily on the left side of the brain. This region soon became known as *Broca's area,* and damage to this area was labeled as Broca's aphasia (Dronkers et al., 2007). Additionally, the trend of speech stemming from the left hemisphere became known as lateralization. Ten years later, Carl Wernicke (1848–1905), a German psychiatrist and neurologist, discovered a similar area in the brain that plays a part in speech production. He did extensive studies in the superior gyrus of the temporal lobe (Wernicke's area), discovering that it was responsible for speech comprehension and reception of language (Duchan, 2011). Similar to Broca's aphasia, defects in this area are known as Wernicke's aphasia. Wernicke is also well known for his enlightenment in sensory aphasias that affect verbal expression in general. The combination of Broca and Wernicke's findings in the 19th century provided a significant basis for understanding the neurological process of speech production.

Scientists progressively discovered more in these areas—discovering that the lateral sulcus in the left hemisphere contains a neural loop that allows the brain to understand and produce verbal expression. The frontal end is Broca's area, which directs language output, and the posterior end is Wernicke's area, which integrates language input. These regions are connected by nervous fibers known as the *arcuate fascilicus,* which direct pathway communication between the two areas. The progression of speech discovery has revealed many mysteries regarding the complexities of the brain, and has set a foundation for scientists to better understand lesions and disorders today.

Current Implications

Due to development in scientific understanding, the process of speech is much better understood today. Scientists have built off Broca's lateralization theory and have found that 97 percent of right-handed people speak from the left hemisphere, 19 percent of left-handed people speak via the right hemisphere, and about

19 percent of them have some language capabilities in both hemispheres (Boeree, 2004). In combining both Broca's and Wernicke's studies, the language process is currently described as the speech loop—information is received (read or heard) and integrated into Wernicke's area, travels into Broca's area to prepare a vocal response, and then loops up into the cortical region to connect to the musculature and execute speech. Interestingly enough, this speech loop stimulation has been witnessed in deaf patients that speak in sign language. Therefore, the loop process is not limited to spoken or heard speech, but rather occurs with communication in general. Wernicke's area is important for social development because, upon hearing speech, it stores verbal and physical patterns so that the brain is able to retrieve the meaning of a word. In regard to reading words, however, the visual cortex receives information, transfers it to the angular gyrus, and then sends the information to Wernicke's area for processing. Wernicke's area is able to put the incoming information into context and send the information via the arcuate fasciculus and into Broca's area for speech pronunciation. Unfortunately, this loop model only covers the basics of language pathways. Because it assumes that each step happens sequentially and in a select order, it fails to truly explain the complex neurological process. The brain is extremely complex and the precise pattern for speech is not extensively understood.

In addition to expanding upon the loop process of speech, scientists have since found more functional roles of Broca's area. As Broca himself discovered, it is responsible for controlling the muscles of articulation, and patients with lesions to that area tend to either be mute or have difficulty producing words. However, more recent studies have questioned the original nomenclature used by Broca while he performed his studies. The area that he believed to be "Broca's area" is only the posterior third of what scientists now refer to as Broca's area (Dronkers et al., 2007). This region, which he believed was critical for speech, was more broad and generalized. Since then, scientists have redefined and expanded upon his original discoveries. Today, Broca's area is seen to deal with speech execution as well as some comprehension of complex sentences, gesture interpretation, and action cognition. This was seen in patients with weak stimulation in Broca's areas while they communicated with nongesturing companions (Skipper et al., 2007). Thanks to Broca's research, scientists have been able to further study this area, causing it to evolve into neuropsychology, speech-language pathology, neurolinguistics, and cognitive neuroscience (Dronkers et al., 2007). His studies have set up a tremendous platform for researchers to better understand the complexity of the networks involved in speech, language, and comprehension.

Another way to understand language via the brain's hemispheres is through analyzing nonverbal language. While the left hemisphere interprets the meaning and structure of the words, the right hemisphere analyzes the emotional context behind the words and nonverbal communication. Appearance, visual attitude, and gestures, all cultivate a certain context that will coincide with the verbal output. Additionally, the speaker's tone, expression, inflection, and emphases further influence the meaning of the words—all of which is interpreted by the right side of the brain. The two hemispheres must work together in order to interpret both the literal (practical) meaning and the suggested (emotional) meaning of the words. As a result, lesions to either of these areas dramatically affect the patient's social comprehension. For example, a lesion on the left side of the brain can alter the person's ability to formulate sentences, speak fluently, or interpret literal verbal language. A lesion on the right hemisphere, however, damages the person's ability to decipher sarcasm, metaphorical language, or expressions. In the meantime, the corpus callosum works to mediate and connect the information processed on each side, and enables them to communicate with each other so that the person may speak with clarity and understanding. Speech comprehension is essential for effective verbal performance, and is important for scientific study so that doctors may better understand and treat speech disorders.

Similar to bihemispherical coordination, neurological analysts have recently found that the right side of the brain is even involved in the verbal process of speech as well. The study's subjects were asked to repeat made-up words "kig" and "pob" while being examined with specialized internal electrodes to measure impulses and stimulations. The results displayed that nonwords stimulated the right hemisphere, while actual English words stimulated the left side in concordance with Broca's theory. Thus, the scientists were able to differentiate between language (left) and speech (left and right) in the brain (Cogan et al., 2014). However, the left side is still considered the dominant hemisphere that controls speech because without it, the patient would be completely unable to speak. It also relates more to verbal execution and language interpretation—causing it to be the key player in speech and communication.

Speech pathologists have even discovered speech function beyond Broca's area. Contrary to Broca's findings that the inferior frontal gyrus of the frontal lobe was the area responsible for speech, recent studies in lesion patients have indicated otherwise. Such studies reveal that the brain is able to process and execute language even after damage to Broca's area due to stored patterns and the plasticity of the brain. Because the brain is a dynamic organ (neural plasticity), it is able to retrieve previously stored information as well as recover from trauma. This takes place in the right hemisphere (Plaza et al., 2009).

Although Broca's and Wernicke's areas are in separate regions, the arcuate fascilicus allows them to connect efficiently so that communication is possible. Damage to these fibers, however, typically results in a condition known as conduction aphasia. Patients with this aphasia are able to comprehend language, but they struggle in speaking fluently and in repeating words or sentences (Boeree, 2004).

Similarly, the angular gyrus, located halfway between Wernicke's area and the visual cortex of the occipital lobe, is responsible for allowing the person to read and write. As a result, trauma to this region can lead to problems such as alexia (inability to read), dyslexia (difficulty with reading), and agraphia (inability to write; Boeree, 2004). While the angular gyrus is not directly an actor in the correspondence process, it is a significant contributor in its enabling of the brain to speak through script and to receive communication.

Finally, the last primary actor in speech is the primary motor cortex. Located in the posterior region of the frontal lobe, the primary motor cortex is responsible for voluntary motor control. Although it controls all general musculature, it is able to target the muscles of speech, specifically. Upon receiving stimulation from Broca's area, the motor cortex causes the vocal organs to respond according to the command. Damage to this area may affect speech abilities, but the difficulties become more anatomical and less neurological due to the motor cortex's direct relationship with the muscles. Neurologically speaking, however, the primary motor cortex is the final important step in producing speech and language. Without any of the key regions, communication would be nearly impossible.

In future research, scientists are aiming to better articulate the specificities in the loop model, and the overlapping of steps. Because the brain is so intricate and complex, the individual processes of speech can easily become convoluted and difficult to differentiate. While research studies have shed light on the issue, there is much more to be explored. The issue of bilateral stimulation also falls into this category. Tremendous discoveries have been made in regard to deciphering which regions associate with certain social situations, but the details of the neural circuitry still remain a mystery. Scientists may never fully understand all the ways the brain is able to integrate and store such information—but the approaches thus far have substantially improved clinicians' ability to diagnose and treat those who suffer from speech dysfunction. Most importantly, speech is important to study because of its significance in human interaction and development. Its influence on culture, relationships, and humanity as a whole is something neither science nor history can ever overlook.

Brianna Lynch

See also: Agraphia; Alexia; Aphasia; Broca's Area; Dyslexia; Language; Motor Cortex; Wernicke's Area

Further Reading

Boeree, C. G. (2004). Speech and the brain. *Webspace.* Retrieved from http://webspace .ship.edu/cgboer/speechbrain.html

Cogan, G. B., Thesen, T., Carlson, C., Doyle, W., Devinsky, O., & Pesaran, B. (2014). Sensory-motor transformations for speech occur bilaterally. *Nature.* doi: 10.1038/nature12935. [Epub ahead of print].

Dronkers, N. F., Plaisant, O., Iba-Zizen, M. T., & Cabanis, E. A. (2007). Paul Broca's historic cases: High resolution MR imaging of the brains of Leborgne and Lelong. *Oxford Journal, 130*, 1432–1441. doi:10.1093/brain/awm042.

Duchan, J. (2011). A history of speech—language pathology. *Buffalo.edu.* Retrieved from http://www.acsu.buffalo.edu/~duchan/new_history/hist19c/subpages/wernicke.html

McGill University. (n. d.). *Broca's area, Wernicke's area, and other language-processing areas in the brain.* TheBrain.McGill.ca. Retrieved from http://thebrain.mcgill.ca/flash/d/d_10/d_10_cr/d_10_cr_lan/d_10_cr_lan.html

Plaza, M., Gatignol, P., Leroy, M., & Duffau, H. (2009). Speaking without Broca's area after tumor resection. *Neurocase, 4*, 294–310. doi: 10.1080/13554790902729473.

Skipper, J. I., Goldin-Meadow, S., Nusbaum, H. C., & Small, S. L. (2007). Speech-associated gestures, Broca's area, and the human mirror system. *Brain and Language, 3*, 260–277.

Spina Bifida

Spina bifida, also known as cleft spine or open spine, is a birth defect that is a type of a neural tube disorder. The neural tube in the embryo is the precursor to the central nervous system, which includes the brain and spinal cord. Spina bifida occurs when the neural tube does not close properly during the fourth week of pregnancy. This causes the spinal cord and nerves to be damaged because the vertebrae are not properly fused together. In extreme cases, the spinal cord can protrude through the opening and be exposed to the external environment. If this occurs, the spinal cord is usually encased in a fluid-filled sac.

Within the United States, there are 1,500 babies born with spina bifida each year (CDC, 2013). It has the highest rate of incidence in Hispanic communities and internationally in the Irish and Welsh communities. The rate of spina bifida has been on the decline since the implementation of pregnancy screenings and the development of performing restorative surgery in utero (NINDS, 2013).

History

The history of spina bifida spans numerous centuries, as different medical technologies were developed to treat the condition. In the 1600s, Dutch physician Nicolaes Tulp (1593–1674) was the first person to describe the signs and symptoms of the disorder as well as coin the term spina bifida. During the 1950s, spina bifida was mainly associated with one of its symptoms, hydrocephalus

SPINA BIFIDA

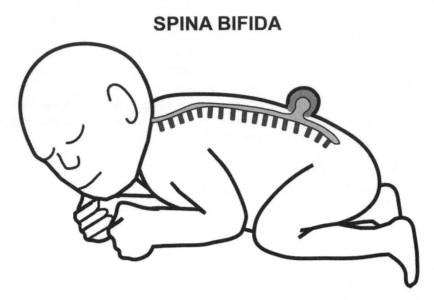

Spina bifida is a congenital condition affecting the spine and is caused by an incomplete closure of the neural tube during fetal development. (ABC-CLIO)

(abnormal increased amounts of cerebrospinal fluid in the brain). Treatment was to implant a valve to shunt the excess fluid; however, these valves were inept and irritated the body. In 1955, hydraulics engineer James A. Holter (1916–2003) had a son Charles Case Holter (1955–1960) who was born with spina bifida. When Holter saw the type of valve that was used to treat his son, he decided to invent his own valve that would improve the technology. Holter collaborated with Eugene Bernard Spitz (1919–2006), a pediatric neurosurgeon at the Children's Hospital in Philadelphia, and created the Spitz-Holter shunt. This device is still used today and it is estimated that 15,000 shunts are implanted yearly.

In 1967, pediatric surgeons at The Children's Hospital in Sheffield, United Kingdom, realized that treating patients early in life with aggressive surgery resulted in better long-term outcomes for the child. However, the optimism in treating children with spina bifida began to generally decrease in the late 1970s to early 1980s. Researchers began to argue that a child's quality of life decreased so much that it would be better for them to not live at all. Unfortunately, this debate was occurring at the same time treatment was improving due to technological advances. To this day, a natural pessimism toward children diagnosed with spina bifida exists in the medical community. However, recent strides from the families of children with spina bifida and even those with the disorder are now speaking out. They can conclude that it is possible for individuals with spina bifida to lead successful and healthy lives.

Types and Symptoms

There are four main types of spina bifida based on the severity of the damage done to the spinal cord. The first type is *occult spinal dysraphism* (OSD). This is usually seen as a dimple or a red mark on an infant's back. Physiologically this indicates that the spinal cord did not grow properly in embryonic development, which can result in serious complications. The second type is *spina bifida occulta,* or "hidden spina bifida." This type typically does no harm and usually the individual does not even know that they have this condition. It may not result in pain or other neurological conditions, and it is diagnosed by X-ray. The third type is *meningocele* and has a physical attribute. In this type, a sac of nervous fluid is found on the outside of the body. Fortunately, there is no major nerve damage and there are only minor disabilities involved. The final and most debilitating type is *myelomeningocele.* In this type, there is an external sac filled with damaged nerve endings and even the spinal cord. Another symptom is abnormal fluid buildup in the brain. Both of these symptoms can cause severe disabilities affecting loss of sensation in the lower limbs, and including difficulty in using the bathroom.

The more common symptoms associated with spina bifida are *paralysis, bladder control issues, deformed bones, irritated skin,* and *abnormal eye movements.* Neurological complications can also result in trouble with executive functioning. Damage to the central nervous system can prohibit the different parts communicating with each other effectively. For example, the corpus callosum can be damaged or underdeveloped. This results in poor coordination between the left and right hemispheres of the brain, which leads to difficulties in problem solving, mobility, and integrating emotions and experiences. It has also been seen that individuals with spina bifida have difficulty with academics and socializing with their peers. However, even with all of these difficulties it is essential to know that these individuals have still been able to become educated and enjoy their lives.

Treatments and Outcomes

Today, significant research is performed on preventing and screening for the syndrome. Although no one knows what causes spina bifida, it has been discovered that expectant mothers can greatly decrease the chance that their child will be born with the disease with the intake of folic acid. Scientists have yet to discover how this works; however, it has proven to be so effective that the United States has mandated folate-enriched grain products as of 1998. There are also three primary screenings that all pregnant women are encouraged to have. The most effective screening is the alpha-fetoprotein (AFP) screening, which looks for the abundance of AFP. Higher occurrences indicate that the fetus has spina bifida.

For children that are born with spina bifida it is highly important that their doctors take aggressive measures as soon as possible, even within 12 to 24 hours of the child's birth. Depending on the severity of the disability, different physical therapies and surgeries can be utilized to help treat the patient.

Future

There is much promise in the field of spina bifida. As advocacy and treatment options have grown, the outlook for individuals diagnosed with spina bifida have gotten much better. The biggest problem is now making the transition from pediatric to adult health care. As the mortality rate decreases and the quality of life increases, it is imperative that these individuals be afforded the opportunity to successfully continue their lives.

Cynthia M. Joseph

See also: Cerebrospinal Fluid; Embryonic Development of the Nervous System; Hydrocephalus; Neural Tube

Further Reading

Center for Disease Control and Prevention (CDC). (2013). *Spina bifida.* Retrieved from http://www.cdc.gov/ncbddd/spinabifida/facts.html

Liptak, G. S. (2012). *What is spina bifida?* Retrieved from http://www.spinabifidaassociation.org/site/c.evKRI7OXIoJ8H/b.8277225/k.5A79/What_is_Spina_Bifida.htm

National Institute of Neurological Disorders and Stroke (NINDS). (2013). *Spina bifida fact sheet.* Retrieved from http://www.ninds.nih.gov/disorders/spina_bifida/detail_spina_bifida.htm

Spinal Cord

The *spinal cord* is an important component of the central nervous system. It provides two major functions for the body. First, it is the structure that connects and integrates the brain with the rest of the body through the transmission of action potentials (nerve impulses) to and from the brain and the periphery. Second, the spinal cord is the location of *spinal reflexes* which provide the body with a mechanism to respond quickly and automatically to external stimuli. The spinal cord is a continuation of the *medulla oblongata* of the *brainstem*. It begins at the *foramen magnum* (a natural large opening) of the skull and travels through the *vertebral foramen*, which are the large openings found in the posterior aspect of all the vertebral bodies of the bony spinal column. It is approximately 17 inches in length and ends at the level of the second lumbar vertebral body where it becomes the *cauda equina*, a collection of axons that projects from the tip of the spinal cord called the *conus medullaris*. The spinal cord is composed of *tracts* or large bundles of axons that carry sensory information from the body to the brain (*ascending tracts* or *afferent tracts*), tracts that carry motor information from the brain to the rest of the body (*descending tracts* or *efferent tracts*), and as a coordination center for many involuntary spinal reflexes. It is protected by three tissues layers called the *meninges*, which include the outermost layer called the *dura mater*, a middle layer called the *arachnoid mater*, and the innermost layer called the *pia mater*.

Location and Segmentation of the Spinal Cord

The human spinal cord is approximately 17 inches (43 centimeters) in length. It is divided into the *cervical region* (C_1–C_8), the *thoracic region* (T_1–T_{12}), and the *lumbar region* (L_1–L_2 as the spinal cord, and L_3–L_5 as the cauda equina). There are two areas of the spinal cord that are enlarged in diameter. These include the *cervical enlargement* which extends from C_3 to T_2 and is where nerves that innervate the upper extremities exit and enter the spinal cord, and the *lumbar enlargement* which extends from L_1 to S_3 and is where nerves that innervate the lower extremities exit and enter the spinal cord. The spinal cord passes through the *vertebral foramen* of each of the vertebral bodies of the vertebral column. Projections known as *spinal nerves* enter and exit the spinal cord at each vertebral level and carry information to and from the body and the spinal cord.

Nerves of the cervical region of the spinal cord control the muscles of the neck, shoulder, upper arm, lower arm, hand, and wrist. The diaphragm, which is critical for breathing, is also controlled by nerves from the cervical region of the spinal cord. Nerves from the thoracic region of the spinal cord control the muscles of the chest, especially those related to breathing (the *intercostal muscles*) as well as the muscles of the abdomen. Nerves from the lumbar region of the spinal cord control the muscles of the hip, thigh, lower leg, ankle, and foot.

The Meninges and Spaces of the Spinal Cord

The spinal cord is surrounded by three tissue coverings that serve to protect the spinal cord and create specific spaces that also serve to support the spinal cord. These coverings and spaces include:

- The *dura mater,* which is the outermost covering of the spinal cord. It is composed of fibrous connective tissues and acts to protect the spinal cord as well as help anchor it in place within the vertebral foramen. The region between the dura mater and the bone of the vertebral body is called the *epidural space* and is filled with *adipose tissue* (fat) that has many blood vessels within it. The space below the dura mater and the underlying arachnoid mater is known as the *subdural space.*
- The *arachnoid mater,* which is the middle tissue layer of the spinal cord. The arachnoid is very vascular and provides vascular support to the tissues surrounding the spinal cord. The space below the arachnoid and the underlying pia mater is known as the *subarachnoid space.* The subarachnoid space is where *cerebrospinal fluid* is located. Cerebrospinal fluid bathes the spinal cord and brain and helps provide both nutritive support as well as protection.
- The *pia mater,* which is the innermost tissue layer of the spinal cord. The pia mater lies directly against the nervous tissues of the spinal cord and also serves to provide protection and vascular support to the spinal cord.

Major Tracts of the Spinal Cord

The spinal cord carries information to and from the brain and the rest of the body. This is accomplished through a series of *tracts* or large bundles of axons that travel through the *white matter* of the spinal cord. The white matter of the spinal cord is located peripherally in the spinal cord and is composed of the (1) *dorsal columns,* which carry sensory information from the body to the brain; (2) *lateral columns,* which also carry sensory information from the body to the brain; and (3) *anterior columns,* which carry motor information to the body from the brain.

Sensory Pathways

The sensory tracts of the spinal cord are composed of three neurons in sequence. These neurons are known as the (1) *first-order neuron,* which delivers sensory information from the periphery to the spinal cord. The bodies of these neurons are located in the *dorsal root ganglion,* which is located peripheral to the spinal cord in the *dorsal root* of the *spinal nerve;* (2) *second-order neuron,* which transmits sensory information from the first-order neuron to the *thalamus* located within the *diencephalon* of the midbrain. The second-order neuron is the neuron that makes up the tract proper; and (3) *third-order neuron,* which will travel from the thalamus of the midbrain to the *primary sensory cortex* of the *cerebral hemispheres* in the brain.

The posterior columns are composed of the (1) *fasciculus gracilis,* which transmits information about fine touch, pressure, vibration, and *proprioception* from the abdomen, pelvis, and lower extremities to the brain; and (2) *fasciculus cuneatus,* which transmits information about fine touch, pressure, vibration, and proprioception from the chest and upper extremities to the brain.

The spinothalamic tracts are composed of the (1) *lateral spinothalamic tract* (located in the lateral columns) which transmits information about pain and temperature from the body to the brain, and (2) *anterior spinothalamic tract* (located in the anterior columns) which transmits information about crude touch and pressure to the brain.

The spinocerebellar tracts are composed of the (1) *posterior spinocerebellar tract* that transmits information about proprioception to the cerebellum of the brain, and (2) *anterior spinocerebellar tract,* which also transmits information about proprioception to the cerebellum.

Motor Pathways

The motor tracts of the spinal cord are composed of two neurons in sequence. These neurons are known as the (1) *upper motor neuron,* which delivers motor information from the *primary motor cortex* in the cerebral hemispheres to the spinal cord; and (2) *lower motor neuron,* which carries information from the spinal cord to an effector in the body. The spinal cord is composed of two major motor tracts which include the (1) *corticospinal tracts* and (2) *subconscious tracts.*

The corticospinal tracts are composed of the (1) *corticobulbar tracts* that transmit motor information for control of the eyes, jaw, and face muscles from the primary motor cortex to these structures; (2) *lateral corticospinal tracts* (located in the lateral columns) that transmit information about conscious control of all skeletal muscles from the primary motor cortex to the various muscles associated with voluntary movement; and (3) *anterior corticospinal tracts* (located in the anterior columns) that also transmit information about voluntary motor control from the primary motor cortex to the muscles.

The subconscious motor tracts are composed of the (1) *vestibulospinal tracts,* which send information from the inner ear and *cochlea* to the *vestibular nuclei* to regulate the muscles of the neck and extremities to help regulate posture; (2) *tectospinal tracts,* which carry information from the *superior colliculi* (which integrate visual information) and the *inferior colliculi* (which integrate auditory information) to the muscles of the head, neck, and upper extremities to respond to visual and/or auditory stimuli; (3) *reticulospinal tracts* that carry information for eye movement as well as respiration; and (4) *rubrospinal tracts* that carry information to the various muscles of the body associated with flexion and extension.

Spinal Nerves

Information passes into and out of the spinal cord to the rest of the body through the *spinal nerves* that are located on each side of the spinal cord. As a spinal nerve approaches the spinal cord, it is a single structure that contains neuronal axons of both motor neurons and sensory neurons. However, as it nears the spinal cord, it will split into two separate structures known as the *dorsal root* of the spinal nerve and the *ventral root* of the spinal cord. The dorsal root of the spinal nerve will connect to the spinal cord along the dorso-lateral aspect of the spinal cord. The dorsal root has a structure called the *dorsal root ganglion* that contains the cell bodies of all the sensory neurons associated with the spinal cord at a given spinal level. Axons of the sensory neurons will enter the *dorsal gray horn* (or *dorsal horn*) of the spinal cord from the dorsal root of the spinal nerve. The ventral root of the spinal nerve serves as the exit point for the axons of the lower motor neurons. Axons of the motor neurons will exit the *ventral gray horns* (or *ventral horn*) of the spinal cord, enter the ventral root of the spinal nerve, and then join with the dorsal root to form the spinal nerve.

Spinal Reflexes

In addition to transmitting information from the brain to the body, the spinal cord is also the location of *spinal reflexes,* which allow for the rapid and automatic response to unexpected stimuli from the environment. Spinal reflexes require five major components consisting of:

- A *receptor* that is usually associated with the *dendritic end* of a *sensory neuron* and receives information about environmental stimuli such as pain, temperature, or other sensory input.
- A *sensory neuron* that conducts receptor input from the peripheral aspects of the body to the spinal cord. This sensory neuron has its cell body located within the *dorsal root ganglion* located in the *dorsal root* of the spinal nerve.
- An *integration center* which is located within the spinal cord proper. This integration center is where the sensory neuron and the *motor neuron* synapse to complete the reflex arc. In some instances, a sensory neuron only synapses on one motor neuron and this is called a *monosynaptic reflex arc.*

In other instances the sensory neuron may synapse either directly or indirectly through an *interneuron* on more than one motor neuron. This is called a *polysynaptic reflex arc*.

- A *motor neuron* which will exit the spinal cord through the *ventral root* of the spinal nerve and terminate in an effector of some type, such as a muscle or an *exocrine gland.*
- An *effector* which is the region or part of the body innervated by the motor neuron. Action potentials generated in the central nervous system will cause a response of some sort in the effector in response to the original stimulus.

Reflex arcs are often used in physical exams to determine whether there has been injury to the spinal cord or some other component of the reflex arc. Some of the more common reflexes evaluated in a medical exam might include the (1) *patellar reflex* (knee jerk), (2) *Achilles reflex* (ankle jerk), (3) *biceps reflex* (forearm jerk), and (4) *triceps reflex* (also a forearm jerk).

Charles A. Ferguson

See also: Axon; Cerebrospinal Fluid; Lumbar Puncture; Meninges; Motor Neurons; Nerves; Neurological Examination; Reflex; Spinal Cord with Vertebra—Building with Clay Activity

Further Reading

Bear, M. F., Connors, B. W., & Paradiso, M. A. (2007). *Neuroscience exploring the brain* (3rd ed.). Baltimore, MD: Lippincott Williams & Wilkins.

Bican, O., Minagar, A., & Pruitt, A. (2013). The spinal cord: A review of functional neuroanatomy. *Neurologic Clinics, 31*(1), 1–18.

Moore, K. L., & Dalley, A. F. (1999). *Clinically oriented anatomy* (4th ed.). Baltimore, MD: Lippincott Williams & Wilkins.

Rezania, K., & Roos, R. (2013). Spinal cord: Motor neuron diseases. *Neurologic Clinics, 31*(1), 219–239.

Summers, P., Lannetti, G., & Porro, C. (2010). Functional exploration of the human spinal cord during voluntary movement and somatosensory stimulation. *Magnetic Resonance Imaging, 28*(8), 1216–1224.

Stem Cell Therapy

Stem cells are undifferentiated (nonspecialized) cells that have the ability to rapidly divide into more stem cells and differentiate (specialize) into different cells. Stem cells exist in a variety of places within the adult human body: bone marrow, adipose

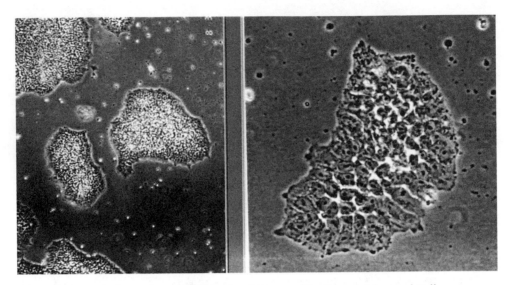

A photo of stem cells in clusters, enlarged at 10x magnification, at Advanced Cell Technology in Worcester, Massachusetts. (AP/Wide World Photos)

tissue (fat), and blood. Within the adult human, stem cells perform repair functions. Stem cells are also found in developing embryos where they are responsible for differentiating into every cell in the body. The ability for a stem cell to rapidly divide into many new cells without worry of damage to the genetic material and to differentiate into almost any cell in the human body is why *stem cell therapy* (SCT) is so heavily researched by the scientific community. Contrary to popular belief, the stem cells used in SCT are generally harvested from its sources in the adult human body or, rarely, from umbilical cord blood taken right after birth. Nonetheless, there are ethical decisions that researchers, physicians, and the general public need to make to ensure the proper and ethical use of stem cells in specific therapies or experiments.

History

The idea that cells are able to divide and produce new "daughter" cells has been known since the 19th century. However, the first documented report regarding this ability was published in 1961 by Canadian researchers James Till (1931–) a biophysicist and Ernest McCulloch (1926–2011) a cellular biologist. For their discovery of stem cells, they are considered the fathers of SCT. Till and McCulloch's work at the Ontario Cancer Institute showed that in a mouse model certain cells were able to reproduce or self-renew over and over, and these new cells were viable and could be used in different regions of the body. Since these initial findings, stem cell research has expanded exponentially.

Stem Cell Techniques and Uses

SCT is a medical procedure where stem cells are introduced into damaged tissues to help treat various diseases. SCT is still mostly in experimental stages as it is costly and highly controversial; however, many medical researchers believe that SCT is a good option to help relieve the suffering caused by many diseases. Even though SCT is in experimental stages, bone-marrow transplantation has been widely used to treat cancers of the blood (types of leukemia) and bone marrow. The range of diseases that SCT could potentially treat is huge; however, much more research needs to be performed before it is a viable option in a clinical setting. Some of the diseases that SCT could treat are cancer, diabetes (type 1), Parkinson's disease, heart damage, damage to the spinal cord, deafness, baldness, Huntington's disease, and Celiac disease.

Riannon C. Atwater

See also: Deafness; Huntington's Disease; Parkinson's Disease

Further Reading

Shetty, A. K. (2014). Hippocampal injury-induced cognitive and mood dysfunction, altered neurogenesis, and epilepsy: Can early neural stem cell grafting intervention provide protection? *Epilepsy Behavior.* pii: S1525–5050(13): 631–8.

Till, J. E., & McCulloch, E. A. (1961). A direct measurement of the radiation sensitivity of normal mouse bone marrow cells. *Radiation Research, 14,* 213–222.

Stereotaxic Surgery

Stereotaxic surgery uses precision and highly technical equipment for several different brain operations. Such surgeries range from mapping the brain to identify regions and their functions to surgical resection to remove damaged regions caused by seizures or tumors. Neuroscientists use this technique to learn about local circuitry (networks of neighboring neurons) in the brain and how these local circuits affect other local and global networks. Neurosurgeons use stereotaxic surgery in only extreme cases to treat epilepsy, subdural hematomas—active bleeding under the dura that was caused by severe brain injury, and to remove tumors that are unresponsive to chemotherapy and/or radiation. To prepare for surgery, a stereotaxic frame is attached to the head, aligning the skull so that it is in a level plane. The fused bones of the skull (sutures) are then used to calculate the distance from one point to another to find underlying brain regions.

Using stereotaxic surgery, neuroscientists are identifying mechanisms that are associated with learning and memory, long-term potentiation (increased neuronal responses that last for more than 24 hours), short-term potentiation (increased neuronal responses lasting for a few hours), synchrony (when neurons fire action potentials at the same time), behavioral tasks (how the brain functions during specific behaviors) as well as mechanisms that are associated with neurological diseases. For example, neuroscientists use stereotaxic surgery to implant indwelling electrodes into the hippocampi (regions of the brain associated with learning and memory) of both epileptic and control, normal, untreated rats. From these chronic recordings of epileptic and normal rat brains, neuroscientists were able to examine the potential differences in a neuron's ability to weaken and strengthen its communication to its neighboring neurons through synapses. Furthermore, the study was able to measure changes in the neuron's firing and in the local circuitry following the dosing of the rats with antiseizure medication. The advantage of using chronically implanted electrodes is that the animal is able to behave normally and the researchers are able to record the activity of the brain during these normal behaviors, like eating, drinking, sleeping, exploring, sniffing, and grooming. These recordings are the best way to understand brain activity in a freely behaving animal.

For neurosurgeons, stereotaxic surgery provides the best results from a complicated operation. Doctors then use the information about location and function of different brain regions from the indwelling electrode experiments completed by neuroscientists. Knowing what part of the patient's brain that controls speech, language, and motor movements like holding a pencil or walking, the surgeons are able to avoid that area as much as possible when trying to remove the damaged brain section. However, every person's brain is different such that language areas may be in the same general region, but the neurosurgeon must map the damaged area prior to resection. Since the brain does not have any pain receptors like the surrounding tissue does (skull, muscle, and skin), the patient is woken up and asked questions to answer or to respond by moving a part of their body. The surgeon slowly lowers the operating tools into the damaged brain region while at the same time the patient is answering questions or performing a task. If the patient has difficulty, then the surgeon knows that part of the brain needs to be saved.

Jennifer L. Hellier

See also: Neurologist

Further Reading

University of Rochester Medical Center. (2013). *Stereotactic brain surgery.* Retrieved from https://www.urmc.rochester.edu/neurosurgery/for-patients/treatments/stereotactic-brain-surgery.aspx

Strabismus

Strabismus is the medical term for crossed eyes. This is when a person's eyes will not look at the same place at the same time. One eye may be turned inward (esotropia), outward (exotropia), upward (hypertropia), or downward (hypotropia) compared to the other eye. Strabismus occurs when the six extraocular muscles are weakened and have poor motor control or when a person has severe farsightedness. The extraocular muscles are controlled by three cranial nerves: *oculomotor* (cranial nerve III), *trochlear* (cranial nerve IV), and *abducens* (cranial nerve VI).

In general, strabismus is the result of an underlying systemic disease, damage to the cranial nerves serving the eye muscles, or inherited. Some diseases resulting in strabismus include but are not limited to cerebral palsy; Down syndrome; stroke; and, trauma to the head. Persons with strabismus may have the same eye always turned the same direction. This can be present all the time or only occur when the person is tired or ill. In other cases, some patients will have their eyes alternate in turning.

Strabismus can cause double vision or *diplopia* in both eyes (binocular diplopia). This occurs because the extraocular muscles do not align the eyes properly so that convergence cannot occur. Here during focusing, one eye may be turned inward or outward compared to the other eye, resulting in the image being on different regions of the two retinas.

Treatment for strabismus depends on the cause of the crossed eyes. The underlying cause must be treated first for best results. Many persons with strabismus are prescribed eyeglasses or contact lenses to correct the farsightedness. An optometrist may also prescribe eye exercises (vision therapy), prism lenses (to reduce the amount of light into the eye so that it does not turn as much), and/or eye surgery (for severe cases).

Jennifer L. Hellier

See also: Abducens Nerve; Diplopia; Down Syndrome; Oculomotor Nerve; Stroke; Trochlear Nerve

Further Reading

Blumenfeld, H. (2010). *Neuroanatomy through clinical cases*. Sunderland, MA: Sinauer.

Stroke

Stroke is a neurological disorder originating from a vascular defect or disorder, such as an aneurysm (tear in an artery) or an obstruction of blood flow. The two main causes of stroke are: hemorrhage (active bleeding) and ischemia. Ischemic strokes are due to a lack of blood in the brain, while hemorrhagic strokes are due to an excess of blood in the brain. In 2009 and 2010, 2.6 percent of adults in the United States suffered from stroke. In 2008, about 41 individuals out of every 100,000 died of stroke. The general symptoms of a stroke are often sudden and include weakness or numbness on one side of the body, impairment of vision, headache, and confusion especially in regards to speaking or understanding speech.

Wallenberg's Syndrome

Wallenberg's syndrome is a result of a stroke or infarct of an artery that supplies the brainstem. Specifically, it is a stroke in the *vertebral* or *posterior inferior cerebellar artery (PICA)*. A German neurologist, Adolf Wallenberg (1862–1949), was the first to describe the clinical findings and the injury to the brainstem when he performed an autopsy on a person with a stroke to the PICA. This is how the syndrome originally received its name. Today, Wallenberg's syndrome is now named for the damaged regions and is termed *lateral medullary syndrome*.

When the blood supply is reduced or blocked to areas of the central nervous system a lack of function occurs. The symptoms that follow an infarct of the PICA result in difficulty in swallowing (dysphagia), hoarseness and change in vocal quality (dysphonia), slurred speech (dysarthria), dizziness (vertigo), nausea and vomiting, involuntary and rapid movement of the eyes (nystagmus), difficulty with balance, double vision (diplopia), and Horner syndrome. Horner syndrome is a combination of dysfunctions including drooping of the affected eyelid (ptosis), constriction of the pupil (miosis), and inability or decreased sweating of the face on the affected side (anhydrous). These symptoms are caused by the damage to the neurons of the vagus nerve (cranial nerve X) that are located in the lateral medulla.

The main treatments for Wallenberg's syndrome are to alleviate the symptoms, provide rehabilitation, and to teach the patient how to deal with the psychological loss of nerve function to the face and voice. If the patient can no longer swallow, a feeding tube may be required until symptoms improve. Patients may be placed on an aspirin regiment for the rest of their lives as well as other medications (like a statin for controlling cholesterol) to reduce the risk of stroke in the future. Depending on the size of the damaged area, persons with Wallenberg's syndrome may recover completely within a few months or may have symptoms for years.

Jennifer L. Hellier

See also: Stroke

Further Reading

National Institute of Neurological Disorders and Stroke (NINDS). (2007). *NINDS Wallenberg's syndrome information page.* Retrieved from http://www.ninds.nih .gov/disorders/wallenbergs/wallenbergs.htm

Pathophysiology, Types, and Symptoms

Hemorrhagic Stroke

In animals, adult skulls are unable to expand, and excess blood in the cranial cavity quickly increases pressure on brain tissue. The increase in pressure, if left untreated, can damage brain tissue and impair brain function. Hemorrhagic stroke is much less common than ischemic stroke, but the consequences can be more severe. Magnetic resonance imaging (MRI, a machine used to view the body and head) is usually used to diagnose and confirm hemorrhagic strokes as well as their causes.

Hemorrhagic strokes can be further categorized into intracerebral hemorrhage (ICH, meaning within the brain) and subarachnoid hemorrhage (SAH, meaning below the arachnoid mater of the meninges). ICH is a collection of blood in brain tissue itself, while SAH is a collection of blood in the cerebrospinal fluid, which surrounds the brain and spinal cord. ICH accounts for 10–15 percent of all strokes. High blood pressure, trauma, ruptured aneurysms, protein deposits in blood vessels, structural defects in vessels, or cocaine use are common causes of ICH. High blood pressure is the most common cause of ICH strokes. Continuous high blood pressure can damage blood vessels in the brain. However, sudden spikes in blood pressure cause strokes, even from causes as simple as exercise. The increase in blood pressure causes blood vessels to break and fluid to pour into the brain tissue. Likewise, protein deposits and structural defects can make blood vessels more brittle, leading to breakage. The blood that collects is referred to as a hematoma. Hematomas gradually increase in size based on blood flow and intracranial pressure. Because they are gradual in nature, ICH strokes also have a gradual onset of symptoms over the course of minutes or even hours. Symptoms of ICH strokes begin with impairment of motor or sensory skills based on the location of the hemorrhage. If the hemotoma grows large enough to affect the pressure of the entire intracranial space, the individual may experience headache and impairment of consciousness or other generalized symptoms. If the bleeding is not contained or otherwise stopped, the individual may die.

On the surface of the brain, there are three layers of membranes called the meninges that are essential for protecting the brain tissue. Starting from the outermost layer, the membranes are named the dura mater, arachnoid mater, and pia mater. Between the pia mater and arachnoid mater is cerebrospinal fluid. In SAH, blood collects in the space between the pia mater and arachnoid mater. The most common cause of SAH is a ruptured aneurysm, while other causes are the same as those for ICH. SAH produces a sudden release of blood, which usually stops quickly. However, the bleeding triggers a widespread increase in intracranial pressure. The individual will immediately experience a severe headache, as well as a possible loss of memory or consciousness. If SAH is not treated immediately, the risk of death and coma are very high.

Ischemic Stroke

Ischemia accounts for 70 percent of all strokes. The three types of ischemic strokes are thrombosis, embolism, and systemic hypoperfusion (decreased blood flow to the brain). Thrombosis refers to a localized blood blockage. An issue in the cerebral blood vessels causes this blockage. The most common obstruction is atherosclerosis, which is a disease of the arteries where fat builds up on the walls. Generally, only an isolated section of the brain is affected producing symptoms that are related to the location of the thrombosis. In order to treat thrombosis, the exact cause and location must be discovered. Surgery and angioplasty are common treatments for thrombosis.

Embolism is when a cerebrovascular blockage originates in another part of the body. For example, a blood clot in the leg could travel through the cardiovascular system to the brain and become fastened in a vessel obstructing blood flow. As with thrombosis, symptoms are based on the location of the embolism. Because the blockage is traveling from another part of the body, multiple parts of the brain may be affected. Surgery may also be used in the treatment of emboli. However, it is important to discover the source of the embolic material to ensure the individual does not have another stroke. For example, a blood clot may be cleared by surgery, but if the individual continues to produce blood clots in their legs, the clots may continue to travel to the brain and cause repeated strokes. If the patient is put on medication to stop blood clots, the risk of a second stroke is considerably decreased.

Systemic hypoperfusion occurs when not enough blood is being pumped into the brain. Cardiac arrest, irregular heartbeat, and lung (pulmonary) embolism are possible causes. Symptoms for systemic hypoperfusion are often generalized, although symptoms tend to originate from areas between the major arteries in the brain. Symptoms include sweating, weakness, and trouble seeing. Treatment depends on the initial cause of low blood supply.

Transient ischemic attacks (TIAs) can, in some ways, be thought of as partial seizures. TIAs can be caused by any of the same causes of ischemic strokes. However, TIAs usually disappear within a few minutes. Often, TIAs are caused by both local and systemic factors. For example, an individual may have a damaged artery that only lets limited amounts of blood though. This may not be an issue most of the time, but if they are severely dehydrated and their blood is thicker, the heart may be incapable of pumping sufficient amounts of blood through the given artery. TIAs cause minor damage, if any. On occasion, TIAs will foreshadow a full stroke, because they have similar causes. It is important to diagnose a TIA so that the cause can be treated before a stroke occurs.

Categorizing Strokes

Strokes may also be categorized based on their location in the brain and the symptoms that occur. The anterior cerebral arteries provide blood for both frontal lobes and most of the parietal and temporal lobes. Strokes involving the anterior cerebral arteries are referred to as either total or partial anterior circulation strokes (TACS and PACS, respectively). TACS display impairment of movement and sensation for over two-thirds of the face, arms, and legs as well as impairment of speech. TACS also results in loss of half of the vision in each eye determined by a vertical line. PACS present two of the symptoms of TACS or just motor or speech impairment.

Posterior cerebral arteries provide blood to the cerebellum and the rear portions of the cerebral cortex. Dysfunctions in the posterior cerebral arteries may result in posterior circulation infarction (POCI). POCI results in drooping of one or both sides of the face, trouble moving both eyes together, difficulty with motor functions, and impairment of speech.

Lacunar stroke is a condition initiated by multiple small infarcts in and near the basal ganglia, particularly in smaller vessels (not arteries or veins). Lacunar infarction (LACI) may present with (1) weakness, numbness, or tingling on one side of the body; (2) both weakness and numbness on one side of the body; or (3) clumsiness on one side of the body. In LACI, the symptoms generally affect two-thirds of the face, arm, and leg on that side of the body where the LACI occurred.

Treatment

Since strokes restrict blood flow to or put extra pressure on the brain, areas of brain tissue may become damaged and no longer functional. After having a stroke, many individuals continue to have physical and psychological problems. Up to 79 percent of people who have had a stroke struggle with urinary incontinence. The first few days after a stroke often provide difficulties with bowel incontinence, but this may improve over time. An individual who has had a stroke may have trouble walking, turning their head, doing basic tasks such as dressing, or even moving at all. Depending on which part of the brain was damaged from the stroke, the individual may have trouble using any of their five senses. Additionally, cognitive functions such as memory, attention, and speech may be impaired. Occupational therapy is often used to help stroke victims recover from all of these physical difficulties. Nonetheless, about 33 percent of people who have experienced a stroke will have depression, which is partially due to the physical limitations that accompany stroke.

Despite damage to brain tissue, 60 percent of stroke survivors are able to live independent lives. However, only 20 percent of individuals who have had ICH strokes return to an independent lifestyle. Tests show that individuals who have suffered a stroke have decreased brain activity on the side of stroke even after recovery. For example, if an individual loses the ability to move their right hand, then regains the ability through occupational therapy, the left side of the brain which controls right hand movement will not show activity while moving the right hand. This shows that the part of the brain that was damaged does not regain function. However, the right side of the brain does show activation while moving the previously paralyzed right hand. This demonstrates that the brain has been remapped to accommodate the damaged tissue. The ability to reorganize brain functions is referred to as neuroplasticity.

One of the most common and effective preventive measures for strokes is aspirin. Aspirin is often given to an individual after they have a stroke, because it prevents blood clots, which often cause ischemic strokes. Aspirin is especially used in the emergency room to treat patients at the first sign of a stroke. A tissue plasminogen activator (TPA) may be injected into a vein to destroy blood clots that have already formed and caused a stroke. This treatment is used within the first four-and-half hours that stroke symptoms begin. While TPA is usually injected through a vein in the arm, doctors may insert a tube through a groin artery into the brain to deliver the TPA directly to the brain. In the case of an emergency, a mechanical device may directly remove the clot. In order to prevent clots that lead to strokes, a surgeon may remove fatty deposits from or use a balloon to expand blocked carotid arteries. In the case of a hemorrhagic stroke, a clamp may be placed close to an aneurism to stop bleeding. Coils may also be placed near the aneurism to reduce blood flow and cause blood clots.

Diagnosis and Risks

It is important for everyone to learn the signs and symptoms of stroke. An easy mnemonic device, a learning technique to help retain information, for the signs of possible stroke is FAST. F stands for face. Ask the person to smile. If one side of their face droops, that is a sign of stroke. A stands for arms. Ask the person to raise both arms above their head. If one arm drifts downward, that is a sign of stroke. S stands for speech. Ask the person to repeat a simple phrase. If their words are slurred or sound strange, that too is a sign of stroke. Finally, T stands for time. If the patient has any of the FAS signs, then immediately get medical help. The faster the patient receives medical attention, the less likely the person will have brain damage.

Risk for stroke is greatly increased by high blood pressure, diabetes, smoking, and irregular heartbeat. Other factors that contribute, but do not have the same level of risk as those just mentioned, are drug usage, obesity, alcoholism, migraines, and many others. Strokes are prevented in two major ways: avoiding causes of cerebrovascular disease and using early diagnosis for those already at risk. Exercise, eating healthy, and avoiding addictive substances such as alcohol, tobacco, and illicit drugs lower the risk of stroke. Additionally, medications may be effective at reducing the risk of stroke in some individuals with high cholesterol or heart disease.

Allison J. Schuster

See also: Cerebrospinal Fluid; Headache; Hematoma (Hemorrhage); Meninges; Neuroplasticity

Further Reading

Bogousslavsky, J. (2006). *Stroke: Selected topics.* New York, NY: Demos.

Edmans, J. (2010). *Occupational therapy and stroke.* Hoboken, NJ: Wiley-Blackwell.

Mayo Clinic Staff. (2012). *Stroke: Treatments and drugs.* Retrieved from http://www.mayoclinic.com/health/stroke/DS00150/DSECTION=treatments-and-drugs

Silverman, I. E., & Rymer, M. M. (2010). *Hemorrhagic stroke.* Oxford: Clinical Publishing.

U.S. Department of Heath and Human Services, Centers for Disease Control and Prevention. (2011). *Health, United States, 2011: With special feature on socioeconomic status and health.* Washington, DC: U.S. Government Printing Office.

Williams, J., Perry, L., & Watkins, C. (2010). *Acute stroke nursing.* Hoboken, NJ: Wiley-Blackwell.

Subconscious

The central nervous system consists of anatomical structures, which are the brain, the brainstem, and the spinal cord. The activity of the brain when a person is awake is called *conscious* or consciousness. This is because the person is aware of their surroundings, aware of themselves, and can focus their awareness. In addition to the conscious state, there is a *subconscious* state, which is part of being conscious but not in the state of focal awareness. The brain can only focus on a limited amount of focal awareness at a time, but it always retains all of its knowledge. When the conscious mind needs information, it draws it from the subconscious mind where information is stored. For example, when a person is writing a letter and needs to spell a difficult word the conscious mind calls on the subconscious for the spelling. The subconscious decides what action the person needs to take from past experiences, will find the correct spelling, and pass this information to the conscious mind. The conscious mind will then move the muscles in the hand to write the word. Finally, the subconscious mind is responsible for controlling the autonomic nervous system, which is made up of the sympathetic and the parasympathetic nervous systems. These are responsible for fight-or-flight response in stress and the digestion of food, respectively. Additionally, the subconscious maintains homeostasis by controlling heart rate, breathing, digestion, and other subconscious activities.

History

The term subconscious was first coined by French psychologist Pierre Marie Felix Janet (1859–1947) and it literally translates as, "below the conscious." This means there is an awareness that lies underneath the conscious layers of critical thought. The subconscious is not the same as being unconscious or completing unconscious activities. However, these two terms are often interchanged, which is incorrect (Miller, 2011). Austrian neurologist Sigmund Freud (1856–1939), who is the father of psychoanalysis, defined the term "unconscious" as part of the brain that has its own purpose and "mind" that cannot be known to the conscious mind. Freud suggests that this is a form of repression that needs to hide socially inappropriate thoughts, wishes and desires, and traumatic events. Through psychoanalysis a person can deal with these feelings and events in a safe manner. Because there is a distinct difference between the terms subconscious and unconscious, psychoanalysis does not use the word subconscious in any of its writings.

Anatomy and Physiology

The conscious mind uses a small amount of the mind's capacity and is capable of only one thought at a time. It focuses on the "here-and-now" situations. When awake the conscious mind is active, and is able to make decisions, rationalize, analyze, and has some control over the voluntary actions of the muscles. The subconscious mind uses the remaining capacity of the mind to absorb everything that is going on around the person. In addition, the subconscious mind controls the autonomic nervous system that controls the automatic functions of heart rate, breathing rate, food digestion, and organ and gland activities to allow the body to remain in homeostasis. These actions are important for the body to run and if the conscious brain had to control all of these functions, it would not be able to have critical thoughts.

The subconscious mind stores all information and experiences that a person has acquired during their lifetime. Much of this information is learned in the first few years of life, but additional experience will obtain new information that will also be stored. The subconscious stores everything that a person sees, hears, smells, and experiences, even if it may not be rational. This is because the conscious mind may need to access this information later in life to protect the person or for retrieval for survival situations. It is posited that some of this information is used in instinct and "gut feelings."

American security expert Gavin de Becker (1954–) describes this action of the subconscious in his 1997 book entitled *The Gift of Fear: Survival Signals That Protect Us from Violence.* In situations when a person "feels" something is not right, many of them will ignore this signal from the subconscious and can become victims of a crime. When people do not ignore this signal, they allow their conscious mind to respond to the subconscious signal to protect them.

Disease

When the autonomic nervous system becomes damaged, specifically the nerves that carry the information from the brain and spinal cord to the organs, it results in a condition called autonomic neuropathy. The subconscious cannot process the autonomic nervous system actions appropriately in these situations. The person may have signs of sudden fatigue, being lightheaded or feeling faint, changes in bowel and bladder activity, and feeling of nausea. Additionally, they may have excessive sweating, abnormal blood pressure, and changes in heart rate (either increased or decreased heart rate at rest). Some causes of autonomic neuropathy are alcoholism, diabetes, multiple sclerosis, and Parkinson's disease, to name a few.

Treatment to reverse nerve damage is usually not possible and the goal is to prevent further damage. Thus, treatments for autonomic issues are first to help the underlying cause of the autonomic neuropathy. For example, patients with diabetes focus on controlling the person's blood sugar. Additional self-care for managing symptoms is suggested.

Patricia A. Bloomquist

See also: Autonomic Nervous System; Conscious and Consciousness; Diabetes Mellitus; Homeostasis; Learning and Memory; Multiple Sclerosis; Parkinson's Disease

Further Reading

de Becker, G. (1997). *The gift of fear: Survival signals that protect us from violence.* Boston, MA: Little, Brown and Company.

Dougherty, P., & Tsuchitani, C. (1997). Central control of the autonomic nervous system and thermoregulation. In *Neuroscience Online, an electronic textbook for the neurosciences* (Chap. 3). Open-access educational resource provided by the Department of Neurobiology and Anatomy at the University of Texas Medical School at Houston. Retrieved from http://neuroscience.uth.tmc.edu/s4/chapter03.html

Miller, M.C. (2011). Ask the doctor. I've always used word subconscious when talking about thoughts that are buried. But someone corrected me recently and said unconscious is the correct term. Have I been using the wrong word? *Harvard Health Letter, 36*(12), 8.

Substance Abuse

Substance abuse, which might also be used synonymously with drug abuse, is a pattern of behavior in which the user (1) consumes more of a drug than is recommended; (2) uses a drug for a purpose other than a recommended purpose; and (3) does so without the supervision or approval of a medical professional. Substance abuse is not just the overuse of illegal or prescription drugs, but could also be used to refer to use of a drug for sports performance enhancement, such as steroids, or to the abuse of alcohol. It might even refer to the misuse of substance like inhalants and solvents, caffeine, nicotine, and over-the-counter medications, if these substances are used in excess. Theoretically, almost any substance has the potential for abuse. Abuse is characterized by a compulsive need for the substance, a tolerance to the substance, and the presence of withdrawal symptoms if use of the substance is stopped or diminished.

Many people experiment with recreational or prescription drugs, including alcohol and tobacco. Drug use and experimentation often begin in adolescence, and the majority of people will phase out drug use before it becomes a problem. For those who do not phase it out, the costs to society, to the individual, and to the family can be great. The National Institute on Drug Abuse estimates that the cost of drug abuse, in terms of health care and crime, is around $100 billion annually in the United States. However, the social and economic costs, in terms of broken homes, lost jobs, and lost lives, are difficult to determine.

There is much debate about the difference in use and abuse. Most people would define abuse as continuing to use the substance, despite psychological or physical harm to the user. Compulsive or repetitive use may result in dependence, and the user may become dependent on the substance, and suffer withdrawal if reducing or discontinuing the use of the substance. Substance abuse affects people of all ethnicities, socioeconomic groups, and age groups.

History

Since ancient times, many cultures used mood altering drugs or hallucinogens and viewed these as an aid to spiritual experiences. There are many depictions of drug use in other cultures, but experts believe that these cultures did not suffer from addiction because they were able to self-regulate the use. Many experts and scientists view substance abuse mostly as a modern-day problem. For example, it was in 1956 when the American Medical Association officially declared that alcoholism was a disease. For the many years since then, scientists and researchers have viewed addiction as a brain disease. Substances are readily available on the street, and substance use and abuse is an ever-growing problem in all societies.

Signs and Symptoms

Many people experiment with drugs, but very few become addicted. They take drugs for different reasons; they want to feel better or they want to be better. They might just be curious about the drugs. There may be peer pressure or social pressure to use substances. Maybe they are suffering from acute or chronic pain. They may have a mental illness. They may turn to drugs to enhance their performance in certain sports. Whatever the reason, substance abuse begins with experimentation and sometimes progresses to more aggressive use.

Environmental factors play a large role in substance abuse. The user must have access to the substance or substances of choice. It is well documented that some aspects of family life and relationships can influence substance use and abuse as well. Family practices, like poor supervision of children, ineffective discipline, and poor communication, can be factors in the initial experimentation and continued use of drugs. Family attitudes and behaviors toward substances can also contribute to the misuse of substances. Initiating and continuing illegal drug use appear to be strongly influenced by both societal norms and peer pressure.

Community issues, such as lack of educational resources, high crime rates, and poor role models can have some bearing on substance abuse. Sometimes, the lack of other diversions or pleasurable resources within a community can contribute to extensive drug use.

Adolescents are particularly susceptible to the attraction of substance abuse, due to the dramatic biological and psychological changes that occur during adolescence. Many believe the adolescent brain may be more susceptible to the effects of drugs, which may encourage greater use. One of the brain areas still maturing during adolescence is the frontal cortex, which controls the ability to assess situations and make good decisions. This may have longer-lasting consequences for adolescent drug users. Issues of a poor self-image, low self-esteem, coupled with a desire to become independent from parents and limited coping strategies, may also increase vulnerability to substances and their abuse. Incidents of depression, anxiety, conduct disorder, and attention-deficit and hyperactivity can also lead to drug use and abuse.

Physical indications of substance abuse could include unexplained weight loss, frequent unexplained injuries, red eyes or enlarged pupils, frequent illnesses, chronic cough, needle tracks, blank stares, scratch marks, and excessive acne. Academic indicators might include the loss of short-term memory, failing grades, frequent absences, suspension or expulsion, poor judgment, and conflicts with teachers and others in authority. Behavioral indicators might include risky behaviors, such as stealing or trading sex for drugs, extreme mood swings, loss of interest in other activities, disturbed sleep patterns, lying, altered appetite, and poor hygiene.

Using recreational drugs causes a surge of dopamine in the brain, which triggers pleasure sensations. Dopamine is a natural chemical in the brain that controls emotion, pleasure, and motivation. Most drugs target the pleasure center of the brain, and can interfere with the way the brain sends and receives messages. Repeated and extensive use can cause actual changes in the brain, affecting the way the brain looks and feels and responds to pleasure. Tolerance may develop, and may require more of the substance to affect the same change. These changes can affect the ability to make decisions and to control the quantity and frequency of drug use.

Treatment

Treatment programs for substance abuse focus on stopping the use of substance, recovery, and avoiding relapse. Treatment may involve a variety of methods, from individual counseling, to group counseling, to family counseling. Effective treatment will address the many aspects of the user's life that have been affected by the addiction, from lifestyle changes to health issues.

Brief interventions have been successfully used with many substance abusers. Usually initiated by family members with the assistance of a professional, brief interventions consist of asking the user to consider quitting on their own or attending a self-help group, like Alcoholics Anonymous or Narcotics Anonymous to help them quit.

According to the National Institute on Drug Abuse, there are some key principles of effective treatment programs. No single treatment is effective or even appropriate for all substance abusers. The treatment must attend to the multiple needs of the user, and is more than just stopping the use of the substance. It is critical that the addict remains in treatment for an adequate amount of time, and that his or her treatment plan be constantly assessed and monitored to make sure that it meets the ever-changing needs of the addict. Health concerns, such as the presence of infectious diseases such as HIV (human immunodeficiency virus), AIDS (acquired immunodeficiency syndrome), tuberculosis (TB), or hepatitis must be assessed and treated, as well as any mental health issues of the addict.

Future

Today, the world is permeated with both illegal and legal substances that are often misused and abused. What constitutes the difference in use and abuse or misuse may be a matter of opinion. Readily available drugs, coupled with dysfunctional families and crumbling neighborhoods, may increase drug use and abuse, especially among vulnerable adolescents.

The fifth edition of the American Psychiatric Association's *Diagnostic and Statistical Manual of Mental Disorders* has proposed eliminating "substance abuse" and "substance dependence" as disorders, and replacing them with a single category "addictions and other related disorders" to outline the difference between dependence, tolerance, and addiction. Prior to this, each addiction was categorized by substance, like "alcohol use disorder." There will be the addition of drug craving as criteria for diagnosing addiction, and it will drop criminal encounters of the user, mainly due to the inconsistency of state laws throughout the United States. There will be the addition of a category for behavioral addiction, currently with only a single category, gaming addiction. Both behavioral and basic science will have to research and resolve other behavioral addictions in the future.

Lastly, it is important to note that addiction is no longer just about substance use and abuse, but a disease that encompasses all compulsive behavior and cravings that are associated with poor impulse control and problems with the reward circuitry in the brain.

Terri Blevins

See also: Addiction; Alcohol and Alcoholism; Attention Deficit Disorder/Attention Deficit Hyperactivity Disorder; Behavioral Health; Depression

Further Reading

Molintas, D. (2006). A history of addiction. *Power and control.* Retrieved from http://powerandcontrol.blogspot.com/2006/11/history-of-addiction.html

National Institute on Drug Abuse. (2009). *DrugFacts: Treatment approaches for drug addiction.* Retrieved from http://www.drugabuse.gov/publications/drugfacts/treatment-approaches-drug-addiction

Rowe, C., & Liddle, H. (2003). Substance abuse. *Journal of Marital and Family Therapy, 29*(1), 97–120.

Sulcus (Sulci)

The central nervous system is made up of the brain, brainstem, and spinal cord. In mammals, the brain is more developed compared to reptiles (snakes, turtles, lizards, etc.) and avians (birds). This is clearly seen by the complex shape the brain has as well as the increase in surface area. By increasing the surface area, many more neurons (brain cells) can be packed into the brain, allowing more integration and processing of sensory and motor functions. This is seen by the invaginations and bumps of the cerebral cortex. An invagination or depression is called a *sulcus* (pronounced \'səl-kəs\) while a bump or ridge is called a *gyrus.* The term *sulcus* is Latin for "furrow" and the plural form of the term is *sulci* (pronounced \'səl-kəs\). The word *gyrus* is Latin for "circle" and the plural form is *gyri.*

The characteristic appearance of the cerebral cortex is made by sulci and gyri. The development of the sulci and gyri begins in humans around five months old and generally finishes within the first year of birth (Hoffman, 1989). For each gyrus there is a sulcus on either side. In fact, it looks like a sinusoidal wave that is made up of brain tissue. The sulci are different throughout the cerebral cortex. Some are very deep while others are shallow. The deeper sulci are used to divide the brain into its four main lobes within each cerebral hemisphere: the frontal, parietal, temporal, and occipital lobes. In fact, these deep sulci are usually called fissures. The deepest furrow that divides the two cerebral hemispheres is not called a sulcus. It is known as the *interhemispheric fissure.*

Although there are many sulci within the brain, for this encyclopedia entry we will focus only on a few. The *central sulcus* is the longest and straightest invagination that starts roughly in the middle of the brain. There are two central sulci, one on each hemisphere. They are almost directly across from each other, beginning at the interhemispheric fissure. The sulci then follow the lateral aspect of each cerebral hemisphere. The central sucli are used as landmarks to separate the frontal and parietal lobes. The parallel sulci in front of and behind the central sulcus are called the *precentral* and *postcentral sulci* respectively. These are prominent furrows on the lateral aspect of cerebral hemispheres. The *lateral sulcus* is perpendicular to the central sulcus and divides the temporal lobe from the frontal and parietal lobes. Finally, the parietal and occipital lobes are divided by the *parieto-occipital sulcus.*

This groove runs deep and on the medial surface of the cerebral cortex with a small portion following the lateral surface.

Jennifer L. Hellier

See also: Brain Anatomy; Gray Matter; Gyrus (Gyri); Lissencephaly

Further Reading

Blumenfeld, H. (2010). *Neuroanatomy through clinical cases.* Sunderland, MA: Sinauer.

Hofman, M. A. (1989). On the evolution and geometry of the brain in mammals. *Progress in Neurobiology, 32*(2), 137–158.

Ono, M., Kubick, S., & Abernathey, C. D. (1990). *Atlas of the cerebral sulci.* New York, NY: Thieme Medical Publishers, Inc.

Superior Colliculus

Processing a visual stimulation involves multiple areas of the brain. One important component is the *superior colliculus.* This structure—located deep within the brainstem—helps process both visual and somatic (peripheral tactile sensations). It is involved in specific eye movements called "saccades," head movements, and an interpretation of body position relative to somatic (peripheral tactile) sensation.

Studying this structure across different species, called comparative biology, reveals varying functions of this structure. Certain snakes possess the ability to sense infrared signals. This sense is aided by neurons from the trigeminal nerve (or cranial nerve V, which supplies the head and face) in contrast to the optic nerve (or cranial nerve II) in primates or human. The trigeminal nerve senses stimulations such as touch (tactile), temperature (heat), and pain for the face, and helps to explain how these reptiles are able to detect heat signals.

Anatomy

The superior colliculus is known as the "upper hill." It is located on the uppermost part of the brainstem in the posterior (toward the back) aspect. Surrounding structures include the pineal gland, thalamus, and cerebellum. Piercing through this structure is the cerebral aqueduct (a natural space) responsible for connecting the flow of cerebrospinal fluid from the ventricles to the exterior of the cortex and spinal cord. These surrounding structures are highlighted, as any process causing increased size (such as a tumor) could potentially create problems with the superior colliculus.

Within the structure of the superior colliculus, there exist multiple individual structures. Surrounding the cerebral aqueduct is the periaqueductal gray. This area plays a role in the sensation and modulation of pain signals from the periphery. Additionally, the oculomotor nucleus and the Edinger-Westphal nucleus are present. The oculomotor nucleus is responsible for multiple eye movements facilitated by the medial, superior, and inferior rectus muscles. Also, this area controls the opening and closing of the eyelid. The Edinger-Westphal nucleus is responsible for constricting the eye and aiding in accommodation of the lens (seeing close) and convergence of the eye (ensuring both eyes are pointed in similar directions).

Directly inferior to this structure is the inferior colliculus. It is similar in structure but different in function. The major function is processing of auditory information. The location of a sound source can be triangulated utilizing the shorter relay time from the side a sound originates compared to the longer relay time on the opposite side. Taken together, these two structures are known as the "tectum" or roof of the midbrain. They combine to process important sensory information and facilitate an understanding of the outside world.

Physiology

The visual input from the retina (the photosensitive lining containing sensory receptor cells in the back of the eye) is rapidly conducted via the optic nerve to the occipital cortex, the frontal eye field, and subsequently the superior colliculus. This frontal eye field, also known as Brodmann area 8, is specifically responsive to new visual stimulus. Consider another person walks into the room and in the periphery of a right visual field. More attention is given to this new stimulus and the signal is transmitted to neurons within the superior colliculus.

Before the signal arrives, it first had to cross to the contralateral (opposite) side via the optic chiasm. Similar to the left occipital cortex processing information from the right visual field, the left superior colliculus reflects a map of the right visual field.

The signal from the person walking into the right visual field is processed in the left superior colliculus. At this point, the new stimulus' position is compared to the location of the fovea (an area of highest resolution) in the retina. A calculation of direction and distance is made in order to align the fovea and new visual stimulus. The next step is to initiate rapid movement of both eyes known as a "saccade" and head positioning to facilitate this alignment.

In order for the rightward saccade to occur in a horizontal manner, the paramedian pontine reticular formation (PPRF) is engaged. This structure relays a signal to the right eye lateral rectus muscle to contract allowing for a deviation to the right. Simultaneously, the left eye quickly moves left via a signal relayed by the "median longitudinal fasciculus." This structure signals the left oculomotor nerve to facilitate a contraction of the left medial rectus muscle. Ultimately, this coordinated effort brings the new visual stimulus into the focus of both foveas.

Interestingly, the superior colliculus also directs rapid movement of the head and neck. This process takes place via the "tectospinal tract." Nerve cell bodies responding to the visual or somatosensory signal on the right will again initiate in the left within the superior colliculus. These tectospinal neurons will decussate (or crossover) at an area called the medulla pyramid in the brainstem. The motor signal will exit at the level of the cervical spinal cord toward musculature in the right periphery. At this point, neck muscles quickly contract to help adjust the visual field to the new stimulus.

Taken together, the superior colliculus is a region within the brainstem responsible for reflexive adjustments to new visual or tactile stimulation. Arising from an evolutionarily old portion of the brain (the brainstem itself), it is clear that an animal's survival can be dependent on quickly processing and adjusting to new information.

Diseases

It becomes clear, when considering the close spatial arrangement around the brainstem, that an abnormal enlargement may interfere with the structures near the superior colliculus. One such example is a pineal gland tumor. This type of malady creates a situation called "Parinaud's syndrome" or sylvian aqueduct syndrome.

In this syndrome, both the tumor mass and subsequent disruption of cerebrospinal fluid flow create a situation in which pressure is applied to the superior colliculus. The result is a characteristic inability to gaze upward. Simultaneously, the upper eyelid is retracted and the pupils may abnormally dilate or constrict. Additional symptoms include the inability to focus as objects come nearer (accommodation) and decreased ability to keep eyes pointed in the same direction (convergence).

Another malady affecting the normal functioning of the superior colliculus is stroke, either hemorrhagic or ischemic. It is rare to diagnose an isolated stroke in this region, but it is believed that strokes in different areas in the brain connected to the superior colliculus are responsible for stubborn poststroke symptoms.

One such example is unilateral spatial neglect. This symptom disallows a person from even noticing one part of their visual field. Imagine looking directly at a clock. People with this ailment are only able to see one-half of the clock face. Similarly, these individuals only "see" one-half of their face in a mirror and have been known to completely ignore shaving the unseen side of their face or ignore combing their hair on that same side. It is important to mention there is no problem with the retina, ocular nerve, or occipital cortex. Rather, the problem arises from connections to and from the parietal lobe and possibly within the retino-collicular (retina to superior colliculus) pathway.

Recent studies have shown that unilateral spatial neglect is usually associated with damage to the right parietal lobe. It has a wide range of incidence from 13 to 81 percent of people being affected following such a right parietal lobe lesion (Pierce and Buxbaum, 2002). This is because the integrated pathway between the parietal lobe and the superior colliculus is interrupted. In severe cases, as previously stated, patients will ignore the entire side of their body and objects on the same side, such as the food on their plate. In mild cases, it is usually less noticeable and may not be properly diagnosed. However, these patients have an increased tendency to fall with a poor rehabilitation outcome. Within a year of the injury, the unilateral spatial neglect usually progresses resulting in functional deterioration of everyday activities, like dressing and eating. To date, not many treatment options have been found to improve this disorder. Some studies have shown that eye patching and prism adaption have some promise in helping these patients. Recently, Ogourtsova and colleagues (2010) have been trying to understand the involvement of the superior colliculus in unilateral spatial neglect so that new and more effective treatments can be developed.

Nicholas Breitnauer

See also: Accommodation; Cerebellum; Inferior Colliculus; Occipital Lobe; Oculomotor Nerve; Optic Nerve; Pineal Gland; Retina; Saccades; Thalamus; Ventricles; Visual Fields; Visual System

Further Reading

Alberstone, C. D., Benzel, E. C., Najm, I. M., & Steinmetz, M. P. (2009). *Anatomic diagnosis of neurologic diagnosis.* New York, NY: Thieme Medical Publishers, Inc.

Dragoi, V., & Tsuchitani, C. (1997). Visual processing: Cortical processing. In *Neuroscience Online, an electronic textbook for the neurosciences* (Chap. 15). Open-access educational resource provided by the Department of Neurobiology and Anatomy at the University of Texas Medical School at Houston. Retrieved from http://neuroscience.uth.tmc.edu/s2/chapter15.html

Ogourtsova, T., Korner-Bitensky, N., & Ptito, A. (2010). Contribution of the superior colliculi to the post-stroke unilateral spatial neglect and recovery. *Neuropsychologia, 48*(9), 2407–2416.

Pierce, S. R., & Buxbaum, L. J. (2002). Treatment of unilateral neglect: A review. *Archives of Physical Medicine and Rehabilitation, 83,* 256–268.

Wisconsin University. (2006). *Unit Nº. 2, brainstem: Superior colliculus.* Retrieved from http://www.neuroanatomy.wisc.edu/virtualbrain/BrainStem/23Colliculus.html

Synapse

The *synapse* is a specialized site of interaction or communication among the nerve cells or between a nerve cell and other types of cells. A synapse allows passing of a signal from one neuron to the next cell in an effective way. The communication may be conducted either chemically or electrically. In humans, almost all communications that occur at synapses are of a chemical nature. Specifically, releasing a variety of chemicals, collectively called neurotransmitters, transfers information between the two cells. This chemical signal is then converted into an electrical signal in the postsynaptic neuron (the receiving cell). If the electrical signal is large enough, it will generate an action potential that propagates along the postsynaptic neuron's axon.

A typical synapse is composed of an axon terminal of one neuron that delivers a signal (the presynaptic cell) and a dendrite of another neuron or a specialized receptor site on an effector cell that receives the signal (the postsynaptic cell). The narrow space between the presynaptic axon terminal and the postsynaptic cell membrane is the synaptic cleft. This is the location where neurotransmitters are released and

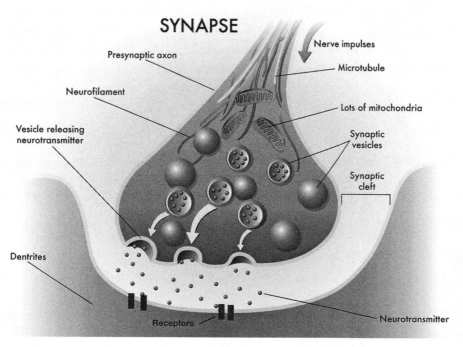

Elements of a typical axon to dendrite synapse, illustrating the release of neurotransmitters. (Dreamstime.com)

diffused across to the postsynaptic cell. The postsynaptic cell membrane contains a high concentration of receptors (specialized proteins) that bind specific neurotransmitters. Furthermore, the site of the synapse is often covered and insulated by supportive glial cells.

Each neuron in the brain is said to have approximately 5,000 synapses, each receiving a variety of signals from the presynaptic neuron. The signals received at the synapse may be excitatory or inhibitory in nature. An excitatory response propagates transmission of the signal through the postsynaptic cell, while an inhibitory response halts the signal. This electrical signal changes the resting potential (the voltage of the cell membrane at rest) of the postsynaptic neuron. These electrical signals are called postsynaptic potentials (PSPs), which are summed together throughout the postsynaptic neuron. If the PSPs are large enough, an all-or-none response is made at the region immediately before the axon, called the axon hillock. This all-or-none response is dependent upon whether or not the change in membrane potential has reached the threshold voltage to fire an action potential down the axon.

The communication through the synapse occurs at an incredibly fast speed with a typical neuron firing signals between 5 and 50 times a second. Once a signal is fired from a neuron, it is transmitted as an action potential through a long, cellular projection of the neuron called the axon. When the action potential reaches the end of an axon, termed the axon terminal or bouton, it triggers the stored vesicles filled with neurotransmitter to be released into the synaptic cleft. Once released, neurotransmitters diffuse across the synaptic cleft toward the postsynaptic cell membrane, which contains numerous neurotransmitter receptors. The specific binding of neurotransmitters to the receptors can generate PSPs and eventually an action potential in the postsynaptic cell, thus propagating the signal throughout the tissue. In case of an inhibitory signal, binding of neurotransmitters to the receptors may hyperpolarize the cell membrane, that is move the membrane potential more negative and away from the threshold potential. Thus, it inhibits the generation of an action potential.

Regardless, the released neurotransmitters in the synaptic cleft must be removed quickly to prevent erroneous signals from being generated in the postsynaptic cell. Some neurotransmitters diffuse away and degrade naturally. Those bound to the receptors on the postsynaptic membrane are engulfed and destroyed by the postsynaptic cell. Most neurotransmitters, however, are recycled and reused when the presynaptic axon terminal reuptakes them via endocytosis. This process reduces the workload on the already metabolically active neurons to ensure that neurotransmitters are not produced in excess.

Synapses also exist between presynaptic axons and their effector cells. For example, the neuromuscular junction is a synapse between a motor axon terminal and a skeletal muscle cell. Here, when an action potential reaches the axon terminal at the synapse, the neurotransmitter acetylcholine is released, which diffuses across the synaptic cleft and binds to acetylcholine receptors concentrated on the muscle cell membrane. An action potential is then generated in the muscle cell membrane, which travels quickly throughout the muscle cell, triggering the contractile mechanism.

Defects in any aspect of the synaptic mechanism may cause a variety of diseases ranging from depression and Parkinson's disease to myasthenia gravis, a progressive muscle-weakening condition.

History and Function

Aristotle (384–322 BC) first described the concept of communication between different parts of the body through a network of regulatory mechanisms, "spirit," or "energy" in the fourth century BC He believed that vital pneuma (ancient Greek for "breath": air, soul, spirit) that was inhaled from the universe traveled through the blood, eventually reaching the muscles, which triggered the muscles contraction. Between the second and third century AD, Galen (130–200 AD) and his pupils observed the importance of the brain and spinal cord as well as the nerves that arise from them. As a result, they elaborated that the inhaled vital pneuma is transported through the blood to the brain where it is converted into psychic pneuma, which is delivered to the muscles via nerve fibers to trigger muscle contractions.

René Decartes (1596–1650), 1300 years later, described that pneuma is converted into animal spirits in the form of fine particles in the brain, which is delivered to the muscle via nerves to initiate muscle contraction. This concept of the particle form of animal spirit being delivered from the nerve to the muscle was carefully scrutinized in the next several centuries. In the 1700s, Luigi Galvani (1737–1798) contested the concept of animal spirit particles, describing that the messages from the brain were being transmitted to the muscles and other organs in the form of electrical transmissions. The existence of electrical transmission was confirmed in the 19th century through the discovery of membrane potential across the nerve cell and localized wave of action potential. In 1879, Charles Sherrington (1857–1952) coined the term "synapse."

Anatomy and Physiology

The synapse is composed of a presynaptic axon terminal, a synaptic cleft, and a postsynaptic cell membrane that belongs to another neuron, muscle cell, or other cell types the neuron innervates. A typical presynaptic axon terminal is dilated and stores numerous vesicles that contain neurotransmitters. The wide variety of neurotransmitters can be classified into three groups of chemicals: amino acids, peptides, and monoamines. Most of the neurotransmitters are produced in the neuron cell body, where they are then concentrated and packaged into vesicles. The vesicles are then transported through the length of the axon to the axon terminals via microtubules that function as a set of transport cables. Once they reach the axon terminal, the vesicles accumulate and are stored until an action potential arrives and triggers their release.

Boutons and Boutons en Passant

Chemical synapses are the main functional connections of neurons to neurons, neurons to muscles, and neurons to secretory cells. The structure of a synapse is very small but is critical for the central nervous system to compute biological information into sensory perception as well as higher thinking. A chemical synapse consists of two cells and a space. The cells are called a *presynaptic neuron* and a *postsynaptic cell* while the space is called the *synaptic cleft*. Specifically, the synapse contains the axon of the presynaptic neuron connecting to the dendrite (branches that receive input signals), soma (cell body), or axon (output of a neuron) of the postsynaptic neuron. The morphology of the terminal end of the presynaptic axon is what made the French to name it a *bouton*, or button. *Boutons en Passant* is French for "buttons in passing" as an axon can be branched and have several boutons along its length. This makes the branched axon look like a string of pearls, or *boutons en passant*.

The presynaptic axon at the synapse becomes enlarged compared to the rest of the axon and look knob-like or button shaped. This is because it contains several organelles, like scaffolding proteins and mitochondria, and chemical packages called vesicles. The chemicals (neurotransmitters) are used to activate the postsynaptic neuron. These swellings of an axon are usually where a synapse will occur. In neuroscience, the terms *bouton, varicosity, en passant terminal,* and *axonal bouton* are generally used interchangeably.

Jennifer L. Hellier

See also: Axon; Synaptic Cleft

Further Reading

Bear, M., Bear, M. F., Connors, B. W., & Paradiso, M. A. (2001). *Neuroscience: Exploring the brain.* Hagerstown, MD: Lippincott Williams & Wilkins.

Frank, C. A., Wang, X., Collins, C. A., Rodal, A. A., Yuan, Q., Verstreken, P., & Dickman, D. K. (2013). New approaches for studying synaptic development, function, and plasticity using Drosophila as a model system. *Journal of Neuroscience, 33*(45), 17560–17568.

When an action potential reaches the axon terminal, the calcium channels in the axon membrane open allowing the influx of calcium ions (Ca^{2+}). The influx of Ca^{2+} triggers the vesicles to fuse with the axon terminal membrane to release neurotransmitters into the synaptic cleft. Neurotransmitters then diffuse across the synaptic cleft and bind to receptors that are present on the postsynaptic cell membrane. Depending on the receptor and the nature of interaction, binding of neurotransmitter will either depolarize (excite) or hyperpolarize (inhibit) the post-synaptic cell membrane. Depolarization refers to the reduction of charge difference between the inside and the outside of the cell membrane. At resting state, the inside of the cell is negatively charged and the outside of the cell positively charged. The charge difference between the inside and outside of the cell is the membrane potential.

When depolarization occurs, positively charged ions rush into the cell through the open membrane channels, reducing the charge difference across the cell membrane. Once the charge difference reaches a certain threshold level, it leads to an eventual reversal of the charge across the cell membrane (positive inside and negative outside), which is called the action potential. Hence, the neurotransmitter-receptor interaction that leads to the generation of an action potential in the postsynaptic cell is considered to be stimulatory. On the other hand, hyperpolarization refers to increasing of the charge difference between the inside and outside of the cell membrane, which makes it more difficult to generate an action potential. Thus, the neurotransmitter-receptor interaction that increases the negative charge in the inside the cell making it more difficult to generate an action potential in the postsynaptic cell is considered inhibitory. Since a single neuron may receive a mixture of signals from thousands of synapses, whether it fires its own action potential or not depends on the accumulating effect of all the signals at any given time.

Neuromuscular junctions, the synapse between an axon and a muscle cell, utilize the neurotransmitter acetylcholine exclusively. The muscle cell membrane at the neuromuscular junction contains a high concentration of acetylcholine receptors. Thus, binding of acetylcholine at the neuromuscular junction is an excitatory response, which leads to contraction of the muscle cell.

Diseases

Depression, addiction, anxiety disorders, autism, and schizophrenia are just a few known diseases that are involved with abnormalities at the synapse. Parkinson's disease is one of the most common brain disorders affecting persons over the age of 50, and is characterized by the loss of dopamine-producing neurons, which is the primary neurotransmitter used to regulate muscle movements. Decreases in dopamine levels and disruptions in synaptic communication among the neurons cause the loss of proper muscle function, leading to a series of irregular movements and other devastating symptoms in patients. Symptoms of Parkinson's disease include tremor, loss of dexterity and coordinated movements, reduced facial expression, constipation, drooling, difficulty swallowing, confusion, memory loss, and dementia. All of these symptoms increase in severity with progression of the disease. Although scientists do not know why dopamine-producing neurons die in Parkinson's disease, a number of genetic factors have been identified. Currently, there is no identified cure for Parkinson's disease and medical treatment is limited to managing symptoms such as reducing tremors, improving coordinated movements, and stimulating autonomic functions for digestion. Common medications for Parkinson's disease are designed to increase dopamine levels in the brain or directly act as dopamine agonists. Since the introduction of medications, the mortality rate in Parkinson's disease patients is reported to have dropped by 50 percent (Luscher and Isaac, 2008).

Another disease affected by abnormal synapses is myasthenia gravis, an autoimmune disease that attacks the neuromuscular junction. In this disease, the patient's own antibodies recognize, destroy, and reduce the amount of acetylcholine receptors on the muscle cell membrane at the neuromuscular junction. This, in turn, results in a reduced action potential generated in the muscle, causing progressive loss of muscle strength and generalized weakness. Researchers have identified synaptic signaling mechanisms at the neuromuscular junctions, thus, making myasthenia gravis one of the most treatable neural disorders. Patients are often treated with cholinesterase inhibitors and immunosuppressive drugs. Cholinesterase inhibitors prevent enzymes from breaking down acetylcholine, thus increasing its concentration and prolonging its presence in the synaptic cleft. Immunosuppressive drugs are designed to reduce the autoimmune recognition and/or destruction of acetylcholine receptors thereby increasing the amount of neurotransmitter that binds to receptors and subsequent action potential generation in the muscle cells. With the combination of these two types of medications, prognosis for patients with myasthenia gravis is quite good.

Depression is perhaps the most common neurological disorder (with a synaptic basis) that affects a large percentage of population but is commonly not diagnosed, misperceived, or treated. A current hypothesis for depression is that there exists an inappropriate interaction, regulation, and sensitivity of neurotransmitters and/or receptors at the synapse. Particularly, the reduction of the neurotransmitter serotonin or its receptors in the brain has been implicated to play an important role in depression. The active ingredients for most antidepressant medications are targeted to increase the concentration of serotonin in the synaptic cleft by inhibiting reuptake of serotonin into the presynaptic axon or inhibiting enzymes that break down serotonin.

A number of harmful drugs such as cocaine and methamphetamines affect the synapses of the brain but in a manner that is harmful and addictive. These drugs block reuptake of dopamine neurotransmitter by the presynaptic cell, prolonging its reward effects in the brain.

Lisa M. J. Lee

See also: Acetylcholine and Its Receptors; Action Potential; Axon; Dendrites— Building with Clay Activities; Dopamine and Its Receptors; Neuromuscular Junction; Parkinson's Disease; Serotonin and Its Receptors

Further Reading

Bennett, M. R. (1999). The early history of the synapse: From Plato to Sherrington. *Brain Research Bulletin, 50*(2), 95–118.

Boness, L. (2010). *Over 130 brain diseases linked to synapse proteins.* Retrieved from http:// scienceillustrated.com.au/blog/medicine/over-130-brain-diseases-linked-to-synapse-proteins/

Hasselbring, B. (n.d.). *How do antidepressants work?* Retrieved from http://health.how stuffworks.com/mental-health/depression/questions/how-do-antidepressants-work.htm

Linden, D. J. (2007). *The accidental mind: How brain evolution has given us love, memory, dreams, and god.* Cambridge, MA: The Belknap Press of Harvard University Press.

Luscher, C., & Isaac, J. T. (2008). The synapse: Center stage for many brain diseases. *The Journal of Physiology, 587*, 727–729.

Ross, M. H., & Pawlina, W. (2011). *Histology: A text and atlas* (6th ed.). Baltimore, MD: Lippincott Williams & Wilkins. http://health.howstuffworks.com/mental-health/depres sion/questions/how-do-antidepressants-work.htm

Synaptic Cleft

The central nervous system connects most of its neurons by chemical signals that travel from one neuron to the other. This forms the *synapse* (the functional connection of two cells) and the *synaptic cleft* (the space between the two cells). The synaptic cleft can also be found between neuronal and nonneuronal cells like muscle or secretory cells. These chemical synapses allow the central nervous system to make complex circuits that modulate signals and compute biological information into sensory perception to higher thinking within the brain. Additionally, chemical synapses connect the central nervous system to other parts of the body.

The synaptic cleft is so small (about 20 nanometers) it cannot be viewed with a light microscope but it has been confirmed to exist by electron microscopy. The synaptic cleft consists of two cells, the *presynaptic neuron* and the *postsynaptic cell,* and the space between the cells. The postsynaptic cell can be a neuron, muscle cell, or a secretory cell. At the synaptic cleft, it is the terminal end of the presynaptic cell's axon that is connecting to the postsynaptic neuron's *dendrite* (branches that receive input signals), *soma* (cell body), or *axon* (output of the neuron). Depending on the location of the synapse—axon to dendrite, axon to soma, or axon to axon—the outcome of the chemical signal can vary greatly.

The axon of the presynaptic neuron contains several little packages of chemicals. These packages are called *vesicles* while the chemicals are called *neurotransmitters*. The vesicles fuse with the presynaptic membrane, releasing the neurotransmitter into the synaptic cleft. Because of its small size, neurotransmitter concentration within the cleft increases quickly. The neurotransmitter crosses over to the postsynaptic cell and binds to the *receptors* that are located within the postsynaptic cell membrane. These receptors are specialized proteins that form a pore or channel, allowing ions to flow into or out of the cell. This action will change the membrane potential of the postsynaptic cell, which can result in producing an all-or-none response called an *action potential.*

To stop the chemical signaling within the synaptic cleft, the neurotransmitter must be cleared from the space. This occurs by three different methods: (1) natural diffusion out of the space, (2) repackaging of the neurotransmitter into vesicles within the presynaptic neuron, and (3) breakdown of the neurotransmitter by enzymes. From these actions, the concentration of the transmitter decreases quickly within the small space of the synaptic cleft. Any neurotransmitter that is bound to the receptor will eventually break loose from thermal shaking. These molecules will also be removed from the synaptic cleft by one or all of the three methods previously stated. This ends the synaptic activity and "resets" the synaptic cleft for its next chemical wave.

Jennifer L. Hellier

See also: Acetylcholine and Its Receptors; AMPA and Its Receptors; Dopamine and Its Receptors; GABA and Its Receptors; Glutamate and Its Receptors; Glycine and Its Receptors; NMDA and Its Receptors; Serotonin and Its Receptors; Synapse

Further Reading

Bear, M., Bear, M. F., Connors, B. W., & Paradiso, M. A. (2001). *Neuroscience: Exploring the brain.* Hagerstown, MA: Lippincott Williams & Wilkins.

Kandel, E. R., Schwartz, J. H., & Jessell, T. M. (2000). *Principles of neural science* (4th ed.). New York, NY: McGraw-Hill.

T

Tardive Dyskinesia

Dopamine and its receptors (specialized proteins in brain cells) are found throughout the brain. The receptor is activated when dopamine is bound, but can be inactivated by drugs called dopamine receptor blockers. *Tardive dyskinesia* (TD) is a condition seen in humans after continuing exposure to dopamine receptor blockers, mainly those used as antipsychotic (to stop psychoses) and antiemetic (to stop nausea) medications such as chlorpromazine. The term *tardive* means "delayed" while the word *dyskinesia* means "abnormal movement." The movements typically seen with TD primarily involve the tongue, lips, and jaw. A combination of tongue twisting and protrusion, lip smacking and puckering, and chewing movements in a repetitive and stereotypic fashion is often observed. This pattern is in contrast to the dyskinesias seen in Huntington's disease, where movements are random and unpredictable. Although usually confined to the orofacial area, dyskinesias may spread to the extremities. The involuntary mouth movements may be readily suppressed by the patients when asked to do so. They can also be suppressed by voluntary actions such as putting food in the mouth or talking. When TD involves the limbs, the legs often move repeatedly, with flexion and extension of the toes and foot tapping while sitting. Commonly, the hands will twist and have splayed "piano-playing" fingers. Respiratory dyskinesias may occur and cause increased or decreased breathing, which is rarely life threatening. The full TD syndrome may take days to weeks to develop and often stabilizes. TD tends to emerge for the first time or worsen when a dopamine receptor blocking agent is reduced or discontinued. Reinstituting or increasing the dose of the offending drug often reduces movements.

History

Dopamine receptor blockers and other antipsychotic drugs were first developed in the 1950s. However, TD was first seen and coined by Faurbye and colleagues

(1964). In this description, Faurbye emphasized that the incidence increased with duration of exposure to dopamine blocking agents.

Pathophysiology

Tardive dyskinesia is primarily seen after long-term use of dopamine blocking agents used to treat schizophrenia, although the symptoms will sometimes be seen after a reduction in dose or the withdrawal of the drug. A few drugs used for nausea, such as metoclopramide or prochlorperazine, exert their effect by blocking dopamine receptors. Thus, TD is seen with extended treatment of these agents as well. Ironically, the agents that cause TD also suppress those same symptoms before they have a chance to manifest.

This raises questions about whether TD is a manifestation of schizophrenia itself, or if it solely dependent on dopamine receptor blockade. TD unfortunately is prolonged and often irreversible even after the cessation of the prescribed drug. It is hypothesized that this occurs because long-term blockade of dopamine receptors results in an increase in receptors that become supersensitive, which leads to changes to brain chemisty. The hypothesis suggests that an imbalance between different dopamine receptors (D1 and D2) in the basal ganglia (deep structures in the brain) may be responsible for TD. According to this theory, traditional antipsychotic drugs like chlorpromazine preferentially block D2 receptors, resulting in excessive activity of D1 receptors. This leads to the D1 receptors having an altered firing patterns and producing the clinical features of TD. This model explains why new second-generation antipsychotics (clozapine and olanzapine) are less likely to cause TD because they do not block D2 receptors completely but also block other dopamine receptors as well as serotonin receptors.

Epidemiology

Overall, the incidence of new TD cases ranges from 3 to 8 percent annually, and the incidence increases to 10–20 percent in those patients over the age of 55 (Dynamed, 2013). The risk of developing TD with the use of second-generation antipsychotics is much lower than first generation, although it is still possible especially with higher doses and long-term use. Some patients require multiple agents to help stabilize their disease and this will increase their risk of developing TD.

Prevention and Treatment

Prevention of TD and the early detection and treatment of potentially reversible cases of TD are of paramount importance. The only certain method of TD prevention is to avoid treatment with antipsychotic drugs and metoclopramide. The use of antipsychotic drugs, particularly for longer than three months, requires careful evaluation of indications, risks-benefits, and should be limited to situations where there is no safer effective therapy. Metoclopramide should not be used continuously for longer than 12 weeks.

While the treatment for TD is currently lacking, the American Psychiatric Association Task Force has the most promising recommendations. They recommend that antipsychotics not be used in other disease states such as depression, anxiety, sleep disorders, and chronic pain. Those requiring antipsychotics should be maintained on the lowest effective dose and should be evaluated every six months to reexamine the need for treatment. With close monitoring, health care providers can recognize early movement disorders that arise before TD, and thus a reduction in dose or drug switch can be made.

The best data for treating TD is seen with prevention and close monitoring; however, there are some pharmacological agents that have been shown promise. Benzodiazepines (a class of drugs used to treat seizures) have some evidence because they increase gamma-aminobutyric acid (GABA). Studies have shown that TD is associated with the depletion of GABA and therefore benzodiazepines are a reasonable choice. The use of clozapine, which is an atypical antipsychotic, has been used because it has the lowest incidence of causing TD than all other agents. Clozapine, however, comes with an extensive list of side effects itself and therefore the decision needs to be made diligently. Other treatments have been tried but they tend to not be as effective. These include (1) switching to second-generation antipsychotics with less TD incidence (olanzapine, risperidone, quetiapine); (2) Botulinun Toxin Type-A (botox); (3) vitamin E; (4) medications affecting acetylcholine and its receptors; and (5) deep brain stimulation. Presently, none of the options have been very successful, and therefore the best approach is to watch patients carefully.

Conclusion

Tardive dyskinesia does not cause physical harm to the patient, but is an extremely debilitating and socially crippling syndrome. Oftentimes, TD can be reversed with stopping the offending drug, yet this decision is not easy if the patient's psychosis is being controlled. TD can be irreversible, thus clinicians must follow these patients carefully to see if TD symptoms start to manifest themselves.

Jeremy E. Brothers

See also: Dopamine and Its Receptors; Schizophrenia

Further Reading

DynaMed. (2013). *Tardive Dyskinesia.* Ipswich, MA: EBSCO Information Services.

Faurbye, A., Rasch, P. J., Petersen, P. B., Brandborg, G., & Pakkenberg, H. (1964). Neurological symptoms in pharmacotherapy of psychoses. *Acta Psychiatrica Scandinavica, 40,* 10–27.

Soares-Weiser, K., & Fernandez, H. (2007). Tardive dyskinesia. *Seminars in Neurology, 27*(2), 159–169.

Taste Aversion

The word *aversion* means a "strong dislike of something"; thus, the term *taste aversion* means a "strong dislike of a certain food," which can last for years. A taste aversion or a *conditioned taste aversion* develops when an animal or a human associates a certain food with symptoms of sickness (vomiting and nausea) that were caused by toxic, poisonous, or spoiled food. Taste aversions can be so strong that it only takes one episode of associating a food with sickness for the taste aversion to develop.

Taste aversions are common in persons receiving chemotherapy, which can be dangerous as each time the patient eats a new food, they develop a new taste aversion. This is because the medicine causes the nausea or vomiting, but the patient associates the sickness with ingesting the food. Eventually, chemotherapy patients do not want to eat, which can slow down their recovery as well as be dangerous to their overall health.

Taste Aversion Experiments

American psychologist John Garcia (1917–2012) was most noted for his conditioned taste aversion experiments performed in the 1950s. Garcia was observing a rat's behavior following a session of radiation. He found that the rat would develop a taste aversion to the food it ate just prior to the radiation treatment. At the time, scientists believed that taste aversions would develop after a single trial with a long delay between the ingestion of the food and the sickness. Thus, to better understand the occurrence of taste aversion, Garcia gave three groups of rats sweetened water and then followed it with Group 1 receiving no radiation, Group 2 receiving mild radiation, and Group 3 receiving strong radiation. He then measured the amount of sweetened water they would drink after the radiation or no radiation session. The rats with both mild and strong radiation drank significantly less sweetened water compared to nonirradiated rats. This finding showed that a long delay was not required to develop a taste aversion and that an event causing nausea could produce the association to the food. Thus, the study of conditioned taste aversion began.

Behavior and Physiology

Survival of a species is a paramount trait that is innate in all animals. Behavioral scientists and psychologists posit that taste aversions are a type of survival mechanism or an adaptive trait that teaches the animal to avoid toxic or poisonous foods, such as poisonous plants (e.g., oleander, floxglove, and rubarb leaves) and berries (e.g., nightshade, holly, and pokeweed berries). By causing the animal to vomit or be nauseated, the animal will stop eating the plant or berry before it causes severe harm or death. This strong association of a food with sickness will protect the animal so that it will avoid other similar plants or berries and ultimately avoid future toxicities or poisonings.

The development of a taste aversion, however, can be unintentional. Specifically, a taste aversion can occur by other events or other substances and not by the food itself. Consider the following example of an event causing the taste aversion. A person at an amusement park eats a hot dog. Right after he eats, the person rides a fast spinning ride like the Tea Cups at Disneyland, which makes him vomit. The spinning ride actually caused the nausea or sickness, but the person associates the hot dog as the cause of the vomiting. For an example of another substance causing a taste aversion, consider a young child with a very loose tooth eating corn on the cob. The child bites into the corn, which results in the tooth falling out and the gum bleeding. The mixture of blood with the corn can cause a sickening taste or feeling. Thus, the child will develop a taste aversion to the corn, when it was the blood that caused the nausea. Both of these types of instant taste aversion can last for years and may never become extinct.

Disease and Treatments

Patients with cancers often receive chemotherapy and/or radiation to treat their disease. As shown by Garcia, this can lead to taste aversions. It is important to note that a person does not need cognitive awareness for a taste aversion to develop. This means that the person does not have to recognize the connection of the cause and the effect or the food and the sickness. As in chemotherapy patients, they are hungry and hope to enjoy their food, but the drugs make them sick and cause their body to reject the food. Thus, research has focused on developing strong antiemetic (anti-nausea and anti-vomiting) drugs to counteract and to prevent the development of taste aversions for cancer patients as well as for motion sickness.

Jennifer L. Hellier

See also: Dizziness and Vertigo; Pavlov, Ivan; Reward and Punishment; Taste System

Further Reading

Bernstein, I. L. (1999). Taste aversion learning: A contemporary perspective. *Nutrition, 15*(3), 229–234.

Carelli, R. M., & West, E. A. (2014). When a good taste turns bad: Neural mechanisms underlying the emergence of negative affect and associated natural reward devaluation by cocaine. *Neuropharmacology, 76*(B), 360–369.

Garcia, J., Kimeldorf, D. J., & Koelling, R. A. (1955). Conditioned aversion to saccharin resulting from exposure to gamma radiation. *Science, 122*(3160), 157–158.

Taste System

Taste, or gustation, is the sensation that occurs when a substance in the mouth, a tastant, reacts chemically with receptors to send a signal to the brain. Taste is to be distinguished from flavor, a term that generally describes a broader experience, which includes gustation, olfaction (smell), trigeminal nerve stimulation (texture, pain, temperature), and even sight and sound. There are five basic categories of taste: *bitter, sweet, sour, salty,* and *umami* (a Japanese word that loosely translates as "savory" in English). Other possible basic tastes, such as fatty acids, calcium, carbon dioxide, and even water, are being investigated.

Taste has evolved to help humans distinguish between nutritious and toxic foods. Foods with sugar have evolved to taste good because sugar is essential for survival. Umami tastes delicious because proteins are essential. Salt is an essential nutrient that must be consumed in a specific amount to maintain proper levels in the body; this is why a little bit of salt tastes good, but too much salt tastes bad. Sour appears to have both aversive and pleasant qualities that function to alert us when foods have spoiled or when plants are not yet ripe, but also to encourage the consumption of sour fruit that contain important vitamins and nutrients. Bitterness has evolved to be a generally aversive taste because most foods that taste bitter tend to be poisonous. However, the bitter molecules in many edible plants are toxic only in high concentrations and these edible plants contain anticarcinogenic (fight against cancer) nutrients. Thus, it makes sense that these edible plants taste pleasant to many people.

Anatomy

Taste stimulants (tastants) are detected via taste organs, called taste buds, which are located in the mucosa of the tongue, soft palate (roof of the mouth), inner cheeks, pharynx, and epiglottis. It is important to note that taste buds are *not* the bumps on a person's tongue; these are called papillae. Each person has about 3,000–10,000 taste buds, most of which are on the surface of the tongue (Bartoshuk and Snyder, 2013). Each taste bud is a cluster of 50–100 elongated epithelial cells arranged like the segments of an orange. The cells are renewed about every 12 days. They are divided into three main groups: Type I are support cells; Type II are the receptor cells, which contain the G protein-coupled receptors that bind sweet, bitter, and umami

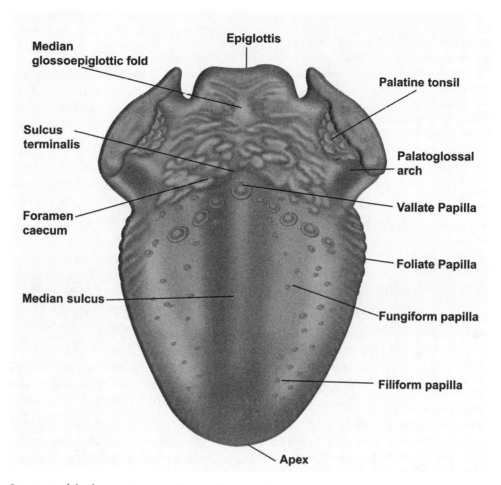

Structure of the human tongue. (Dreamstime.com)

tastants; and Type III react to sour stimuli, which involve ion channels. Type III are also known as presynaptic cells because, unlike Type II, they have they have identifiable synapses with the nerve fiber and release neurotransmitters, such as serotonin and GABA (gamma-aminobutyric acid), onto the afferent nerve fiber. The mechanism that Type II cells use to excite the nerve fiber is unknown; however, it is speculated that ATP (adenosine triphosphate) acts as a transmitter. The cells that contain receptors for salty taste have not been clearly delineated.

The receptor proteins are located in the plasma membrane of long microvilli called gustatory hairs that extend from the taste cells through a taste pore to the surface of the papillae. The taste pores are filled with saliva, which transports the dissolved tastants to the receptors. The epithelial taste cells then generate impulses in the sensory nerve fibers that innervate them.

Most taste buds are contained in papillae. There are three types of papillae: the relatively large circumvallate, found at the back of the tongue in an arc; foliate, found on the edges of the medial tongue; and fungiform, found at the tip of the tongue. The taste pores containing the protrusions of the microvilli are located on the surface of the fungiform papillae and buried in the sides of the circumvallate and foliate papillae. In order for food molecules to be tasted, they must be dissolved in saliva because only then can they flow into the taste pores.

The popular tongue map that shows each of the five tastes being perceived on a certain region of the tongue, specifically bitter on the back, sweet on the tip, is a successfully propagated myth that was started in 1942 by a textbook author who misunderstood a research paper on the subject. Contrary to this popular belief, all five tastes can be perceived anywhere there are taste buds.

To the Brain

Taste information travels to the brain via three cranial nerves, which serve sensory and motor function to the face, head, and neck. The chorda tympani branch of the facial nerve (cranial nerve VII) carries impulses from taste receptors in the anterior two-thirds of the tongue; the glossopharyngeal nerve (cranial nerve IX) from the tongue's posterior third and pharynx; and the vagus nerve (cranial nerve X) from the few taste buds on the epiglottis and lower pharynx. These three cranial nerves synapse in a nucleus (a group of cell bodies) in the medulla called the *solitary nucleus*. From there, impulses are transmitted to the *ventral posterior medial nucleus* of the thalamus and then to the gustatory area of the cerebral cortex in the *insula lobe*. The orbitofrontal cortex receives projections from the insular cortex, as well as information about touch, temperature, and smell, suggesting it is an integration area for flavor. The three nerves partially inhibit one another. This provides a means to retain taste perception if one nerve is damaged, for the other two nerves will have amplified signals. When a nerve is damaged, this delicate inhibition process is tampered with and this can sometimes result in "phantom taste."

The lingual branch of the trigeminal nerve (cranial nerve V) has nerve endings surrounding taste buds. It sends sensory information about touch, temperature, and pain. These nerves can be irritated by certain chemicals, such as capsaicin, and send a signal of pain and heat to the brain, giving us the sensation of spiciness, or pungency. Menthol works the same and elicits a feeling of coolness. These are both chemesthetic sensations.

Theories of Transduction

There are two theories that explain how taste sensations are encoded from receptor to brain: the *labeled line hypothesis* and *pattern coding theory*. Labeled line theorizes that each individual nerve fiber encodes only one of the five basic tastes. Pattern coding, also known as across fiber coding or population coding, theorizes that nerve fibers receive information from more than one of the five tastes, and the overall pattern of many nerve fibers firing is interpreted by the brain to be a particular taste or tastes.

In fungiform papillae, the nerve fibers that innervate taste cells branch so they innervate multiple cells, and each cell can also be innervated by multiple different fibers. Recordings show that the taste cells innervated by branches of the same taste fiber have similar specificities to tastants. This supports the labeled line theory. However, recordings also show that nerve fibers can respond to more than one taste class, evidence supporting the pattern coding theory. A general consensus is beginning to arise that both theories are partially correct: nerve fibers are "best" at transducing one taste. So while they may weakly respond to another taste, "sucrose" best fibers, for example, are best at sending the "sweet" message to the brain.

Bitter

Bitterness is a "bad" taste that is believed to have developed to preserve life, as many bitter foods are poisonous. Thus, when a person or animal eats something that is bitter, they do not like the taste and spit it out. Substances that are bitter include coffee, beer, aspirin, quinine, peels of citrus fruits, and many vegetables. There are about 25 different known receptor proteins that bind with bitter tastants. They are called the T2R receptors and are encoded from a family of genes called *Tas2r,* which are located on three different chromosomes: chromosome 5, chromosome 7, and chromosome 12. Some of the receptors have known ligands; however, most of the bitter stimuli humans encounter have not yet been linked to their receptors. The bitter molecule— quinine, which is often used in taste studies—has been shown to stimulate nine different receptors. The brain does not distinguish between different types of bitter ligands; the brain perceives all bitters as the same one bitter taste. This is true for all five tastes.

In 1932, a chemist discovered that a particular molecule, phenylthiocarbamide (PTC), tastes bitter to some people but is tasteless to others. A chemically similar molecule, propylthiouracil (PROP), was later identified to elicit the same responses. The TR2 receptor involved in binding these molecules, called TAS2R38, was identified during the Human Genome Project along with all the other T2R receptors. People with two recessive copies of the gene *TAS2R38* cannot taste PTC and PROP, while those with at least one copy of the dominant allele can generally taste them. The bitter molecule in cruciferous vegetables such as broccoli and brussel sprouts is detected by the TAS2R38 protein receptor. Children, who have stronger senses of taste than adults, often strongly dislike these vegetables because, if they have a dominant allele of the gene, they can taste the bitterness. It is speculated that "taste blindness" to this bitterness was selected for in some regions of the world because those that eat vegetables, gain the anti-cancer benefits of them and are more likely to survive.

In the early 1990s, the term "supertaster" was coined by American psychologist Linda Bartoshuk (1938–) to describe people who reported an intense sensitivity to the bitterness of PROP. In a 1994 study, Bartoshuk found a correlation between PROP supertasters and a high fungiform papillae count as well as increased sweetness and capsaicin sensations. This subsequently led to the use of the term supertasters by the media and general public to include those that have a hypersensitivity to all tastes. Since the two definitions are different, and because the association of fungiform papillae density to PROP sensitivity is no longer uniformly accepted in the field (Fischer et al., 2013), the term hyperguesia has been suggested to describe those that have hypersensitivity to taste.

Sweet

Sweetness is the taste of simple carbohydrates (sugar), which are the body's source of energy. It is important for survival and eating sweet foods signals reward pathways in human brains so that everyone is encouraged to eat these energy-rich foods. There are about 25 variants of the T2R bitter receptors but only 3 variants of the T1R G protein–coupled receptors for sweet and umami. This makes sense, for while there are many different molecules that are poisonous, there are only a few different carbohydrates that are biologically important to humans. In order for most sweet molecules to be detected, the T1R2 and T1R3 receptors must unite to form a heterodimer. This receptor has several binding positions for each different sweet molecule. The T1R3 receptor can also act alone; it binds sucrose.

Umami

Umami (Japanese for "deliciousness") was recognized as a basic taste in the 1980s (although it was identified by a Japanese scientist in the early 1900s). It is a savory taste that is elicited by the amino acid glutamate that is found naturally in meat, aged cheeses, and tomatoes. In its salt form, glutamate is the flavor enhancer monosodium glutamate, or MSG. There was controversy about the safety of MSG, but the consensus today is that aside from a few sensitive people, MSG is safe. The umami receptor is a G protein–coupled receptor that is a heterodimer of the T1R1 and T1R3 receptors.

Salty

Saltiness is the taste elicited by salts, which are molecules made up of oppositely charged particles. The salt humans most often ingest is table salt, sodium chloride (NaCl). NaCl dissolves into positively and negatively ions, Na^+ and Cl^-, when in water. Sodium ions enter taste cells through sodium ion channels and depolarize the taste cells, causing them to transduce signal to the afferent nerve fiber.

Sour

Sour is the taste of acid, such as hydrogen chloride (HCl) or organic acids, such as lactic acid and citric acid. Sour foods include many fruits, especially citrus fruits, vinegar, yogurt, and spoiled dairy, such as cheese and sour cream. Acids release hydrogen ions (H^+) that interact with ion channels on taste cells and depolarize them. The exact mechanisms of H^+ detection are not completely understood. One mechanism that plays a role is the blockage of potassium channels in taste cell membranes by H^+, preventing the release of K^+ from the cell and causing depolarization and neurotransmitter release.

Emma Boxer

See also: Chorda Tympani Nerve; Cranial Nerves; Facial Nerve; G Proteins; Glossopharyngeal Nerve; Ion Channels; Sensory Receptors; Trigeminal Nerve; Vagus Nerve

Further Reading

Bartoshuk, L. M., & Snyder, D. J. (2013). Taste. In D. W. Pfaff (Ed.), *Neuroscience in the 21st century, from basic to clinical* (pp. 781–813). New York, NY: Springer Science+Business Media LLC.

Fischer, M., Cruickshanks, M., Schubert, C., Pinto, A., Klein, R., Pankratz, N., . . . Huang, G. (2013). Factors related to fungiform papillae density: The beaver dam offspring study. *Chemical Senses, 38,* 669–677.

Hayes, J. E., & Keast, R. S. (2011). Two decades of supertasting: Where do we stand? *Physiology and Behavior, 104*(5), 1072–1074.

Mueller, K. L., Hoon, M. A., Erlenbach, I., Chandrashekar, J., Zuker, C. S., & Ryba, N. J. (2005). The receptors and coding logic for bitter taste. *Nature, 434,* 225–229.

Yarmolinsky, D. A., Zuker, C. S., & Ryba, N. J. P. (2009). Common sense about taste: From mammals to insects. *Cell, 139*(2), 234–244.

Tay-Sachs Disease

Tay-Sachs disease, also known as *GM2 gangliosidoses* or *Hexosaminidase A* deficiency, is an autosomal recessive genetic disease that causes a progressive and irreversible deterioration of nerve cells primarily in the brain that begins in affected individuals at about six months of age. Nerve cell deterioration is caused by an accumulation of *gangliosides* (complex biological molecules) due to the lack of the enzyme *hexosaminidase A,* which is responsible for the enzymatic breakdown of *fatty acids* into other metabolic by-products. Symptoms consist of the gradual development of deafness, blindness, and difficulty with swallowing as the muscles of the neck and throat become weakened. Death usually occurs by the age of four. At this point in time, there is no known treatment for Tay-Sachs disease. Treatment consists of providing medical and nonmedical support for patients affected by this disease.

Historical Perspective

Tay-Sachs disease was first reported by British ophthalmologist Waren Tay (1843–1927) and Jewish-American neurologist Bernard Sachs (1858–1944) in 1884. Both physicians observed the specific symptoms of this disease that were clearly different from other nondescript neurological diseases of the time. Tay-Sachs disease was first observed in the eastern European Ashkenzai Jewish population and Dr. Sachs was the first to recognize that there was a familial basis for this disease. In 1969, researchers Shintaro Okada (n.d.) and John S. O'Brien (n.d.) showed the molecular and genetic basis for this disease and were able to demonstrate that it is caused by a deficiency in hexosaminidase A and the resultant buildup of gangliosides in neurons (specialized cells that transmit electrical impulses) of the brain.

Genetics

Tay-Sachs disease is an autosomal recessive genetic disease that is the result of a defect in the gene needed for the synthesis of the enzyme hexosaminidase A, which normally helps with the breakdown of fatty acids in cells. Individuals affected by this disease have two copies of the defective gene (recessive), one from each parent. The specific gene affected is known as the HEXA gene, which is located on chromosome 15. At this point in time, researchers have found over 100 different mutations of this gene. The more common mutations include *single base insertions* or *deletions* where single *nucleotide bases* (segments of deoxyribonucleic acid, DNA) have been removed or added. This results in a defective polypeptide, and *missense mutations* where single nucleotide bases have been replaced by another base, rendering the gene defective.

Today, Tay-Sachs disease is one of the many disorders that newborn children are screened for at birth. This is done through the testing of a blood sample from a person suspected of having this disease. In this blood test, hexosaminidase A activity is tested and if present, it is assumed that the genetic mutation that causes this disease is not present.

Pathophysiology

The most common form of Tay-Sachs disease is known as *infantile Tay-Sachs* disease. In infantile Tay-Sachs disease, infants appear to be symptom free for three to six months after birth. As a child continues to mature, they begin to exhibit delayed maturity and development of specific "milestones" associated with normal development. Infants will begin to develop symptoms of nervous system dysfunction that can include the development of a generalized decrease in response to mental and/or physical stimuli, seizures, and general *lethargy* (decreased physical activity, depressed emotional state, and/or listlessness). Infants often show delayed development of specific motor skills such as sitting, turning over, or crawling. As children become older, they also begin to exhibit decreased coordination, which can lead to difficulty walking, difficulty maintain their balance, issues with speech, and often difficulty with swallowing and breathing. These complications are all related to decreased function of motor neurons in the nervous system as a result of the buildup of gangliosides in the cells. One very specific diagnostic sign of Tay-Sachs disease is the presence of a *cherry-red spot* in the retina. The relationship between this finding and the overall effects of the disease are still unclear.

Although much less common, individuals can develop symptoms of Tay-Sachs disease as adults as well. Adults who develop Tay-Sachs disease often show a much milder form of the disease. The most common symptoms include muscle weakness, *ataxia* or the loss of muscle coordination, and speech issues. While adult onset of Tay-Sachs does not directly cause a rapid death, individuals affected with adult onset Tay-Sachs disease do often become very dependent on wheel chairs and other assistive devices for completion of normal daily activities.

Because this disease tends to remain in families, it is possible today to help prevent or reduce the incidence of Tay-Sachs disease in a family. These include (1) the use of prenatal diagnosis, which is often used when both parents are known *carriers* of the defective HEXA gene (meaning they each have one copy of the defective gene); (2) *preimplantation genetic diagnosis* (PGD) where eggs from the mother are fertilized via *in vitro* fertilization and the fertilized egg is then tested to see if the gene exists in the egg; or (3) mate selection where individuals consciously select mates who have been shown not to carry the gene for Tay-Sachs disease.

Future Research

Significant research is being done to gain a better understanding of the pathophysiology of Tay-Sachs disease as well as trying to develop treatments for patients affected by this disease. While there is no definitive treatment for Tay-Sachs disease as yet, significant progress is being made toward the further understanding of how this disease progresses over time. Current research directions include:

- *Substrate reduction:* Researchers are investigating the use of several enzymes similar to hexosaminidase in an attempt to help neurons in the brain breakdown accumulating gangliosides. One enzyme that has shown an ability to degrade gangliosides is called *sialidase*. However use of sialidase is still very experimental.

- *Hexosaminidase A activity stimulation:* Investigators are working with a drug called *pyrimethamine,* which has been shown in preliminary experiments to potentially increase the activity of hexosaminidase A. Unfortunately, at this point in time, this drug has not shown the desired outcome to make it an effective treatment.
- *Enzyme replacement:* Studies are being done to see if providing patients with *exogenous* hexosaminidase A through injection into the vascular system (the veins) or into the *cerebrospinal fluid* that surrounds the brain and spinal cord may be a way to help patients affected with Tay-Sachs disease metabolize increased gangliosides more easily. Early results, however, indicate that this is probably not a valid treatment path as the enzyme itself is too large to be able to pass through the walls of blood vessels or to get through to the neurons of the brain.

Summary

Tay-Sachs disease is an autosomal recessive genetic disease that results in the failure of the enzyme hexosaminidase to be produced and to degrade fatty acids as part of the normal cellular metabolism of neurons. The failure of hexosaminidase to be synthesized is due to mutation of the HEXA gene located on chromosome number 15 in humans. Common symptoms of infantile Tay-Sachs disease include muscular weakness, particularly of the throat and neck, difficult swallowing, problems with balance, and speech issues. Most individuals affected by this disease do not live past the age of four on average. Patients who exhibit adult onset Tay-Sachs disease often have similar symptoms as patients with infantile Tay-Sachs, but to a much lesser degree.

At this point in time, there is no significant treatment or cure for Tay-Sachs disease. Researchers are experimenting with several techniques that would either replace the missing enzyme allowing normal breakdown of fatty acids, or finding a similar enzyme that might be able to replace hexosaminidase activity and prevent this disease. Some early experiments are being done to investigate the possibility of using gene replacement therapy, but those studies are in their initial stages and many years from human use or trials. Treatment at this point in time consists of using assistive devices to overcome muscular weakness and other therapy to assist with the normal activities of daily living.

Charles A. Ferguson

See also: Ataxia; Gene Therapy; Seizures

Further Reading

Chavancy, C., & Jendoubi, M. (1998). Biology and potential strategies for the treatment of GM2 gangliosidoses. *Molecular Medicine Today, 4*(4), 158–165.

Fernandes Filho, J. A., & Shapiro, B. E. (2004). Tay-Sachs disease. *Archives of Neurology, 61*(9), 1466–1468.

Maegawa, G. H., Stockley, T., Tropak, M., Banwell, B., Blaser, S., Kok, F., . . . Clarke, J. T. (2006). The natural history of juvenile or subacute GM2 gangliosidosis: 21 new cases and literature review of 134 previously reported. *Pediatrics, 118*(5), 1550–1562.

Mahuran, D. J. (1999). Biochemical consequences of mutations causing the GM2 gangliosidoses. *Biochimica et Biophysica Acta, 1455*(2–3), 105–138.

Montalvo, A. L., Filocamo, M., Vlahovicek, K., Dardis, A., Lualdi, S., Corsolini, F., . . . Pittis, M. G. (2005). Molecular analysis of the HEXA gene in Italian patients with infantile and late onset Tay-Sachs disease: Detection of fourteen novel alleles. *Human Mutations, 26*(3), 282.

Neudorfer, O., Pastores, G. M., Zeng, B. J., Gianutsos, J., Zaroff, C. M., & Kolodny, E. H. (2005). Late-onset Tay-Sachs disease: Phenotypic characterization and genotypic correlations in 21 affected patients. *Genetics in Medicine, 7*(2), 119–123.

Telencephalon

In vertebrate development, different regions of the neural tube give rise to the structures of the central nervous system (the brain, brainstem, and spinal column). These are the forebrain (*prosencephalon*), the midbrain (*mesencephalon*), and the hindbrain (*rhombencephalon*). The *telencephalon* is the region of the neural tube that makes up what is called the cerebrum, which is the largest and superior (meaning by direction as in toward the top) part of the brain. Along with the diencephalon, the telencephalon makes up the forebrain. In the adult brain, the telencephalon sits above the diencephalon (comprised of four sub-structures including the *epithalamus, thalamus, subthalamus,* and *hypothalamus*) and above the brainstem (*midbrain, pons,* and *medulla oblongata*). The telencephalon is divided into the ventral (toward the chin) and dorsal (toward the top of the skull) sections. The ventral telencephalon becomes the basal nuclei or the subpallidum, while the dorsal telencephalon becomes the cerebral cortex or pallidum. The pallidum is what most people see in popular pictures of the brain. The term *telencephalon* is derived from Greek, meaning the "last brain" as it is the last portion of the brain to develop fully. During this final development, the mammalian cerebrum consists of gyri (plural; gyrus, singular form) and sulci (plural; sulcus, singular form). Together these make up the bumps and grooves, respectively, that give the brain a convoluted and unique shape.

The cerebrum is divided into two hemispheres that are joined by a large bundle of white matter (axons of neurons that are covered in a protective insulation called myelin). This bundle is called the corpus callosum, which allows the two hemispheres to "talk to each other." In addition, the cerebrum is divided into four main lobes with one on each hemisphere: frontal lobe, parietal lobe, temporal lobe, and the occipital lobe. Each lobe has been shown to have specific functions to serve the sensory and motor activities of the body.

Frontal Lobe

The frontal lobe is rostral (toward the nose) to the parietal lobe and dorsal to the temporal lobe. The central sulcus is the demarcation between the frontal and parietal lobes. Similarly, the lateral or Sylvian fissure separates the frontal lobe from the temporal lobe. The central sulcus is a prominent landmark in the mammalian brain as it is the longest, uninterrupted, "straight" groove on the lateral aspect of the cerebral hemisphere. The frontal lobe is generally associated with complex activities such as voluntary movement, planning, speech, and making decisions. In addition, it constitutes a large portion of the human brain and plays a complex role in personality and cognitive functions. Finally, language is an important function of the frontal lobe, and is located on the left hemisphere for most humans.

Parietal Lobe

The parietal lobe has three distinct anatomical boundaries. First, the central sulcus separates the parietal lobe anteriorly from the frontal lobe. Second, the parieto-occipital sulcus divides the posterior portion of the parietal lobe from the anterior portion of the occipital lobe. Lastly, the Sylvian fissure separates the ventral region of the parietal lobe from the dorsal region of the temporal lobe. The parietal lobe is generally associated with integrating sensory information as well as spatial orientation. It has also been shown to be important for processing language and spirituality. As with the frontal lobe, language processing in the parietal lobe tends to occur in the left hemisphere in most humans.

Temporal Lobe

The temporal lobe is found near the ear at an oblique angle. It is inferior (below) to the frontal and parietal lobes, rostral to the occipital lobe, and lies below the Sylvian fissure. The temporal lobe is generally associated with processing sensory input from other lobes, learning, forming and storing new memories, retaining visual memories, understanding language, and emotions.

Occipital Lobe

The occipital lobe is located in the most posterior region of the cerebral cortex and sits superior to the cerebellum (which is not considered part of the cerebrum). This lobe is involved with vision and contains the primary visual cortex and the association visual cortices. Thus, the occipital lobe recognizes size, shape, color, light, motion, and dimension of objects.

Jennifer L. Hellier

See also: Brain Anatomy; Brain Build with Clay: Cerebellum, Cerebral Cortex; Frontal Lobe; Gyrus (Gyri); Parietal Lobe; Occipital Lobe; Sulcus (Sulci); Temporal Lobe

Further Reading

Bear, M. F., Connors, B. W., & Paradiso, M. A. (2007). *Neuroscience exploring the brain* (3rd ed.). Baltimore, MD: Lippincott Williams & Wilkins.

LangBrain. (2000). Telencephalon. In *Language and brain: Neurocognitive linguistics.* An online resource provided by Rice University, Houston, Texas. Retrieved from http://www.ruf.rice.edu/~lngbrain/cglidden/telen.html

Purves, D., Augustine, G. J., Fitzpatrick, D., Hall, W. C., LaMantia, A.-S., McNamara, J. O., & Williams, S. M. (Eds.). (2004). *Neuroscience* (3rd ed.). Sunderland, MA: Sinauer Associates.

Temporal Lobe

The mammalian brain (or cerebrum) is made up of *gyri* (plural; *gyrus,* singular form) and *sulci* (plural; *sulcus,* singular form). Together these make up the bumps and grooves that give the brain a convoluted and unique form. The cerebrum is divided into four major divisions with the *temporal lobe* being located near the ear at an oblique angle. It is inferior (below) to the frontal and parietal lobes and anterior (toward the front) to the occipital lobe. Specifically, it lies below the *lateral* or *Sylvian fissure.* The temporal lobe is generally associated with (1) processing sensory input from other lobes, (2) learning, (3) forming and storing new memories, (4) retaining visual memories, (5) understanding language, and (6) emotions. Because there are two hemispheres of the brain, there are two temporal lobes present, both with the same functions.

Anatomical Divisions and Functions

The cerebrum is divided into four lobes that are named after the bones that overlie them: *frontal, parietal, temporal,* and *occipital* lobes. Each lobe has its own distinct function but in general the cerebral cortex of the lobes is organized in a similar way with six horizontal layers. It is important to note that in humans and monkeys, the directional terms dorsal (back) and ventral (front) are different in the head compared to other mammals. This is because during development, the brain rotates forward. Thus, dorsal is the top of the skull while ventral is under the chin.

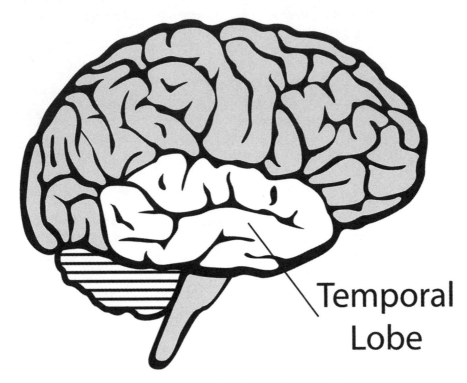

Diagram highlighting the temporal lobe of the brain. (Shutterstock)

The temporal lobe has two sulci: the *superior temporal sulcus* and the *inferior temporal sulcus.* These sulci divide the temporal lobe into three distinct gyri: the *superior temporal gyrus,* the *middle temporal gyrus,* and the *inferior temporal gyrus.* These gyri lie at an oblique angle on the surface of the cerebral cortex. At first sight, the inferior temporal gyrus may seem small. However, it wraps around its ventral surface medially and extends deep into the brain. Two additional gyri are located inferior and medial to the inferior temporal gyrus. These are the *fusiform gyrus* and the *parahippocampal gyrus.* Together they are separated from each other by the *collateral sulcus.*

The upper and caudal (toward the back) surface of the superior temporal gyrus, which includes the surface enfolding medially into the lateral fissure, is the *transverse temporal gyrus of Heschl* or *Brodmann areas 41 and 42.* It is the primary auditory cortex that is important for processing sounds. The most caudal portion of the superior temporal gyrus, which encloses around the lateral fissure and extends upward to the parietal lobe, are *Brodmann areas 22, 39, and 40.* It is also known as *Wernicke's area,* which is essential for understanding language. The number order for Wernicke's area may seem strange to the reader. This is because when German anatomist Korbinian Brodmann (1868–1918) first sectioned the brain, he did so at an oblique angle. The first area he studied was named *Brodmann area 1,* which is part of the somatosensory cortex (the postcentral gyrus). As Brodmann continued his research, he continued to number the regions based on the order he studied them. This is why Wernicke's area has three nonconsecutive numbers.

Moving to the most rostral region of the superior temporal gyrus lays the *temporopolar area* or *Brodmann area 38.* This region includes the most rostral part of the middle temporal gyrus as well. Its function is believed to bind complex, highly processed perceptual inputs to visceral emotional responses. In other words, this may be when a person follows their "gut" in response to their perception of a situation. It is usually the first area that is affected by Alzheimer's disease as well as the earliest start of temporal lobe seizures.

The middle temporal gyrus is *Brodmann area 21.* Although its precise function is unknown, the middle temporal gyrus has been associated with: distance planning, identifying and recognizing faces that are known to the person, and retrieving word meanings when the person is reading.

The most ventral portion (the bottom surface of the brain) of the temporal lobe is the inferior temporal gyrus or *Brodmann area 20.* It is a visual association cortex making its function to process high-level visual information received from the visual cortex (Brodmann areas 17 and 18). In addition, this region is involved with recognition memory.

The *fusiform gyrus,* previously named the *occipitotemporal gyrus,* is part of the inferior section of the temporal lobe and the rostral portion of the occipital lobe. It is found medially between the inferior temporal gyrus and the parahippocampus gyrus. The fusiform gyrus is *Brodmann area 37* and is important for visual and cognitive processing. It is associated with processing color information from the occipital lobe, recognizing faces, recognizing words, and identifying if an object belongs in a certain category (such as an eagle belongs in the bird category). Most neuroanatomists consider this region as the *ventral stream of vision* (the vision of "what" or "how"), while the *dorsal stream of vision* (the vision of "where" something is) projects to the parietal lobe.

The parahippocampal gyrus is in the medial portion of the temporal lobe. It surrounds the hippocampus. The hippocampus has been extensively studied, as it is associated with long-term potentiation, learning, and memory. The hippocampus consists of two interlocking gyri that physically look like a small letter "c" hooked into a capital letter "C." Together these interlocking C's specific cell layers make up the tri-synaptic circuit, which means there are three major synapses that occur within the hippocampus. The first synapse is at the granule cell layer located within the small letter "c." This is called the *dentate gyrus.* The output of the granule cells projects to the hilus (or CA4) and to the pyramidal cell layer of the *Cornu Ammonis* (or Ammon's horn), which makes up the capital letter "C." The pyramidal cell layer is divided into three regions called the CA1, CA2, and CA3. The CA3 is closest to the hilus and the dentate gyrus. It is the second synapse of the tri-synaptic circuit. These pyramidal cells then project to the CA1, which is the third synapse. The axons of the CA1 are the output of the hippocampus (forming the subiculum) and terminate in the opposite hippocampus as well as other limbic structures. The hippocampus is part of a larger structure of the brain called the limbic system, which is thought to be part of the neural system involved in emotion. It also plays a very important role in memory (especially the process of integrating short-term and long-term memory), learning, and spatial learning strategies. Even with its important functions, the hippocampus is one of the regions of the brain first affected in some disease processes such as Alzheimer's disease and general aging; schizophrenia—a mental disorder that is characterized by a loss of understanding reality and having hallucinations; long-term stress; temporal lobe epilepsy; and global transient amnesia.

Diseases and Disorders

Based on its location in the skull, the temporal lobe is prone to trauma following a head injury, particularly the rostral portion. Additionally and as previously stated, the temporal lobe is often the first sight of diseases and disorders of the central nervous system. Since it is the seat of both auditory and visual processing, learning and memory, processing of emotions, and understanding written and spoken language, damage to this lobe can be rather devastating for humans. In this entry, only a few disorders are discussed and the reader should know this is not a complete list of diseases and/or disorders that affect the temporal lobe.

Damage to the primary auditory cortex can produce *auditory verbal agnosia, auditory agnosia,* and *cortical deafness.* Auditory verbal agnosia is called *pure word deafness* because it is the inability to understand language, repeat words, and write from dictation. However, the patient can still produce spontaneous speech and is able to read and write. In *auditory agnosia,* the brain is unable to process the meaning of a sound. Thus, a person cannot recognize or differentiate between sounds. This means that the person can physically hear the sound but will describe the sound in unrelated terms because they cannot recognize what it means. For example, the person may hear a meowing sound but cannot correlate that sound with a cat. Cortical deafness occurs when there is bilateral damage to both primary auditory cortices. The person's anatomy and physiology of the ear and its vestibulocochlear nerve are unaffected such that they have the ability to receive sound and that sound is converted to a nerve impulse. However, the brain cannot process the auditory input and the sound cannot be perceived. Thus, cortical deafness can be thought as a combination of auditory verbal agnosia and auditory agnosia. Nonetheless, cortical deafness is a rare condition and usually occurs from a bilateral embolic stroke to Brodmann areas 41 and 42.

If the left temporal lobe is injured particularly in Wernicke' area, it may result in a form of *aphasia*. Aphasia occurs when a person is unable to communicate. This means they cannot be understood by their audience, nor are they able to express themselves with writing. This is a condition known as *Wernicke's aphasia*, or *receptive aphasia* and the words spoken by the patient flow freely but they are nonsensical and difficult to interpret. Wernicke's aphasia was originally described by German physician Karl Wernicke (1848–1905). In 1874, Wernicke published his results of studying two patients with profound deficits in their comprehension of the spoken language. Though these patients had no problems forming sounds, the sounds that they formed did not resemble any words in German or any other language. This has been described more recently as "cocktail chatter." Further, the patients did not appear to notice that anything had been disrupted with their speech patterns. Upon examination of one of the patient's brains at autopsy, Wernicke noticed a lesion in the left hemisphere, just posterior to, or behind, the primary auditory cortex. This portion of the brain has been shown to be responsible for sound processing and ultimately hearing.

Lastly, *complex-partial seizures* (spontaneous abnormal electrical activity) originating in or involving the mesial temporal limbic structures are the most common type of seizures, and the most common cause is *temporal lobe epilepsy*. Most patients with temporal lobe epilepsy have had some prior brain injury such as trauma to the head from riding a bicycle or a car accident, febrile convulsions (seizures caused by fever), or status epilepticus (uncontrollable seizures that last for more than five minutes). Temporal lobe epilepsy is usually a permanent condition with variable seizure frequencies within a population of afflicted individuals. The seizures will commonly evolve into secondarily generalized seizures that may last for a minute or two. There is anatomical evidence that these seizures cause cell death within the dentate gyrus, which turns to scar tissue called *mesial temporal sclerosis*. Additionally, the cells that survive are disconnected from the hippocampal circuitry and will sprout their axons to be reconnected. However, many of the new connections produce abnormal recurrent excitatory circuits that may help propagate the next spontaneous seizure. Seizures located in the temporal lobe often result in changed perceptions of reality where common items may appear to be foreign or foreign objects may appear to be familiar.

Jennifer L. Hellier

See also: Aphasia; Auditory System; Broca's Area; Brodmann Areas; Cerebral Cortex; Epilepsy; Hippocampus; Learning and Memory; Seizures; Somatosensory Cortex/Somatosensory System; Visual System; Wernicke's Area

Further Reading

Bear, M. F., Connors, B. W., & Paradiso, M. A. (2007). *Neuroscience: Exploring the brain.* Baltimore, MD: Lippincott Williams and Wilkins.

Dafny, N. (1997). Overview of the nervous systems. In *Neuroscience Online, an electronic textbook for the neurosciences* (Chap. 1). Open-access educational resource provided by the Department of Neurobiology and Anatomy at the University of Texas Medical School at Houston. Retrieved from http://neuroscience.uth.tmc.edu/s2/chapter01.html

Hellier, J. L., White, A., Williams, P. A., Edward Dudek, F., & Staley, K. J. (2009). NMDA receptor-mediated long-term alterations in epileptiform activity in experimental chronic epilepsy. *Neuropharmacology, 56*(2), 414–421.

Kandel, E. R., Schwartz, J. H., Jessell, T. M., Siegelbaum, S. A., & Hudspeth, A. J. (Eds.). (2012). *Principles of neural science* (5th ed.). New York, NY: McGraw-Hill.

Lah, S., & Smith, M. (2014). Semantic and episodic memory in children with temporal lobe epilepsy: Do they relate to literacy skills? *Neuropsychology, 28*(1), 113–122. doi:10.1037/neu0000029.

Thalamic Nuclei

The brain and spinal cord serve as the system in humans that allow us to sense our environment through numerous receptors and specialized senses and to respond to these stimuli through the activation of our muscles and other effectors. There is a tremendous amount of sensory information that comes into the brain and must be interpreted and passed on to other areas of the brain for integration and response. The region of the human brain that receives almost all sensory information is called the *thalamus* and is found in an area of the brain called the *midbrain*. It is in the same region of the brain as the *hypothalamus* and the *epithalamus*. The thalamus is the "grand central station" of the human brain and acts as a routing center for incoming sensory information. This is done through the use of various *nuclei* that are found in the brain. These nuclei are divided into several types, based on their overall function. These include the (1) *specific relay* nuclei, which include the *lateral geniculate nucleus*, the *medial geniculate nucleus*, the *ventral posteromedial nucleus*, the *ventral lateral/ventral anterior nucleus*, the *anterior nucleus*, and the *ventral posterolateral nucleus;* (2) *association* nuclei, which include the *pulvinar*, *lateral posterior nucleus*, and the *dorsomedial nucleus;* (3) *subcortical* nuclei, which include the *reticular nucleus;* and (4) *nonspecific* nuclei, which include portions of the *ventral anterior nucleus* and the *intralaminar nucleus*. All of these nuclei receive sensory information from very specific regions of the body and route that information to other regions of the brain for further integration and response.

The lateral, medial, and anterior groups are named by their location relative to a large collection of axons called the internal medullary lamina. The system of lamellae is made up of myelinated fibers that separate the different subparts of the thalamus. The intralaminar, midline, and reticular groups are considered nonspecific thalamic nuclei. The lateral nuclei are further divided into two tiers: *the ventral* and *dorsal.* The ventral tier of the lateral nucleus is further divided into six nuclei, which are named for their location within the ventral tier. These consist of relay neurons that receive limited sensory and motor input and project this information to specific sensory and motor cortical regions. The dorsal tier of the lateral thalamus and the medial group project to association cortices and thus are both considered association nuclei. The anterior group receives specific neuronal impulses and relays this information to the hypothalamus and the cingulate gyrus of the cerebral cortex. The intralaminar group is made up of a cluster of nuclei that are intermixed within the internal medullary lamina. The reticular group is found on the lateral aspect of the thalamus and the midline group is located on the dorsal wall of the third ventricle, which is a natural space found in the brain for the flow of cerebrospinal fluid.

The Specific Relay Nuclei

The specific relay nuclei include the following nuclei:

- The *lateral geniculate* nucleus which receives information from the eye (specifically the axons of the ganglion cells located in the retina) via cranial nerve II or the *optic nerve.* Information from the eye is then passed on to the *visual cortex,* which is found primarily within the *occipital lobe* of the cerebral hemispheres of the brain. There is evidence that the lateral geniculate nucleus also sends information to the *superior colliculus,* which is found in a region of the brain called the *corpora quadrigemmina* within the brainstem.
- The *medial geniculate* nucleus which receives information from the ears (specifically the axons of the hair cells located in the cochlea) via cranial nerve VIII or the *vestibulocochlear nerve.* Information from the ear is then passed on to the *auditory cortex,* which is found primarily in the *temporal lobe* of the cerebral hemispheres of the brain. There is evidence that the medial geniculate nucleus also sends information to the *inferior colliculus,* which is found in a region of the brain called the *corpora quadrigemmina.*
- The *ventral posterolateral nucleus* (*VPL*) which is a major integration region for sensory information coming to the brain from all parts of the body. In particular, this nucleus receives sensory information from the periphery (extremities) of the body regarding pain, pressure, temperature, touch, and discriminative touch. It receives most of the information from the body via the *spinothalamic tract* found in the spinal cord as well as the *medial lemniscus* which is a tract found in the brainstem.
- The *ventral posteromedial nucleus* (*VPM*) which, like the ventral posterolateral nucleus, receives significant input from the body. This nucleus also receives information from the *trigeminothalamic tracts* that carries information from cranial nerve V (trigeminal nerve) about the face, head, and neck.

- The *ventral lateral/ventral anterior nucleus* (*VL/VA*) integrates with regions of the brain associated with motor control of the muscles of the extremities and trunk of the body. Tracts from the *cerebellum* and the *basal nuclei* connect to the VL/VA to help with the subconscious "smoothing out" of muscle movement in the body. This nucleus also sends axon tracts to a region of the brain called the *motor* and *premotor cortex* in the brain, which assists with motor control.
- The *anterior nucleus* which, like the VL/VA nucleus, has connections to the *mammillothalamic tract* (from the mammillary bodies that are part of the hypothalamus) as well as the *cingulate gyrus* (which is part of the limbic system) to regulate both conscious and subconscious motor control of the muscles and organs of the body.

The Association Nuclei

The specific association nuclei include the following:

- The *pulvinar nucleus,* which plays an important role in vision, receiving input from the *retina* of the eye as well as the *superior colliculus.* This nucleus sends information on to the *parietal-occipital-temporal association cortex* in the cerebral hemispheres of the brain to integrate visual sensory information with other senses of the body.
- The *lateral posterior nucleus* (*LP*) which also receives significant neural input from the superior colliculus. The lateral posterior nucleus then sends fiber tracts to the *parietal association area* of the cerebral hemispheres to help integrate visual information with other somatosensory information for response.
- The *dorsomedial nucleus* (*DM*), which receives information from several regions of the midbrain and brainstem including the *amygdala,* and the *olfactory cortex.* This nucleus is important in the integration of smell and information about emotion and mood by sending information to the *prefrontal cortex.*

The Nucleus of the Subcortical Region

There is only one nucleus associate with the subcortical region of the thalamus. This nucleus is the *reticular nucleus,* which is not as well studied as others within the thalamus. Histological data indicates that this nucleus may be an internal "relay station" for other incoming neural information from other nuclei within the thalamus.

The Nonspecific Nucleus of the Thalamus

There is one primary nucleus of the thalamus that is classified as being "nonspecific" in its function. This nucleus is known as the *intralaminar nucleus.* It receives neural input from several major regions of the brain including the *reticular formation* which controls many of our subconscious actions, the *basal ganglia* which play a major role in voluntary motor function, the *cerebellum* which makes up a large part of the brainstem and is the structure that leads to the first segment of the spinal cord. The cerebellum helps to find motor control and many of the *somatosensory* pathways of the brain. This nucleus has connections to virtually all regions of the brain that deal with voluntary/conscious sensory and motor functions.

Neurotransmitters of the Thalamus

The neurons of the thalamus are important for receiving, modulating, and transmitting incoming sensory information to all regions of the brain for further interpretation and response. The modulatory function of the thalamus is accomplished in part by the presence of a significant number of *inhibitory interneurons* that help relay information from one region of the thalamus to other regions of the brain. These interneurons use *GABA* (gamma-aminobutyric acid) as a neurotransmitter which acts to slow down or prevent neurons from propagating a neuronal signal to the next neuron. By doing this, the thalamus can help regulate the intensity and frequency of a neuronal signal to other regions of the brain for a potential response.

Summary

The thalamus is a structure located within the brain that together with the hypothalamus, form the diencephalon. The thalamus is the central location for sensory input from the rest of the body and is composed of numerous *nuclei* or collects of neuronal cell bodies that receive this sensory information and then route that sensory information to the rest of the brain for evaluation and response. These nuclei are divided into several types based on their overall function. These include the (1) *specific relay* nuclei, which deal primarily with visual and auditory sensory information; (2) *association* nuclei, which receive information from the extremities of the body; (3) *subcortical* nuclei, which most likely act as an internal "router" for information coming into the thalamus; and (4) *nonspecific* nuclei, which receive information about mood, emotion, and subconscious sensory input.

Charles A. Ferguson

See also: Diencephalon; Motor Cortex; Somatosensory Cortex/Somatosensory System; Thalamus

Further Reading

Guillery, R. W., & Sherman, S. M. (2011). Branched thalamic afferents: What are the messages that they relay to the cortex? *Brain Research Reviews, 66*(1–2), 205–219.

Schiff, N.D., Nauyel, T., & Victor, J.D. (2014). Large-scale brain dynamics in disorders of consciousness. *Current Opinion in Neurobiology, 25,* 7–14.

Temel, Y., Blokland, A., Steinbusch, H.W., & Visser-Vandewalle, V. (2005). The functional role of the subthalamic nucleus in cognitive and limbic circuits. *Progress in Neurobiology, 76*(6), 393–413.

Vukadinovic, Z., Herman, M.S., & Rosenzweig, I. (2013). Cannabis, psychosis and the thalamus: A theoretical review. *Neuroscience & Biobehavioral Reviews, 37*(4), 658–667.

Watanabe, Y., & Funahashi, S. (2012). Thalamic mediodorsal nucleus and working memory. *Neuroscience & Biobehavioral Reviews, 36*(1), 134–142.

Wurtz, R.H., McAlonan, K., Cavanaugh, J., & Berman, R.A. (2011). Thalamic pathways for active vision. *Trends in Cognitive Sciences, 15*(4), 177–184.

Thalamus

The central nervous system consists of the brain, brainstem, and the spinal cord. Within the brain, there are a few deep structures that are essential for normal brain functioning. One of these structures is the *thalamus,* which is located on the midline of the brain and consists of two symmetrical halves. It is part of the diencephalon as it is the posterior portion of the forebrain, which includes the epithalamus, thalamus, hypothalamus, subthalamus (or ventral thalamus), and the third ventricle (a natural space in the brain where cerebrospinal fluid flows). The word *thalamus* is derived from Greek, meaning "chamber" or "inner room" as it receives almost all sensory and motor information. Thus, the thalamus is generally believed to act as a relay station between a variety of subcortical areas and the cerebral cortex.

History

The first known documentation of the thalamus is attributed to Roman physician Galen of Pergamon (130–200) in the first century. It was believed at the time that the brain held the "spirits" of the body and that the thalamus was a reservoir for the "vital spirit." Galen posited that the vital spirit would travel from the thalamus through the optic nerve and end in the eyes. Thus, this was the first connection of the thalamus to the eye that has been known for centuries. At one point, the French named the thalamus as the "optic thalamus" as it was suggested that only visual information was projected here.

In the 14th century, the thalamus was defined as the larger part of the diencephalon and not just the lateral bumps where Galen spoke of in his writings. The first extensive anatomical drawing of the thalamus was completed by English physician Thomas Willis (1621–1675) in the 17th century; however, the function of the thalamus was not truly understood until physicians noted patients with distinct injuries to the thalamus. Thus, it was realized that the thalamus was involved with sensory processing. In 1889, the nuclei (distinct groups of brain cell bodies) of the thalamus were identified and named by German neuropathologist Franz Nissl

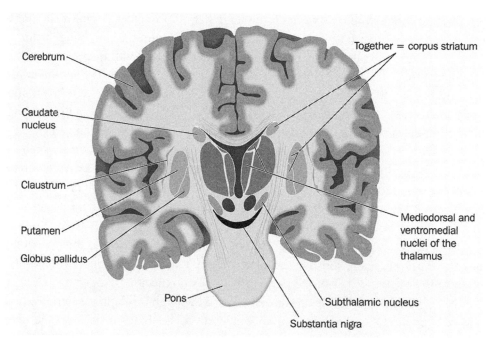

Drawing of the brain showing the basal ganglia and thalamic nuclei. (Dreamstime.com)

(1860–1919). Specifically, Nissl used a stain that he developed, which would mark the rough endoplasmic reticulum within neurons (brain cells). Thus, Nissl was able to distinguish neurons from glia, which are the supporting brain cells.

Today, the thalamus is known to receive all sensory and motor information, except for olfaction. Because of its significant role in sensation and motor function, extensive research has been performed on the thalamus and its interconnections.

From the 1940s through the 1970s, physiological studies of the thalamus were performed using microelectrode techniques. This allowed the thalamus to be mapped for sensory and motor functions. It resulted in a topographical sensory representation of the body surface, visual field representation in the sensory relay nuclei, auditory representation in the sensory relay nuclei, and the stimulus-response activity of neurons within these thalamic nuclei. These studies also verified the connections of the cerebral cortex to the thalamus (the corticothalamic loop), which have shown to be essential for the conscious state of the brain, for sleep-wake cycles, and cognition.

Anatomy and Physiology

There are three main parts of the diencephalon: the hypothalamus (which literally translates as less than the thalamus), the subthalamus (which carries impulses from the basal nuclei to the thalamus then on to the hypothalamus), and the thalamus.

All three of these structures work closely together, as a nuclear complex, in many different bodily functions. The hypothalamus controls temperature, hunger, thirst, fear, anger, and the pituitary gland. The hypothalamus acts with the portion of the reticular system in the midbrain to keep the brain alert, and awake. The subthalamus acts like a train depot where it carries impulses from the basal nuclei to the thalamus, and then to the hypothalamus. It is important for transporting and modulating neural impulses used for coordinating movements. Finally, the thalamus is a center that delivers or relays sensory impulses to the surface of the cerebrum, such as impulses from the cerebellum to the cerebral cortex. The thalamus provides input about ongoing movement to the motor areas of the cerebral cortex. It also contains a special part of the reticular system that helps coordinate sensory messages and helps regulate the activity of the brain.

Overall, the thalamus is the main part of the diencephalon, and is the regulation of consciousness, sleep, and alertness. It is found at that most superior portion of the brainstem, near the center of the brain. It is highly connected by fiber tracts (large bundles of white matter, or axons that are covered with an insulating material called myelin) that bind it to the overlying cerebral cortex. The thalamus is about the size, and shape of a walnut, and is located obliquely and symmetrical on each side of the third ventricle. There are two thalami, one in each brain hemisphere, and the superior medial surface of each thalamus makes up the lateral walls of the third ventricle. The thalami are also connected to each other on the midline by the interthalamic adhesion.

The thalamus receives blood from the branches of the posterior cerebral artery. Specifically, these branches are the polar artery (posterior communicating artery), paramedian thalamic-subthalamic arteries, inferolateral (thalamogeniculate) arteries, and posterior (medial and lateral) choroidal arteries. In a rare anatomic version, both sides of the thalamus may also receive blood from the Percheron artery, which is a single arterial trunk arising from the posterior cerebral artery. From this large blood supply, it is easy to see how metabolically active the thalamus is for the brain. However, if any of these blood vessels become damaged by a stroke or an aneurysm, it is clear how it can result in specific damage to the thalamus and/or diencephalon and cause specific sensory or motor signs.

Thalamic Nuclei

The thalamus consists of six functionally distinct nuclei, which are the lateral (ventral tier and dorsal tier), medial, anterior, intralaminar, midline, and reticular nuclei. The lateral, medial, and anterior groups are named by their location relative to a large collection of axons called the internal medullary lamina. The system of lamellae is made up of myelinated fibers that separate the different subparts of the thalamus. The intralaminar, midline, and reticular groups are considered nonspecific thalamic nuclei.

The lateral nuclei are further divided into two tiers: the ventral and dorsal. The ventral tier of the lateral nucleus is further divided into six nuclei, which are named for their location within the ventral tier. These consist of relay neurons that receive limited sensory and motor input and project this information to specific sensory and motor cortical regions. The dorsal tier of the lateral thalamus and the medial group project to association cortices and thus are both considered association nuclei. The anterior group receives specific neuronal impulses and relays this information to the hypothalamus and the cingulate gyrus of the cerebral cortex. The intralaminar group is made up of a cluster of nuclei that are intermixed within the internal medullary lamina. The reticular group is found on the lateral aspect of the thalamus and the midline group is located on the dorsal wall of the third ventricle. Because of the intricacies of the thalamic nuclei, another entry in this encyclopedia is dedicated to this topic.

Connections and Functions

Because of how integrated the thalamus is in almost all neurological functions, there are several connections and functions that are involved with these structures. An easy way to understand this is first by grouping the thalamic functions and then identifying the responsible connections. The functions are grouped by limbic, motor, somatic sensation, hearing, and vision. For limbic functions, which include emotional expression, the main inputs are from the mammillary body of the hypothalamus (making the mammillothalamic tract), the cingulate gyrus, the amygdala, the hypothalamus, and the reticular formation of the brainstem. The output fibers for limbic function terminate in the cingulate gyrus, the prefrontal cortex, and the basal forebrain.

Motor information is brought to the thalamus by the globus pallidus of the basal nuclei and the dentate nucleus of the cerebellum. The major output for motor function ends in the premotor (Brodmann area 6) and the motor cortices (Brodmann area 4). This helps modulate ongoing movement and sends this appropriate information to the motor areas of the cortex. Sensory information of the body (such as pain, temperature, touch, discriminative touch, and pressure) is received from the dorsal column and medial lemniscal pathways from the spinal cord (making the spinothalamic tract) as well as the sensory nuclei of cranial nerve V (trigeminal nerve that serves the head and face). This sensory information is then relayed to the somatosensory cortex (Brodmann areas 3, 1, and 2). Research studies have shown that the somatosensory cortex and its association cortices (located in the superior colliculus, temporal lobe, parietal lobe, occipital lobe, and the primary visual cortex—or Brodmann area 17) also project back to the thalamus to further integrate sensory information. This information is then projected to the temporal, parietal, and occipital lobes.

Neurons involved with hearing project to the thalamus via the inferior colliculus. The thalamus then modulates these signals and sends them to the primary auditory cortex (Broadmann areas 41 and 42) within the temporal lobe. Vision is transferred to the thalamus via the retinal ganglion axons that make up the optic nerve (cranial nerve II) and the optic tract. The thalamus then modulates these signals and sends them to the primary visual cortex (Broadmann area 17) within the occipital lobe. Finally, studies have also shown that the thalamus modulates its own activity. This is done through the reticular nucleus. It receives information from the cerebral cortex and the other thalamic nuclei and projects this information after modulation of the signal back out to the remaining thalamic nuclei.

In addition to the functions listed previously, the thalamus is important for regulating sleep, arousal, and wakefulness. In fact, the shared connections with the cerebral cortex (the thalamo-cortico-thalamic circuits) are involved and activated during consciousness. Thus, damage to the thalamus has been implicated in producing a permanent coma (a state of unconsciousness where a person cannot be awakened, respond to painful stimuli, or have voluntary movement).

In the role of memory formation, neurological studies have shown that the thalamus is functionally connected to the hippocampus, as part of the limbic system via the anterior nuclei. Here the anterior nucleus helps with understanding spatial memory, which is integrated into episodic memory for humans. Other studies have shown that the mesial temporal lobe is interconnected with the thalamus and is accessed during recollective memory and familiarity memory.

Finally, the thalamus is connected to the basal nuclei and cerebellum and helps regulate motor movement. It seems that the function of the thalamus here is to receive motor information from the basal nuclei and cerebellum and integrate this information together before sending it out to the motor cortices.

Disease

Thalamic syndrome is caused by a cerebrovascular accident, such as a stroke, to the thalamus. Characteristic signs include burning sensations to one side of the body that are accompanied with mood swings. Another condition that includes the thalamus is Korsakoff's syndrome, where the mammillary bodies are damaged, which causes a disruption of the mammillothalamic tract. This is usually caused by a deficiency of vitamin B1 (or thiamine) from alcohol abuse and/or severe malnutrition. Karsakoff's syndrome produces a type of dementia and psychosis. Both anterograde amnesia (inability to make new memories) and retrograde amnesia (inability to recall formed memories) are common in Karsakoff's syndrome as is confabulation (invented memories to fill gaps in memory), lack of content during conversation, and apathy (where the person easily loses interest in activities and things).

Treatments for these issues are to treat the underlying cause as well as the signs of the syndromes. In the cause of cerebrovascular accidents, patients may be placed on an aspirin regimen to reduce the chance of future strokes. Vitamin B1 supplements are helpful for treating Karsakoff's syndrome.

Patricia A. Bloomquist

See also: Auditory System; Basal Nuclei (Basal Ganglia); Discriminative Touch; Hypothalamus; Motor Cortex; Olfactory System (Smell); Pain; Sensory Receptors; Somatosensory Cortex/Somatosensory System; Stroke; Thalamic Nuclei; Touch; Visual System

Further Reading

Haber, S. N., & Calzavara, R. (2009). The cortico-basal ganglia integrative network: The role of the thalamus. *Brain Research Bulletin, 78*(2–3), 69–74.

Hebb, A. O., & Ojemann, G. A. (2013). The thalamus and language revisited. *Brain and Language, 126*(1), 99–108.

Jones, E. G. (2003). History of neuroscience: The thalamus. In *IBRO history of neuroscience*. Retrieved from http://ibro.info/wp-content/uploads/2012/12/The-Thalamus.pdf

Kandel, E. R., Schwartz, J. H., Jessell, T. M., Siegelbaum, S. A., & Hudspeth, A. J. (Eds.). (2012). *Principles of neural science* (5th ed.). New York, NY: McGraw-Hill.

Minagar, A., Barnett, M. H., Benedict, R. H., Pelletier, D., Pirko, I., Sahraian, M. A., Frohman, E., & Zivadinov, R. (2013). The thalamus and multiple sclerosis: Modern views on pathologic, imaging, and clinical aspects. *Neurology, 80*(2), 210–219.

Thermal Sense (Temperature Sensation)

Temperature for living organisms is essential to maintain health and homeostasis (physiological balance within the body). Animals, and particularly humans, have the ability to sense heat and cold from the environment around them, which allows them to respond in an appropriate manner. Furthermore, the brain helps maintain the animal's core temperature so that the body can protect itself during extreme temperature situations. In animals, temperature and pain sensations travel together in the nervous system. Specifically, these sensations are mediated by the same fiber types within the peripheral nervous system, travel in the spinal cord within the same pathway, and are perceived within the somatosensory cortex (postcentral gyrus of the brain). Regulation of body temperature is mediated by the hypothalamus, a deep brain structure located below the thalamus.

Anatomy and Physiology

The body's sensory systems deal with temperature information being delivered to the nervous system by neurons that have special receptors for temperature stimuli that are generally not too painful, not too hot, and not too cold. These receptors are called *thermoreceptors,* which are free nerve endings found throughout the skin, cornea (the covering of the eye), and the bladder. There are two fiber types used to sense temperature: *C-fibers* and *A delta fibers.* C-fibers are usually unmyelinated, meaning they lack a covering of insulation (myelin, produced by Schwann cells) around their axons. Thus, nerve impulses (action potentials) do not travel as fast in these types of fibers. A delta fibers are lightly myelinated, meaning they have a covering of insulation around their axons allowing action potentials to travel quicker. For warm temperatures between 32 and 48 C (or 90 and 118 F), C-fibers will increase their firing rate of action potentials in response to being warmed. For cool or cold temperatures between 10 and 30 C (or 50 and 86 F), both C-fibers and A delta fibers are activated. Specifically, the C-fibers reduce their firing of action potentials when cooled, while A delta fibers increase their firing rate of action potentials. Nociceptors (pain receptors) can act as thermoreceptors to determine pain from temperature, such as when a person burns his hand. Additionally, nociceptors are activated as thermoreceptors when temperatures are too cold and cause pain.

Temperature signals travel within the C-fibers and A delta fibers to the spinal cord where they synapse on to neurons located in the dorsal horn. These neurons then project some of their axons to the same side (ipsilateral) and the majority of their axons to the opposite side (contralateral) of the spinal cord where they join the *anterolateral system,* the second major ascending (afferent) pathway that ends in the somatosensory cortex. By having temperature and pain information traveling on both sides of the spinal cord, it acts as a backup system so if part of the spinal cord is damaged, not all temperature and pain sensation is lost. For the head and face, temperature information travels through cranial nerve V (trigeminal nerve), synapses in the trigeminal nucleus in the brainstem, and then terminates in the somatosensory cortex.

A body's core temperature is regulated by the hypothalamus in response to peripheral and central input. The set point for human body temperature ranges from 36.4 to 37.2 C (or 97.5 to 99 F) and is called *normothermia.* Temperature regulation works by a feedback system that detects changes between peripheral thermoreceptors in the skin, spinal cord and viscera, and central thermoreceptors in the anterior section of the hypothalamus. The central thermoreceptors in the hypothalamus change their firing rate based on the temperature of the blood or their local temperature. The hypothalamus then integrates temperature information from the autonomic nervous system, endocrine system, and skeletal muscles to determine if the core temperature is too hot (*hyperthermia*) and sweating needs to begin to cool down the body or if the core temperature is too cold (*hypothermia*) and shivering needs to begin to burn energy and make body heat.

Jennifer L. Hellier

See also: Pain; Sensory Receptors; Somatosensory Cortex/Somatosensory System

Further Reading

Kambiz, S., Duraku, L. S., Holstege, J. C., Hovius, S. E., Ruigrok, T. J., & Walbeehm, E. T. (2013). Thermo-sensitive TRP channels in peripheral nerve injury: A review of their role in cold intolerance. *Journal of Plastic, Reconstructive, and Aesthetic Surgery.* pii: S1748–6815(13): 00676–1.

Kandel, E. R., Schwartz, J. H., Jessell, T. M., Siegelbaum, S. A., & Hudspeth, A. J. (Eds.). (2012). *Principles of neural science* (5th ed.). New York, NY: McGraw-Hill.

Purves, D., Augustine, G. J., Fitzpatrick, D., Hall, W. C., LaMantia, A.-S., McNamara, J. O., & Williams, S. M. (Eds.). (2004). *Neuroscience* (3rd ed.). Sunderland, MA: Sinauer Associates.

Tolerance, Drug

Addiction and *tolerance* are intertwined. Addiction is the seeking of a thrill like the emotional rush from drinking alcohol or drag racing cars, while tolerance is the physiological state of where the same amount of drug or action no longer produces the same emotional rush. A basic principle that governs brain function is balance or *homeostasis*. The brain is made up of multiple structures and systems that vie for dominance and so it "seeks" balance between the structures and systems. To understand addiction, the two systems that vie for dominance are the *rational* (the frontal lobe) and *emotional networks* (the limbic system). Drugs work on the emotional systems, and rationality warns of the consequences of drug usage. It can be described as a pathological imbalanced brain where the emotional dominates the rational. One of the key reasons addicts continue to use drugs is that addicts overstress the short-term emotional benefits and undervalue the rational consequences despite repercussions. This eventually results in anatomical, structural, and physiological changes of the brain that can be reversible. There are other nondrug addictions such as *gambling, overeating, sex, shopping, tanning, technology,* and *thrill seeking.* Thus, addiction is a progressive disease of irrationality and pathological imbalance.

Anatomy and Physiology

Neurons are brain cells that are unique because they transmit neural signals between each other in a space called the *synaptic cleft*. Specifically, *neurotransmitters* (natural chemicals used in signal transduction) are released from presynaptic neurons and travel in the synaptic cleft to postsynaptic neurons to send messages from one brain cell to another. The neurotransmitters will bind to specialized proteins (called receptors) within the postsynaptic neuron's membrane. Scientists have shown that dopamine is a natural neurotransmitter that is part of the reward system (associated with the limbic system) in the brain and is necessary for "feeling good." When manmade drugs are abused (e.g., when excessive amounts of drug are ingested over a period of time), it changes the balance of dopamine. Drugs alter the balance in favor of the emotional reward over rational thought. Specifically, if the reward system is excessively stimulated over a long period of time, the neurons learn that the over stimulation has become the "new norm" and attempts to return to homeostasis. In order for this to happen, the neurons in the reward system reduce the number of receptors available in the postsynaptic membrane, which in turn reduces the ability for dopamine to bind to available receptors. It is like removing extra seats in a game of musical chairs while keeping the same number of players. Thus, fewer players are able to get a seat. With fewer receptors for dopamine to bind with, the less stimulation occurs for a neuron, which blunts the effect or "high" of the drug. This results in the person needing to increase the dose or frequency of the drug or thrill seeking activities to obtain the same "high."

These physical changes in the addict's brain are the "new normal" with a less efficient reward system. Without the dopamine boost from drugs, addicts suffer a dopamine deficit that causes withdrawal symptoms and depression. The addict now needs to have the drug not to give the euphoria the addict experienced before, but to maintain the "new normal" now required for a drug-induced dopamine boost. Furthermore, the addict now needs drugs to stave off withdrawal symptoms.

Addiction is a chronic relapsing disease, because long-term drug use alters the brain's structure and function. These brain changes can last as long as months or years after the last use of the drug, which can explain the high rates of relapse after treatment. The disruption and alteration of the dopamine pathways lead to the decrease of feeling good, which pushes the addict to take drugs to compensate. This also may explain why drug addicts lose interest in things, activities, and people they once cared about before sliding into addiction.

Patricia A. Bloomquist

See also: Addiction; Dopamine and Its Receptors; Reward and Punishment

Further Reading

Hingson, R., & White, A. (2014). New research findings since the 2007 surgeon general's call to action to prevent and reduce underage drinking: A review. *Journal of Studies on Alcohol and Drugs, 75*(1), 158–169.

Pava, M.J., & Woodward, J.J. (2012). A review of the interactions between alcohol and the endocannabinoid system: Implications for alcohol dependence and future directions for research. *Alcohol, 46*(3), 185–204.

Touch

In mammals and particularly in humans, *touch* is the oldest, most primitive, and pervasive sense. In the uterus as early as eight weeks of gestation, touch is the first of the five sensory systems to develop and respond to stimulation. Additionally, it is the first sense humans experience as infants. Touch helps babies to grow and bond with mothers, fathers, and other caregivers, while helping animals and humans to learn about the world around them. Touch also plays an integral role in biological, cognitive, and social development. It is the physical contact of the somatosensory system (the skin—providing tactile sense—that covers the entire body, head, and face, and functions as the touch receptor organ) to the outside world. It allows people to learn shapes and hardness of objects through this sense.

There are several million points on the human body that register cold, heat, pain, or touch. These points that register the four basic cutaneous senses (touch and everything else felt through the skin) are mapped within the central nervous system to the somatosensory cortex (postcentral gyrus). This map is called the somatosensory homunculus ("little man"). Thus, touching an object can give the feeling of warmth, cold, pain, and pressure and that information is sent to the brain for processing. There are many kinds of touch organs, called tactile corpuscles, in the skin and mucous membranes. These touch organs are found everywhere on and within the skin: near hair, in hairless areas (like the palm and finger tips), and in deeper tissues.

History

During the ancient Greek period, touch was first described by Aristotle (384–322 BC), a Greek philosopher. Specifically, he defined touch as one of the five human senses and defined the sense of touch as *palpable*. At this time, it was believed that the four physical elements—earth, fire, water, and air—were essential to all beings on the planet. Aristotle considered that the human senses—hearing, sight, smell, taste, and touch—were closely related to the four elements. Since the properties of the elements are palpable (dry, wet, cold, and hot), he attributed touch to the classical elements. It took more than a thousand years before touch was notably studied again. A Catholic priest Albertus Magnus (1193/1206–1280) classified such qualities as hard, soft, rough, cold, and warm. Several hundred years later in 1890, further progress was made in experimental physiology where touch was applied to help define the shape and definite nature of objects.

In 1962, American psychologist James J. Gibson (1904–1979) began to study the difference between active and passive touch. He termed this, "The great cookie-cutter experiment." In this study, participants could not see what object was being used for them to identify. In one group, an experimenter pushes a cookie cutter onto a participant's palm to test passive touching. These participants were able to correctly identify the object, as a cookie cutter, about 49 percent of the time (Gibson, 1962). In the next group, participants were allowed to actively feel the cookie cutter with their hands, testing active touching. These persons correctly identified the object 95 percent of the time (Gibson, 1962). These results demonstrated that active exploration is essential in a person's ability to perceive objects in the physical world.

In 1987, American and Canadian psychologists Susan J. Lederman and Roberta L. Klatzky (1947–) expanded on this research and used an exploratory procedure to describe how humans use touch in stereotypical ways to understand the relevant perceptual information. For example, *texture* is identified when a person uses lateral motion of their fingers to feel the surface. *Pressure* can identify hardness of an object while enclosing the hands around the object will produce information about its *global shape and volume. Temperature* is realized by static contact, by holding the hand steady for a few seconds to determine the difference in temperature of the hand and the object. *Weight* is determined by unsupported holding, meaning allowing the gravity of the object push against the hands. Finally, by allowing the hands to follow the contours of an object, its *shape* is identified.

Anatomy and Physiology

The somatosensory system mediates many sensations received by the skin and body. This system informs the animal about the external environment and movement of the body. There are four main modalities of the somatosensory system: *pain, proprioception* (a sense used to identify parts of the body's location in space and the strength of the pressure being applied), *temperature,* and *touch.* These modalities can be further divided into submodalities. For pain, it includes aching, burning, and cutting pains, while proprioception includes position and movement. For temperature, it is divided into warm versus hot and cool versus cold sensations. Finally, touch includes crude touch—with itch and tickle—and discriminative touch.

Together these modalities make up haptic perception. The term *haptic* is derived from Greek, meaning "to touch." Thus haptic perception integrates somatosensory information in recognizing objects. Texture, hardness, and temperature are material properties that are mediated through touch. It is also important to note that touch and proprioception are integrated sensations as they transmit their signals to the brain via the same pathway within the spinal cord and brainstem, the *medial lemniscus.*

Touch is a peripheral nervous system function that transmits its information to the central nervous system. This means that the cell bodies of the neurons live in the dorsal root ganglion and the axon divides into a peripheral axon and a central axon. The peripheral axon ends in the joint, muscle, skin, or tendon while the central axon ends in the spinal cord of the central nervous system. The skin is the main touch receptor organ while joint, muscle, and tendon tissues are used in proprioception. Proprioceptive stimuli are internal forces that are made by the position or movement of a body part. Proprioception is different from *exteroception,* which perceives the outside world, and it is also different from *interoception,* which perceives pain, hunger, and the movement of internal organs. Instead, proprioception uses static forces on the joints, muscles, and tendons, which keep the limb in position against the force of gravity, to denote the position of the limb. The movement of the limb is due to the changes in these forces. Proprioception is important in posture and balance, and its receptors are located in joint capsules, joint ligaments, skeletal muscles, and tendons.

The sensations of touch are represented by neurons that exhibit modality specificity. Modality specificity occurs when a somatosensory neuron is stimulated, which results in a perceived sensation that is specific to the information processed by the neuron. For example, if an object is warm, the sensation registered by the specific neuron will only respond to warmth to the skin, it will not respond to cool or to touch that does not warm the skin. If the object is hot, then free nerve endings in the tissue give the sense of pain in addition to the sense of temperature.

The somatosensory receptor and its central connections determine the modality specificity of the neurons forming the somatosensory pathway. This means that sensory information travels along different anatomical pathways depending on the information carried. The medial leminscus tract within the posterior column of the spinal cord is the pathway for sending fine or discriminative touch and proprioceptive information to the cerebral cortex of the brain; and the main sensory trigeminal pathway carries discriminative touch and proprioceptive information from the face to the cortex. Temperature and pain are also cutaneous senses. The archi-, paleo-, and neo-spinothalamic pathways carry temperature and all types of pain from the body to the cerebral cortex, while the spinal trigeminal tract carries temperature and pain from the face to the cortex.

Crude versus Discriminative Touch

The skin identifies two types of touch: crude (least sensitive) and discriminative (most sensitive) touch. The form of touch where localization is not possible is called crude touch. Crude touch or nondiscriminative touch is a sensory modality which allows the body to sense that something has touched them, without being able to localize exactly where the body was touched. For example, if a person were touched five inches below their left shoulder, they would say they were touched on their back on the left side and would not be able to give the exact location. Fine touch, then, is able to localize where the body was touched. Fine and crude touch do work in parallel, meaning a person will be able to localize touch until fibers carrying fine touch have been disrupted. When that happens, the body will feel the touch, but will be unable to identify the exact location where it was touched.

The sensation of touch begins when an object comes in contact with the sense organ and presses it out of shape, or touches a nearby hair. The sense of touch is more sensitive in some parts of the body compared to other parts. The lips, tongue, fingers, feet, and genitals are the most sensitive. The least sensitive is the back. The reason for the difference is due to the fact that the end organs for touch are not scattered evenly over the body, but instead are arranged in clusters. This keenness of touch can easily be measured by an *esthesiometer*. This instrument looks like a drawing compass with two needlepoints. The tip of the tongue can feel both points when they are 1 millimeter apart. Less sensitive areas feel only one point at this distance. The back of the shoulders feels two points when the points are more than 60 millimeters apart. These differences show that certain body regions respond only to crude or fine touch. The nervous tissues from the sense organs then carry the sensation or nerve impulses to the brain.

Within the skin, there are many types of cutaneous receptors (specialized proteins that are part of neural tissue located in the skin) that are used for touch. These receptors are classified as *unencapsulated* (bare or free nerve endings) and *encapsulated receptors*. The sensory receptors of crude touch, pain, and temperature senses are unencapsulated that do not end on or near specialized tissue. Such free nerve endings of primary sensory afferents are in many muscles, tendons, joints, and ligaments. These unencapsulated receptors are the somatosensory receptors for pain resulting from muscle, tendon, joint or ligament damage and are not part of the proprioceptive system.

For discriminative touch, the receptors are encapsulated receptors, as a thin sheath encapsulates the terminal and the area around the cutaneous tissue. Other encapsulated receptors include the *hair follicle receptor* and the *Merkel complex*. The Merkel cells are the fine tactile receptors of the discriminative touch system and provide cues used to localize and to perceive the edges of shape and form of objects.

Fine or discriminative touch allows the body to sense and localize the touch. Discriminative touch is further subdivided into flutter, pressure, touch, and vibration. These sensations use specific receptors located in specific regions to sense the touch. For example, the *Meissner corpuscle* is found in the dermal papillae (hairless skin) and is considered to be the discriminative touch system's flutter and movement finding receptors in nonhairy locations. The *Pacinian corpuscle* is found in the underlying tissue beneath the dermis, connective tissues of bone, the body wall, and body cavity. Depending on their location, the Pacinian corpuscle can be cutaneous, proprioceptive, or visceral receptors. In the discriminative touch system, the Pacinian corpuscles in the skin are considered to be the vibration or tickle sensitive receptors.

The discriminative touch and proprioceptive systems are most sensitive to mechanical force. Their sensory receptors are of the mechanoreceptor category, which transduce a mechanical force into an electrical charge or electrical potential. These receptors are types of ion channels that react to mechanical distortion. In turn, ions such as potassium and sodium flow into or out of the cell resulting in depolarization (activation of the nervous tissue called terminal endings). This depolarization will last as long as the mechanoreceptor is activated externally. However, there is a subset of terminal endings that do not sustain depolarization and are considered to be rapidly adapting, meaning the sensation becomes not as intense. Terminal endings that sustain depolarization are called slowly adapting and the sensation can remain at the original intensity or become more intense.

Patricia A. Bloomquist

See also: Discriminative Touch; Discriminative Touch Experiment; Homunculus; Sensory Receptors; Somatosensory Cortex/Somatosensory System

Further Reading

Dougherty, P., & Tsuchitani, C. (1997). Somatosensory systems. In *Neuroscience Online, an electronic textbook for the neurosciences* (Chap. 2). Open-access educational resource provided by the Department of Neurobiology and Anatomy at the University of Texas Medical School at Houston. Retrieved from http://neuroscience.uth.tmc.edu/s2/chapter02.html

Gibson, J. J. (1962). Observations on active touch. *Psychological Review, 69*(6), 477–491.

Klatzky, R. L., & Lederman, S. J. (2002). Touch. In A. F. Healy & R. W. Proctor (Eds.), *Experimental psychology* (pp. 147–176). Volume 4 in I. B. Weiner (Editor-in-Chief) *Handbook of Psychology*. New York, NY: Wiley.

Purves, D., Augustine, G. J., Fitzpatrick, D., Hall, W. C., LaMantia, A.-S., McNamara, J. O., & Williams, S. M. (Eds.). (2004). *Neuroscience* (3rd ed.). Sunderland, MA: Sinauer Associates.

Tourette Syndrome

Gilles de la Tourette syndrome or *Tourette syndrome* is a disorder that involves the nervous system. It is a neurological disorder which causes individuals to have uncontrolled movements and vocalizations. These uncontrolled movements and vocalizations are known as *tics*. Tourette syndrome can affect people of all ages but the symptoms are usually first detected in childhood. Both males and females are affected; however, males are usually affected three to four times more than are females (CDCP, 2011). There is no cure for Tourette syndrome, yet individuals tend to live a regular life span. Tourette syndrome can be managed using medications and other forms of treatment, though many times medication is only needed if the tics interfere with daily life.

History

The first case of Tourette syndrome was reported in medical literature in 1825. A French physician named Jean Marc Gaspard Itard (1774–1838) described the condition of a noble woman who would say swear words and yell vulgarities when holding conversations. In 1855, a French neurologist Georges Albert Édouard Brutus Gilles de la Tourette (1857–1904) described the symptoms of uncontrollable twitching and jerking as well as crying and grunting in nine patients. Thus, the condition was named after him. Because most of the patients were males, it was believed that the symptoms in males and females were due to separate conditions. Gilles de la Tourette also found that the disorder usually ran in families. Tourette syndrome was thought to be a psychological condition. It was found to be a neurological condition in the 1960s when neuroleptic drugs effectively treated Tourette syndrome.

Symptoms

The main symptom of Tourette syndrome is tics. Tics are involuntary movements and can be motor or verbal. Symptoms of Tourette's can vary, ranging from slight to severe. Most tics are in the mild range. When tics are severe, they usually end up interfering with daily life, affecting an individual's quality of life. There are two classifications of tics: simple and complex. Simple tics are usually sudden and brief, are repetitive, and usually involve only a small number of muscle groups. Examples of simple motor tics include, eye blinking and darting, jerking of the head, and shoulder shrugging. Examples of simple vocalizations include throat clearing, grunting, or sniffing. Complex tics are patterns of movements that are coordinated and clearly distinct. These tics usually involve numerous muscle groups and seem to be purposeful. Examples of complex motor tics include nose touching or touching other people, hopping, twisting, or offensive gesturing. Examples of complex vocalizations are repeating words and phrases as well as swearing. Some of the most debilitating and dramatic tics are those where an individual causes self-harm. Tics can vary from person to person. When an individual expresses tics, they experience premonitory urges, which is an uncomfortable sensation of the body, such as an itch. Tic expression produces relief of the urges. Some people are able to repress or stop a tic, until they are able to be in a place that is less disruptive. Some individuals with Tourette syndrome will need to express the tic in a certain way or number of times for the urge to go away. Excitement or anxiety can make tics worse. Tics can also be worsened from physical experiences such as tight clothing or certain sounds. During sleep, tics do not disappear, rather they are decreased.

Causes

There is no known cause of Tourette syndrome. Recent research of Tourette syndrome shows it may be related to abnormalities areas in the brain, the circuits that join the areas, and neurotransmitters (natural brain chemicals) used for communication. The causes of Tourette syndrome seem to be complex. Areas of the brain affected could include the frontal lobe and cortex, while neurotransmitters may include serotonin and dopamine. Tourette syndrome may also be caused by a combination of factors: genetic and environmental. It could be a disorder that is inherited, however, the genes that may be involved are not known. There is some evidence from studies of twins and families that show Tourette syndrome could be hereditary. It was originally believed to be an autosomal dominant trait, but now seems to be more complicated. Tourette syndrome could be caused by a few genes with sizable effects, or could be due to a combination of factors such as many genes with few effects with added environmental causes. There are also some risk factors associated with Tourette syndrome. These include family history and being male.

Diagnosis

There is not a specific test that is used to diagnose Tourette syndrome. It is mainly diagnosed by watching the tics. There are several criteria used to diagnose Tourette syndrome, which were determined by the *Diagnostic and Statistical Manual of Mental Disorders (DSM)*. The criteria include (1) having motor and verbal tics, which do not have to occur at the same time; (2) having tics for at least one year, which can occur multiple times a day, almost every day, or sporadically; (3) tics beginning before the age of 18; and (4) that the tics cannot be due to medications, other drugs, or other conditions. Diagnosis can be hindered because of unfamiliar family members and doctors. Individuals diagnosed with Tourette syndrome are often diagnosed with other associated conditions such as obsessive-compulsive disorder (OCD), attention-deficit/hyperactivity disorder (ADHD), learning disabilities, and anxiety disorders.

Treatments

Many people with Tourette syndrome do not require any medication because their tics do not cause any harm. However, there are medications available for those who have symptoms that interfere with daily functions. Medications are used to help manage tics, but do not completely get rid of them. No medication works the same for every individual, and because many with Tourette syndrome have other related disorders, no one course of treatment will be the same. Medications used to treat Tourette syndrome include (1) neuroleptics, drugs that inhibit dopamine levels in the brain; (2) injections of botulinum toxin type A; (3) stimulants; and (4) central adrenergic inhibitors and antidepressants. Neuroleptics have been the most useful in treating tics. Examples of neuroleptics include haloperidol and pimozide. Like with all prescriptions, medications used to treat Tourette syndrome have side effects. Side effects may include tiredness, muscles stiffness, weight gain, and restlessness. Common side effects of neuroleptics include weight gain and sedation. After long-term use, the discontinuation of neuroleptics must be done slowly in order to avoid a return increase in tics and withdrawal dyskinesia (involuntary muscle movements that are similar to tics). These risks can be lowered by using lower doses of the medication and for less amounts of time. There are also effective medications used to treat the related disorders. ADHD symptoms can be decreased in people with Tourette syndrome with stimulant medications. Along with medications, other forms of treatment can be used such as psychotherapy, behavior therapy, and deep brain stimulation.

Outcomes

Individuals with Tourette syndrome can lead relatively normal lives with a normal life expectancy. Even though there is not a cure, Tourette syndrome usually improves, as the individual gets older. However, though the symptoms of Tourette syndrome may improve, associated conditions may last into adulthood. Improvement is usually seen during the late teens and early 20s. Sometimes the symptoms may disappear altogether or the tics are not as bad and medication is no longer needed. This disorder is chronic, but it is not degenerative. It is important for the patients and general population to be educated about tic disorders. The more educated the population is, the better the understanding and tolerance there will be, which is crucially important to those affected by Tourette syndrome.

Future

There are several organizations that are currently conducting further research on Tourette syndrome. The National Center on Birth Defects and Developmental

Disabilities (NCBDDD) is conducting research in order to further understand Tourette syndrome, which includes researching the prevalence of Tourette syndrome as well as the quality of life with those who have Tourette syndrome. The results will be used to advise doctors which will be used to improve the lives of individuals with Tourette syndrome. The National Institute of Neurological Disorders and Stroke (NINDS) is researching on the brain and nervous system. Investigators from the National Institute of Health (NIH) are conducing genetic studies on Tourette syndrome. They are using technology to screen genome wide, which will hopefully help to find a gene or genes associated with Tourette syndrome. Understanding the genetics associated with Tourette syndrome will help in many ways including improving genetic counseling and insight into more effectual therapies and medications. There are a number of clinical trials involving Tourette syndrome. These trials involved, observing stimulate treatment of ADHD in those with Tourette syndrome treatments for diminishing tics. Trials for other medications have also taken place.

Shannen McNamara

See also: Attention Deficit Disorder/Attention-Deficit Hyperactivity Disorder; Behavior; Behavioral Health; Brain Stimulators

Further Reading

Centers for Disease Control and Prevention (CDCP). (2011). *Tourette syndrome: Facts and resources.* Retrieved from http://www.cdc.gov/Features/TouretteSyndrome/

Mayo Clinic Staff. (2014). *Tourette syndrome.* Retrieved from http://www.mayoclinic.org/diseases-conditions/tourette-syndrome/basics/definition/con-20043570

National Institute of Neurological Disorders and Stroke (NINDS). (2012). *Tourette syndrome fact sheet.* Retrieved from http://www.ninds.nih.gov/disorders/tourette/detail_tourette.htm

National Tourette Syndrome Association. (2014). *What is Tourette syndrome.* Retrieved from http://tsa-usa.org/aMedical/whatists.html

OCD-UK. (2013). *The history of Tourette syndrome.* Retrieved from http://www.ocduk.org/tourette-syndrome-history

Transduction and Membrane Properties

The word *transduction* is derived from "transduce," which means to change one thing into another form. Within an animal's central nervous system, transduction is the conversion of a physical energy into a nerve impulse. These nerve impulses, or action potentials, are unique to brain cells (neurons), as this is how the brain integrates senses and motor functions.

The central nervous system uses an electric form of energy to transmit signals through the neuron. However, between neurons, this electrical signal is converted into a release of chemicals, or neurotransmitters, into the synaptic cleft. The process of this chemical signal is then reconverted into another electrical event. In the peripheral nervous system—which senses the external environment—many signals are not electrical, such as light, sound, and touch. For these energies to be transduced into an electrical energy, each sensory system has specialized receptors that convert the signal into an electrical impulse. For instance, in the visual system, the photosensitive lining of the back of the eye—which is called the retina—there are photoreceptors located on the dendrites of neurons. These photoreceptors will be activated when a specific wavelength of white visible light touches it. The wavelength of the light will then be converted into a postsynaptic potential (a change in voltage across a cell's membrane) that may activate the entire neuron. If enough postsynaptic potentials arrive at the same time, their amplitude will summate and ultimately produce an action potential.

To help propagate the newly made electrical signal, the plasma membrane of the neuron has passive properties. This means that no additional energy is needed to "move" the electrical signal from its initiation point to the trigger zone (axon hillock) of the neuronal cell body. These passive properties include the passive resistance and the passive conduction of the plasma membrane. With these two types of passive properties, a simple R-C circuit, or a resistor-capacitor circuit, can easily represent a neuron's ability to conduct a current.

B. Dnate' Baxter and
Jennifer L. Hellier

See also: Axon; Membrane; Membrane Potential: Depolarization and Hyperpolarization; Membrane Potential Experiment—Understand Membrane Properties; Postsynaptic Potentials; Presynaptic Terminals; Sensory Receptors; Synaptic Cleft

Further Reading

Alberts, B., Johnson, A., Lewis, J., Raff, M., Roberts, K., & Walter, P. (2002). *Molecular biology of the cell* (4th ed.). New York, NY: Garland Science.

Dougherty, P., & Tsuchitani, C. (1997). Somatosensory systems. In *Neuroscience Online, an electronic textbook for the neurosciences* (Chap. 2). Open-access educational resource provided by the Department of Neurobiology and Anatomy at the University of Texas Medical School at Houston. Retrieved from http://neuroscience.uth.tmc.edu/s2/chapter02.html

Kandel, E. R., Schwartz, J. H., Jessell, T. M., Siegelbaum, S. A., & Hudspeth, A. J. (Eds.). (2012). *Principles of neural science* (5th ed.). New York, NY: McGraw-Hill.

Purves, D., Augustine, G. J., Fitzpatrick, D., Hall, W. C., LaMantia, A.-S., McNamara, J. O., & Williams, S. M. (Eds.). (2004). *Neuroscience* (3rd ed.). Sunderland, MA: Sinauer Associates.

Transgenic Mice

All behavior is shaped by how genes and the environment interact on a molecular level. Genes carry information pertaining to physical traits, such as eye color or how tall one is in comparison to siblings, as well as genetic traits like color blindness or predisposition to a particular disease. This genetic material is passed onto the next generation from parent to offspring and the process is called hereditary. All living organisms depend upon genes to build, maintain, and pass along genetic information. Each gene is encoded upon strands of DNA (deoxyribonucleic acid), which is stored within chromosomes. DNA contains the genetic blueprints and makeup of each organism and the term used to describe all this hereditary material is called the genome.

Diploid organisms contain two sets of chromosome, one from each parent. Animals are diploid, including mammals. Diploid organisms receive one copy of each gene from the mother and another copy from the father. These single copies are also called alleles, which can have several different forms of the gene. Genes within an organism's genome are not arranged out of sequence, but in a precise order along the chromosomes, each with its own specific site. Similar alleles are termed homozygous because these are two identical alleles that encode for a particular trait, whereas differing alleles are called heterozygous such that these are two different alleles for a particular trait. Proteins are the results of genes being translated. All living organisms are made up of these proteins (large molecules) comprising amino acids chains and are responsible for many metabolic processes as well as regulation of neural circuits. Since genes store vital information, the ability to manipulate them can provide valuable information about particular genes involved in behavior as well as how the proteins that are made from the genes control that behavior.

Rodents, particularly mice, are ideal for *transgenic experimentation* because they are readily available and respond well to many types of behavioral studies within neuroscience. A *transgenic mouse* has had its genome modified by the insertion of foreign DNA. The modified gene is called a transgene. The source of the foreign DNA is often a human gene that researchers want to over or under express in order to observe and study gene function as well as genetic pathways. Genetic material is manipulated by a technique known as "Recombinant DNA Technology," which combines or mixes DNA molecules from different sources like human and mouse into one resulting molecule.

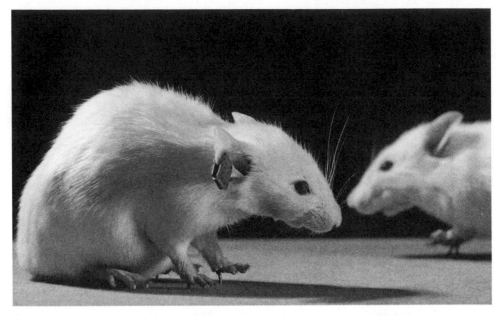

These male mice are direct descendants of the first transgenic mammals to be granted a U.S. patent. Their genes were altered to make the mice more prone to develop cancers by the insertion of an extra piece of DNA taken from a virus. This trait makes this strain of mouse (known as the "oncomouse") particularly useful in cancer research. (Science & Society Picture Library/Getty Images)

If the new, foreign DNA that has been inserted artificially into the mouse genome integrates successfully, the result will be a transgene. The following is a diagram outlining the steps in the creation of a transgene via recombinant DNA technology.

Molecule "**A**"   versus   Molecule "**B**"

→ Break down (digest) the cells with the same restriction endonuclease (an enzyme that cuts DNA at specific nucleotide sequences called restriction sites). Nucleotides are repetitively called the "building blocks" of DNA.

→ The restriction endonuclease cuts the DNA and leaves an overhanging piece called "sticky ends." These sticky ends can pair with DNA molecules that contain complimentary base pairs. Molecule A and B are then mixed together.

→ The molecule mixture is then sealed with DNA ligase (enzyme that joins DNA strands together).

→ The result is recombinant DNA where two sources are incorporated into a single recombinant molecule.

History

The first genetically engineered organism took place in 1973 by two American geneticists, Stanley N. Cohen (1935–) and Herbert Boyer (1936–), cofounders of Genentech. These two scientists gave rise to genetic manipulation techniques as a result of their research combining and transplanting genes. Shortly after the two scientists successfully created an organism that contained genetic material from two different sources, a conference was held to determine and discuss ethical considerations utilizing this new technology. The meeting resulted in the development of strict guidelines governing genetic manipulation techniques to ensure that ethical considerations are being met. In the United States, the National Institutes of Health (NIH) imposes such guidelines for conducting research. Transgenic animals fall under regulation of the NIH's Office of Biotechnology Activities (OBA).

The first transgenic mouse was created by biologist, Rudolf Jaenisch (1942–) in 1974. He is thought to be a pioneer in the field of genetic manipulation and focused his research on studying cancer and neurological diseases. He was the first scientist to successfully insert foreign DNA into the DNA of early mouse embryos resulting in mice that carried the modified gene in all their tissues.

How to Engineer a Transgenic Mouse

There are two routinely used methods for creating transgenic mice: pronuclear microinjection and introduction of DNA into embryonic stem cells. A third method and the least commonly used is called virus-mediated transgenesis.

Method 1: Pronuclear Microinjection

Producing a transgenic mouse can be done via the microinjection of purified foreign DNA into the male pronucleus (precursor of a nucleus contributed by the sperm) of newly fertilized zygotes (early embryo) before they fully mature. Once both pronuclei fuse, that is the normal female portion with the male portion containing foreign DNA combine, the genetically engineered embryos are implanted into donor females that will act as surrogate or foster mothers. The new modified gene containing the foreign DNA (transgene) becomes randomly incorporated into the genome. Since the transgene randomly incorporates itself, only about 10–30 percent of the offspring will contain the foreign DNA within their own chromosomes. The resulting transgenic offspring are identified and bred to produce transgenic mouse lines.

Method 2: Embryonic Stem Cell-Mediated Gene Transfer

This method consists of introducing the foreign DNA by injection into cultured embryonic stem cells (ES) that incorporate into an embryo at the blastocyst stage, which contains a cluster of cells that give rise to embryos, the placenta, and gametes as well as cells needed for development of a healthy fetus. As in the previously mentioned method, the embryos are implanted into donor females that will act as surrogate or foster mothers. The offspring, born of the blastocyst, are called chimera because it is an organism that results from two different early embryos arising from different populations of genetically diverse cells. The chimera contains a mixture of modified ES cells as well as unmodified blastocyst cells.

ES cells often contribute to the germ line cells derived from gametes, which are the reproductive cells. This results in a fully transgenic animal if the sperm carrying the transgene fertilizes a normal egg. As with pronuclear microinjection methods, the researcher needs to test for the presence of the transgene and breed accordingly to propagate the newly developed transgenic line.

Method 3: Virus-Mediated Transgenesis

This method differs from the two previously discussed ones in that a viral packaging system is used to deliver the foreign DNA into a host system. The transfer of the transgene is done by means of using a virus, which is a small, infectious agent that can only replicate in a host environment and can infect all forms of organisms. Gene expression may be significantly increased by using this method due to the ability of the virus to infect host cells. Offspring, as with ES transfers, will be chimeric and the resulting offspring can be tested for transgene presence.

Advantages of Transgenic Mice

The arrival of new advances in genetic engineering gives researchers a unique look at disease progression and an opportunity to observe the system wide damage a disease can have on an organism. Transgenic mouse models are the means by which researchers study human disease and treatments. In agriculture, transgenic models have helped produce disease/insect-resistant crops like rice, cotton, tomato, and potatoes. Weed populations can have a negative impact on agriculture and the toxic herbicides, used to treat damaging weeds, often kills other plant life. Through genetic engineering, researchers can manipulate crops to tolerate some herbicides and prevent the loss of crops.

Advantages of transgenic techniques can be seen in animals as well. For instance, transgenic livestock have been created to improve the functionality of these animals by targeting milk production in cattle, the ability to produce leaner food-animals like cattle, and increasing the quality of marketable textile fibers like wool from sheep. Transgenic cattle can be produced with milk fortified with vitamin A (retinoic acid) and other human proteins, which may play in role in the treatment of emphysema. Other animals are genetically modified to express certain disease characteristics so that researchers can study these models in order to develop feasible treatments. For researchers who study disease models like schizophrenia and diabetes and utilize transgenic genetic manipulation techniques, the advantages outweigh the disadvantages. But, for the communities who reap the rewards of such medical advances, the negative outcomes still need consideration.

Disadvantages of Transgenic Mice

Advances in medical science can be a powerful tool when these techniques are balanced with thoughtful decision making that considers all the ethical dilemmas involved in altering an organism's genetic makeup. Areas that conduct research such as academia, biotechnology, and government need to be concerned with issues of animal welfare as technology grows and changes. Some ethical questions and concerns are outlined in the following.

- When conducting these bioengineering studies, is the science valid? The validation of scientific exploration is a vital role in determining if the research has an outcome that would benefit humankind in a positive way. Without scientific justification, research teeters between unethical and ethical practices.
- Will the organism be harmed and should there be policies to dictate the use of animals in research? Unintentional harm to the organism (usually animals) is a charged subject and one sought after by many animal rights activist groups (e.g., PETA: People for the Ethical Treatment of Animals). The NIH or other federal agencies fund most research in the Unites States. Therefore, the NIH develops policies that outline the humane treatment of animals used in research. Each institution that is federally funded must have an Institutional Animal Care and Use Committee (IACUC) that follows the strict NIH guidelines for animal research.
- Are techniques used to genetically modify organisms (plant or animal based) morally wrong? A survey conducted in 2002 concluded that 64 percent of Americans did believe that cloning was morally wrong and that they would not consume any modified foods. Some believe that although the medical advances allow researchers to clone organisms, it does not mean they should. The controversial debate revolves around how the biomedical advances might negatively impact nature and environments as well as humans.

The moral and ethical concerns are not the only ones to consider when examining the negative impact transgenes have on the organism. Transgenic animals, in particular mice, have lower survival rates (reduction in survival rates among pups) when compared to mice that have not been genetically modified. The inserted foreign DNA may disrupt the function of an existing gene leading to the loss of expression of a characteristic or trait.

In conclusion, transgenic mice provide researchers with a valuable biomedical tool, one that may help create new medicine, new drug strategies, and hope within the disease communities by providing animal models. Like all tools, strict guidelines need to be firmly established to ensure the safety of the animals and research participants so that lines and laws are not crossed for the sake of advances in medical science.

Nicole Arevalo

See also: Behavioral Tests; Diabetes Mellitus; Society for Neuroscience; Retrovirus; Schizophrenia

Further Reading

Alberts, B., Johnson, A., Lewis, J., Raff, M., Roberts, K., & Peter W. (Eds.). (2002). *Molecular biology of the cell* (4th ed.). New York, NY: Taylor and Francis Group.

EndAnimalCloning.org. (2012). Retrieved from http://www.endanimalcloning.org/ethics.shtml

Finger, Thomas E., Silver, Wayne L., & Restrepo, Diego. (2000). *The neurobiology of taste and smell* (2nd ed.). New York, NY: Wiley-Liss.

Kandel, E. R., Schwartz, J. H., & Jessell, T. M. (2000). *Principles of neural science* (4th ed.). New York, NY: McGraw-Hill.

Lodish, H., Berk, A., Matsudaira, P., Kaiser, C. A., Krieger, M., Scott, M. P., Zipursky, S. L., & Darnell, J. (Eds.). (2004). *Molecular cell biology* (5th ed.). New York, NY: W.H. Freeman and Company.

National Health Museum. (2012). *Transgenic mice.* Retrieved from http://www .accessexcellence.org/RC/VL/GG/transgenic.php

Nicholls, J. G., Martin, A. R., Wallace, B. G., & Fuchs, P. A. (Eds.). (2001) *From neuron to brain* (4th ed.). Sunderland, MA: Sinauer Associates Inc.

Transgenic animals. (2012). Retrieved from http://users.rcn.com/jkimball.ma.ultranet /BiologyPages/T/TransgenicAnimals.html

Transient Global Amnesia

When animals learn a new task, such as how to access their food, they form memories. There are two types of memories: anterograde memory and retrograde memory. Anterograde memory means, "to form new memories" and retrograde memory means, "to access already formed memories." When there is an inability to recall or form new memories, it is a condition called *amnesia. Transient global amnesia* is an experience of short-term memory loss that has a sudden onset and is brief, meaning it lasts for less than 24 hours. It is important to note that transient global amnesia is different from *anterograde amnesia* and *retrograde amnesia*. Both of these types of amnesia occur following an injury to the brain and last for more than 24 hours. Transient global amnesia generally only occurs once in a person's lifetime but there is a 4 to 5 percent chance of recurrence (Ardila, 2013). This temporary amnesia causes a loss in short-term memory. This causes patients to keep asking the same questions, usually about where they are or why they are there, repeatedly without remembering the explanation. This does not, however, affect the memory of who you are or your recognition of people you are well acquainted with. This condition may also be associated with a strong emotional response. After the short-lived episode, memories are slowly returned intact, except for those from during the incident. Patients generally do not remember the 24-hour period in which they are experiencing the transient global amnesia (Mayo Clinic, 2011). The occurrences in the United States are 5.2 cases per 100,000 in the whole population and 23.5 cases per 100,000 in individuals over the age of 50 (Ardila, 2013). This shows a correlation to age and the risk of transient global amnesia. Internationally, the estimates on frequency vary greatly between countries, with some having fewer cases and some having more cases than the United States per 100,000 (Ardila, 2013). Despite this variety from country to country, there has been no consistent correlation between race and the risk of transient global amnesia. Likewise, there has been no correlation between gender and increased risk, although men and women have been found to have differing triggers (Sucholeiki, 2012).

Causes

Transient global amnesia is not yet fully understood, and a leading hypothesis is that it may have multiple causes. One of these proposed causes is found in the fact that many cases have reported similar events prior to the episode. In women, this event is usually emotionally linked, such as bad news, conflict, or overwork, whereas in men it is usually physically linked, such as strenuous physical activity, head trauma, or sudden immersion in water of extreme temperatures. There is also a vascular hypothesis that states insufficient blood flow to the brain as a cause. This hypothesis was generally accepted until further research was done and showed that patients suffering from transient global amnesia do not have an increased risk of cerebral vascular disease or stroke on follow up, which would likely ensue if it were caused by ischemia (lack of blood flow to the brain). A history of migraines is also generally associated with transient global amnesia. However, they have not been found to occur prior to or during the episode. Therefore, history of migraines is more recently thought to be a risk factor, as opposed to a cause (Mayo Clinic, 2011).

A recent study has given rise to another possible cause as well. During this study, transient global amnesia was accidentally induced in a patient while undergoing deep brain stimulation for another condition. An electrode was misplaced on the right hippocampus and was therefore subject to high-voltage, high-frequency stimulation. This event indicates that inhibition of local neuronal activity due to high current density within the hippocampus (Baezner et al., 2013). The hippocampus is part of the limbic system and has shown to be important in forming and maintaining memories. These findings correlate with those that show a higher density of hippocampal cavities (a normal fluid collection within the vestigial hippocampal sulcus) in a high-resolution magnetic resonance imaging (MRI) for patients that have suffered from transient global amnesia as compared to the controls. Although further research is necessary to make a conclusion about this correlation, these two studies both seem to indicate that the hippocampus may be part of the cause of transient global amnesia (Sucholeiki, 2012).

Symptoms

The most major symptom of transient global amnesia is the sudden lack of knowledge about what has just happened. This unexpected loss of memory is a symptom also associated with other, more serious, conditions such as a stroke or a seizure, so a more thorough analysis of the symptoms is necessary for diagnosis of transient global amnesia. A stroke, for instance, will often be accompanied by limb paralysis or trouble with speech, and these will not be present in a patient with transient global amnesia. The patient should also retain their identity, be able to recognize familiar objects and people, and follow simple directions. An episode of transient global amnesia should not last longer than 24 hours and the patient will regain their memories gradually as the episode comes to an end (Ardila, 2013).

Diagnosis

Due to the fact that transient global amnesia is still not fully understood, diagnosis is generally accomplished by eliminating illnesses with similar symptoms using a combination of physical exams and imaging. The physical exam includes an analysis of reflexes, gait, posture, muscle tone, and coordination. If the patient is suffering from transient global amnesia, the functions listed above should not be impaired. If this is the case, a stroke can be eliminated as a possible diagnosis, since it would negatively affect some, if not all, of these areas. Electroencephalography (EEG; recording of the brain's electrical activity) can be performed to determine if the memory loss is caused by epilepsy. Even when a seizure is not taking place, people with epilepsy generally have fluctuations in their brain waves. Abnormalities in the brain, such as distortion (stretching or breaking) in blood vessels, could also be a cause for memory loss similar to that of transient global amnesia, so a computed tomography (CT; imaging of the brain displayed as cross-sectional images) image is generally completed to determine whether brain abnormalities are present. Transient global amnesia and transient epileptic amnesia (TEA) manifest with very similar symptoms in the beginning phases, but the episodes that occur in TEA are shorter, generally between 20 and 60 minutes, and are more often recurring. They can, therefore, be differentiated fairly easily based on length of episode. For an accurate diagnosis, the episode must be witnessed by someone who can verify the patient's immediate symptoms and confirm if it was rapid onset (Mayo Clinic Staff, 2011).

Treatment

Transient global amnesia resolves itself and, therefore, requires no treatment. However, if there is a possibility of other conditions as well, such as transient ischemic attack, epilepsy, or migraine, those will be treated accordingly. If the condition does not resolve itself after 24 hours, it is no longer categorized as transient global amnesia. In this case, the most common diagnosis is an ischemic attack or a cranial bleed.

Current Research

Research for transient global amnesia in recent years has had a strong focus on attempting to find a more concrete way to diagnose it. One study used 12 subjects that were "purely" transient global amnesia cases and looked for vascular risk factors, brain MRI findings, and subsequent cerebrovascular or seizure events. "Pure" transient global amnesia indicates that the patients had no history of other conditions. This experiment showed no difference between the control group and the experiment group in terms of vascular risk factors, brain MRI measures, subsequent attacks, or acute brain abnormalities. It was mentioned that a small sample size was used, but, in general, the conclusion stated that transient global amnesia was not related to vascular risk factors of cerebrovascular disease (Romero et al., 2013).

There has also been recent research showing that transient global amnesia is not as benign as originally thought. Experiments have shown an impairment of verbal memory, categorical learning, and attention even months after the episode. This experiment compared age and intelligence quotient (IQ) matched controls with their transient global amnesia patient and found mild yet persistent impairment of both anterograde and retrograde memory (Ardila, 2013). Aside from this new data supporting long-term effects of a transient global amnesia episode, this experiment supports the findings of previous experiments when it comes to triggers (more emotional for women and physical for men), diagnosis (no set symptoms to diagnose definitively), and correlations to risk factors (migraines).

Kathryn Wellman

See also: Epilepsy; Gait; Learning and Memory; Reflex; Seizures; Stroke

Further Reading

Ardila, A. (2013). Transient global amnesia. In *Neurology MedLink*. Retrieved from http://www.medlink.com/medlinkcontent.asp

Baezner, H., Blahak, C., Capelle, H. H., Schrader, C., Lutjens, G., & Krauss, J. K. (2013). Transient global amnesia associated with accidental high-frequency stimulation of the right hippocampus in deep brain stimulation for segmental dystonia. *Stereotactic and Functional Neurosurgery, 91*(5), 335–337.

Mayo Clinic Staff. (2011). *Diseases and conditions: Transient global amnesia.* Retrieved from http://www.mayoclinic.org/diseases-conditions/transient-global-amnesia/basics/definition/con-20032746

Romero, J. R., Mercado, M., Beiser, A. S., Pikula, A., Seshadri, S., Kelly-Hayes, M., & Wolf, P. A. (2013). Transient global amnesia and neurological events: The Framingham heart study. *Frontiers in Neurology, 4,* 47.

Sucholeiki, R. (2012). Transient global amnesia clinical presentation. In *Medscape*. Retrieved from http://emedicine.medscape.com/article/1160964-clinical

Transient Ischemic Attack (TIA)

Transient ischemic attacks (TIAs) are the result of decreased blood flow in the vessels of the brain, spinal cord, or retina of the eye. These attacks are temporary and seldom result in any permanent tissue damage or loss. The most common symptoms of a TIA include visual disturbances, temporary numbness or paralysis on one side of the body, and, in some instances, cognitive problems. Treatment most often consists of treating the symptoms a patient experiences, as well as using drugs such as aspirin or Plavix to reduce blood clot formation.

History

TIAs are considered a neurological disease. TIAs occur in about 5 million individuals in the United States each year (Panagos, 2012). These attacks result when blood flow to a region of the brain, spinal cord, or retina is significantly reduced or stopped for a period of time anywhere from a few seconds to several minutes by an *occlusion* (blockage) of a blood vessel. TIAs are often called "mini-strokes" due to the similarity of the mode of action of TIAs compared to strokes or *cerebrovascular accident* (CVAs). Unlike strokes, which usually result in very significant and often, permanent tissue damage or death, TIAs usually do not result in significant tissue infarction (*death of the tissue*). Nonetheless, TIAs are considered by the medical profession to be a warning sign for future CVAs.

Pathophysiology

Transient ischemic attacks are most often the result of an *embolism* (obstruction of an artery generally by a blood clot or an air bubble) that blocks a major artery in the brain or eye. There are two primary sources of these emboli. The first source is often fatty deposits that develop within the *carotid arteries* called *atherosclerosis* or *plaque*. Atherosclerotic plaques develop most often in the blood vessels of individuals who have diets high in lipids or fats. When these small pieces of plaque break off they form an embolism, which will travel through the carotid arteries, main arteries of the neck and the primary blood vessels that supply the brain with blood, and lodge in smaller vessels in the brain. This results in a temporary decrease in blood flow to the brain. Such a decrease in blood flow results in a decrease in oxygen supply to those areas of the brain supplied by a blood vessel, and that region of the brain does not function correctly as a result.

The second source of an embolus that could cause a TIA is the heart. As humans age, they develop a condition called *atrial fibrillation* which is an uncoordinated, quivering of the heart muscle, specifically the two top chambers of the heart called the left and right *atria*. This often results in the formation of small blood clots in these chambers of the heart. Occasionally, these blood clots break up and produce a *thrombus* or blood clot that is similar to an embolism. These also travel from the heart into the brain and cause a decrease in blood flow to regions of the brain affected by the blocked artery.

Other factors that result in an increased chance of plaque buildup or the formation of clots include *hypertension* (high blood pressure), smoking, increased dietary cholesterol, and *diabetes mellitus* or type 2 diabetes.

Symptoms and Diagnosis

The signs of a TIA can be variable and often overlooked due to their temporary nature. The primary signs of a TIA include (1) a temporary decrease or loss of vision in one eye or the other—it is very rare to have loss of vision in both eyes simultaneously; (2) difficulty speaking (*aphasia*); (3) unilateral *hemiparesis,* which is a general weakness on one side of the body or the other; and (4) general numbness on one side of the body or the other (*parasthesia*). Both hemiparesis and parasthesia will occur on the *contralateral* side (opposite side) of the body from the hemisphere of the brain that is being affected by a decrease in blood flow. Less common secondary symptoms of a TIA include (1) dizziness, (2) difficulty with or loss of balance, and (3) very rarely, temporary loss of bowel and/or urinary bladder control.

The diagnosis of TIAs is often difficult due to the transitory nature of the symptoms. However, when a patient is having prolonged symptoms and seeks medical attention, this diagnosis can be made fairly readily using a number of different radiographic techniques. The technique used will depend, to some extent, on the symptoms a patient is experiencing. To determine if a blood vessel in the brain is occluded, two primary techniques are used. These include (1) *computerized axial tomography* or CAT scanning and (2) *magnetic resonance imaging* or MRI scanning. To determine if there is a significant plaque buildup within the carotid artery in the neck, an *ultrasound* of the neck can be performed, and to determine if blood clots might be present within the atria of the heart, the use of *echocardiography* (an ultrasound of the heart) can be used.

There are a number of other medical conditions which have symptoms similar to TIAs. These include (1) migraine headaches, (2) *parietal lobe* seizures (the parietal lobe is found within the cerebral cortex of the brain), (3) type 1 and type 2 diabetes, (4) *electrolyte* imbalance (electrolytes are ionically charged elements such as sodium, potassium, calcium, and chlorine), (5) hypertensive encephalitis, and (6) brain tumors, to name a few. It is critical that an individual be evaluated by a qualified health care practitioner to determine the exact cause of the symptoms he may be experiencing.

Treatment and Prevention

Treatment of TIA is dependent on the cause. In many cases, primary treatments are centered on controlling the symptoms of the attack. Once symptoms are managed, secondary treatment will then be instituted to decrease the cause of the symptoms. When a patient is having TIAs as a result of thrombi formed by the release of plaque from the carotid artery, the two primary goals are to (1) reduce the formation of plaque and (2) remove plaque, should there be a significant quantity within the carotid artery. Plaque formation can be reduced most easily by maintaining a recommended diet in regard to fat and carbohydrate consumption. When plaque buildup is significant, an *endarterectomy* is commonly performed to help remove this fatty buildup. An endarterectomy is a surgical procedure that is performed to remove excess plaque buildup that has caused the arterial wall to narrow. Commonly, this is performed on carotid arteries.

When a patient is having a TIA as a result of blood clots being released from the atria of the heart, anticoagulants such as aspirin or clopidogrel (Plavix) are used. Plavix has shown to reduce the buildup of blood clots within the atria of the heart as well as help dissolve any clots that may currently exist. However, a physician should always be consulted before using any pharmaceutical methods for treatment of potential symptoms of a TIA.

TIAs can be prevented to some degree by life style choices. Risk factors for increased TIAs include (1) smoking; (2) increased use of alcohol; (3) diets that are high in fat, cholesterol, or carbohydrates; (4) lack of regular aerobic exercise; (5) obesity; and (6) *hypertension* (high blood pressure). Regular exercise, diets high in grains as well as fruits and vegetables, and limited alcohol use or smoking will all work to reduce the risk of TIAs significantly.

Patients who have experienced TIAs have a 30 to 35 percent chance of a recurrence of their symptoms, and a 30 to 40 percent chance of having a full CVA or stroke. It is important to determine the cause of a TIA and to treat this cause to reduce the chance of recurrence and potentially CVA.

Charles A. Ferguson

See also: Aphasia; Diabetes Mellitus; Encephalitis; Headache; Magnetic Resonance Imaging (MRI); Migraine; Paralysis; Stroke

Further Reading

Inoue, T., Kimura, K., Minematsu, M., & Yamaguchi, T. (2004). Clinical features of transient ischemic attack associated with atrial fibrillation: Analysis of 1084 TIA patients. *Journal of Stroke and Cerebrovascular Diseases, 13*(4), 155–159.

National Institute of Neurological Diseases and Stroke. (2013). *NINDS transient ischemic attack information page.* Retrieved from http://www.ninds.nih.gov/disorders/tia/tia.htm

Panagos, P. D. (2012). Transient Ischemic Attack (TIA): The initial diagnostic and therapeutic dilemma. *American Journal of Emergency Medicine, 30,* 794–799.

Shah, K. H., & Edlow, J. A. (2004). Transient ischemic attack: Review for the emergency physician. *Annals of Emergency Medicine, 43*(5), 592–604.

Verbraak, M. E., Hoeksma, A. F., Lindeboom, R., & Kwa, V. I. H. (2012). Subtle problems in activities of daily living after a transient ischemic attack or an apparently fully recovered non-disabling stroke. *Journal of Stroke and Cerebrovascular Diseases, 21*(2), 124–130.

Trauma

The word *trauma* comes from the Greek language meaning "wound." Its origin is placed between 1685 and 1695 and should be pronounced "trou-ma," with the "ou" sounding like *how* ("Trauma," 2013). Trauma is often referred to bodily injury including the feeling of pain, active bleeding, and/or broken bones. However, trauma can mean much more than its obvious definition. When the word was adopted from the Greek language, its base definition was a physical wound. The word trauma came to have a more distinct definition in the medical field as to describe a body wound that was inflicted from sudden physical injury. As time passed, the word continued with the same base definition but different areas of study use the word to describe different examples. In turn, the word trauma came to be used differently in both the fields of medicine and psychology.

Medicine

In medicine, trauma is used to describe a physical injury from a physical wound. In many cases, the injury needs to be attended to quickly and the patient may be admitted to the emergency room or urgent care. Health care providers need to quickly determine how severe the injury is; therefore, several trauma-scoring systems have been developed. The most commonly used scales are the Abbreviated Injury Scale (AIS)—published in 1969, the Glasgow Coma Scale (GCS)—published in 1974, and a Revised Trauma Score (RTS)—published in 1989.

The AIS was revised in 1990 and scores anatomical injury against the probability of survival. It is the core of the Injury Severity Score (ISS) and ranks the severity of an injury from one (minor) to six (unsurvivable). If the patient has a head injury or is unconscious, the GCS is used. This scale determines the level of responsiveness from three quick tests: the eye response, the verbal response, and the motor response. A score is given for each test and summed. A GCS that is less than 9 indicates a severe brain injury, while a GCS that is greater than 12 is a minor brain injury. The RTS includes three measures: the GCS, systolic blood pressure, and respiratory rate. It excludes capillary refill and respiratory expansion from the original Trauma Score, as these tests are difficult to evaluate in the field. Scoring ranges from 0 to 12. A patient with a score less than three is considered dead and should not receive treatment, as they are highly unlikely to survive. A patient with a score between 3 and 10 needs immediate attention, while a person with a score of 11 is considered urgent. Today, the RTS has been expanded for use in triage during mass-causality incidents. The triage-RTS is more sensitive and can better determine if a person may survive if they receive care quickly (Champion et al., 1989).

Today, severe trauma injuries are further classified to describe certain types of injuries seen in the medical field. Some of these include blunt trauma, traumatic cardiac arrest, traumatic asphyxia, penetrating trauma, chest trauma, abdominal trauma, facial trauma, geriatric trauma, pediatric trauma, and *polytrauma*. Polytrauma is when multiple traumatic injuries occur simultaneously, while blunt trauma is a physical injury due to a blunt source. As seen in these two definitions, the word that is placed with trauma simply describes the type or place of trauma. One branch of medicine that studies the wounds inflicted from trauma type sources is called traumatology. Traumatology is not just the study of wounds or injuries but also the study of how to treat traumatic injuries.

Traumatic Brain Injury

Traumatic brain injury (TBI) is a form of acquired brain injury that occurs when a sudden trauma causes damage to the brain. There are two types of TBI: penetrating and closed. For a penetrating injury, the skull is unable to protect the brain from a foreign body, while a closed injury occurs from a sudden and violent contact with the skull. Closed injuries can also consist of a simple blow or jolt to the head that disrupts the normal function of the brain. Patients with severe TBI should be seen by a doctor immediately to reduce the risk of permanent brain damage. The most common type of closed injury occurs during sports, which may result in a concussion. The signs and symptoms of TBI range from mild to severe and may include loss of consciousness for several seconds to minutes, confused or disoriented mental status, difficulty with memory or concentration, headache, dizziness or loss of balance, nausea or vomiting, sleeping problems, mood swings, agitation, slurred speech, convulsions or seizures, dilation of one or both pupils of the eyes, and/or clear fluids draining from the nose or ears.

Psychology Uses

The use of trauma in psychology ranged from trauma model of mental disorders to historical trauma, traumatic experiences leading to disabilities, and psychological trauma. The use of the word as "trauma models of mental disorders" is alternatively known as trauma models of psychopathology. This is the emphasis on the effects of psychological trauma, as the major factor in causing or developing psychiatric disorders (Brenner, 2002). A well-known use of trauma models of mental disorders is post-traumatic stress disorder (PTSD). Historical trauma (HT) is used heavily in social work and refers to cumulative emotional and psychological wounding that proceeds throughout an individual's life span and across generations. Psychological trauma is a psychological injury due to a stressful or life-threatening situation. Recent research on traumatizing experiences such as living with serious illness suggests that the disruption and fragmentation from such experiences serve to establish the same feeling every day. This means that psychological trauma experienced once, could affect an individual every day for the remainder of his life if it is not treated (Crossley, 2000).

Ryan Lerch and
Jennifer L. Hellier

See also: Aneurysm; Coma; Glasgow Coma Scale; Pain; Post-Traumatic Stress Disorder; Seizures; Stroke; Traumatic Brain Injury (TBI)

Further Reading

Brenner, I. (2002). The trauma model: A solution to the problem of comorbidity in psychiatry. *Psychiatric Services, 53*(3), 350.

Champion, H. R., Sacco, W. J., Copes, W. S., Gann, D. S., Gennarelli, T. A., & Flanagan, M. E. (1989). A revision of the Trauma Score. *Journal of Trauma, 29*(5), 623–629.

Crossley, M. L. (2000). Narrative psychology, trauma and the study of self/identity. *Theory and Psychology, 10*(4), 527–546.

National Institute of Neurological Disorders and Stroke. (2012). *NINDS traumatic brain injury information page*. Retrieved from http://www.ninds.nih.gov/disorders/tbi/tbi.htm

Trauma. (2013). Oxford Dictionaries. Retrieved from http://oxforddictionaries.com/us/definition/american_english/trauma?q=trauma

Traumatic Brain Injury (TBI)

Traumatic brain injury (TBI) is a form of acquired brain injury that occurs when a sudden trauma causes damage to the brain. TBI can result from the head suddenly and violently coming into contact with an object (closed injury) or a penetrating injury to the skull with a foreign body entering the brain (penetrating injury). Closed injuries can also consist of a simple blow or jolt to the head that disrupts the normal function of the brain. Patients with severe TBI should be seen by a doctor immediately to reduce the risk of permanent brain damage.

Epidemiology

Each year, approximately 1.7 million people sustain some type of TBI, which contributes to 30.5 percent of all injury-related deaths in the United States (U.S. National Library of Medicine 2012). In 2010, direct medical costs and indirect costs, such as lost work productivity, due to TBI totaled an estimated $76.5 billion in the United States. The costs of fatal TBIs and TBIs requiring hospitalization, many of which are severe, account for approximately 90 percent of the total TBI medical costs (Centers for Disease Control and Prevention, 2012).

Who Is at Risk?

According to the Centers for Disease Control and Prevention (2012), children aged 0 to 4 years, older adolescents aged 15 to 19 years, and adults aged 65 years and older are most likely to sustain a TBI. Children aged 0 to 14 years constitute nearly half a million emergency department visits for TBI annually. The highest rates of TBI-related hospitalization and death occur in patients who are aged 75 years and older. Approximately 18 percent of all TBI-related emergency department visits involve children aged 0 to 4 years of age and 22 percent of all TBI-related hospitalizations involved adults aged 75 years and older. Although men and women are both prone to TBI, the majority of diagnoses occur in males (59%).

During wartime, TBI incidence significantly increases for both military personnel and civilians in and near war zones. The leading causes of TBI for active duty military personnel in war zones are blasts from gunfire, roadside bombs, and grenades to name a few. It is important to note that the Centers for Disease Control and Prevention figures presented above do not include injuries seen at the U.S. Department of Defense or U.S. Veterans Health Administration when considering the burden of TBI-related disease in military populations.

Mechanism of Injury

A blow or other traumatic injury to the head or body causes traumatic brain injury. The severity of injury depends on the nature of the precipitating event, direction, duration, and force of impact. Damage may be localized to the area directly below the point of impact on the skull or it can be more diffuse when a force is severe enough to cause multiple points of damage as a result of the brain moving back and forth against the skull. When focal injuries occur, the function of affected brain tissue is disrupted. The most common areas for focal lesions in nonpenetrating brain injury are the orbitofrontal cortex and anterior temporal lobes, areas which are involved in social behavior, emotional regulation, olfaction (sense of smell), and decision making.

When the head is exposed to extreme rotational forces, cellular structures can be torn. Individuals exposed to blast force resulting from explosion, for example, can cause widespread damage to the brain. A penetrating injury to the skull directly damages brain tissue and blood vessels surrounding the foreign body. After an injury occurs, associated bleeding in and around the brain, swelling, and blood clots can disrupt oxygen supply to the brain, leading to further and possibly permanent damage.

In general, the most common cause of TBI is falls (35.2%), followed by motor vehicle accidents (17.3%), struck by/against events (16.5%), and assaults (10%). Falls cause half of the TBIs among children aged 0 to 14 years of age and 61 percent of all TBIs among adults aged 65 years and older. Motor vehicle crashes are the second leading cause of TBI; however, these result in the largest percentage of TBI-related deaths (31.8%). Finally, the second leading cause of TBI among children 0 to 14 years of age is colliding with a moving or stationary object (Centers for Disease Control and Prevention, 2012).

Concussion

Sports-related concussions are receiving more attention than ever before in the medical community and news media. This results from recognition that concussion are a traumatic brain injury and the fact that return to play too soon after sustaining a concussion can have very serious consequences if the player is "hit" again, which may lead to further injury or death. A concussion is a serious brain injury and should be treated as such with proper medical evaluation. Even if a player receives a "ding" or got their "bell rung," they should be evaluated, given the fact that most concussions occur without a loss of consciousness. Free training courses are available for high school sports coaches and trainers at the Centers for Disease Control "Heads Up" program website: http://www.cdc.gov/concussion/headsup/index.html.

Signs and Symptoms

The manifestations of brain injury can be both physical and psychological. While some symptoms appear immediately following the injury (primary injury), others may surface days or weeks later (secondary injury). Secondary injury is the leading cause of death during hospitalization after TBI. It is mostly related to brain swelling caused by increased intracranial (within the skull) pressure. As the brain swells, decreases in cerebral perfusion occur, leading to ischemia (insufficient oxygenated blood to the region).

Presenting signs and symptoms of TBI vary based on severity of the precipitating injury. TBIs are categorized by severity: mild, moderate, and severe. However, even though the severity of TBI is denoted as "mild," it is still a very serious condition requiring immediate medical attention. The signs and symptoms of mild TBI include:

- Loss of consciousness for several seconds to minutes
- Retention of consciousness, but confused or disoriented mental status
- Difficulty with memory or concentration
- Headache
- Dizziness or loss of balance
- Nausea or vomiting; sensory problems
- Sensitivity to light or sounds
- Fatigue or drowsiness
- Difficulty sleeping
- Sleeping more than usual
- Mood swings
- Feelings of depression or anxiety

The signs and symptoms of moderate to severe TBI Include:

- Any of the symptoms mentioned for mild TBI
- Loss of consciousness from several minutes to hours
- Profound confusion
- Agitation
- Combativeness or other unusual behavior
- Slurred speech
- Inability to awaken from sleep
- Weakness or numbness in the fingers and toes
- Loss of coordination
- Persistent headache or headache that worsens
- Repeated vomiting or nausea
- Convulsions or seizures
- Dilation of one or both pupils of the eyes
- Clear fluids draining from the nose or ears

Given their limited verbal communication, symptoms and signs of TBI are different in children and young infants. Unusual irritability, inability to be consoled, changes in eating and sleep habits, depressed mood, and loss of interest in favorite toys or activities may represent changes resulting from brain injury. Given the fact that the very young age group is disproportionately affected by TBI-related emergency department visits, hospitalizations, and deaths, it is important that health care providers include TBI in their differential diagnosis when a child presents with such symptoms. Shaken baby syndrome is a form of abusive head trauma and is the leading cause of child abuse in the United States. Medical providers must determine if the mechanism of head injury in a child is developmentally plausible given their age or whether nonaccidental trauma may be involved.

Diagnosis

The diagnosis of TBI is based on mechanism of injury, clinical evidence of injury, and a measure of injury based on the Glasgow Coma Score. Imaging tests such as a computed tomography (CT) scan of the head and magnetic resonance imaging (MRI) are often used in the evaluation of TBI. These imaging studies are of limited utility in the evaluation of TBI related to diffuse injury, because the TBI will likely be clinically apparent but not obvious on the CT or MRI scan. Functional MRI, which uses magnetic resonance imaging to measure metabolic changes that take place in an active part of the brain, however, can be useful in assessing damage related to brain injury.

Gradation of Injury

TBI is graded as mild, moderate, or severe on the basis of level of consciousness or Glasgow Coma Scale (GCS) after resuscitation. The GCS is a clinical measure of eye opening, motor response, and verbal response, with a maximum score of 15. Mild TBI receives a GCS score between 13 and 15. This score (GCS 13–15) constitutes the majority of cases of TBI (75%) and mostly results in a full neurologic recovery, although patients may have short-term memory and concentration difficulties. In moderate TBI, the patient receives a GCS score between 9 and 13. These patients generally present as lethargic or stuporous. Finally, the most severe TBI patients receive a GCS score from three to eight. In severe injury, these patients are comatose, unable to open their eyes, and unable to follow verbal commands.

The Abbreviate Injury Scale (AIS), the Trauma Score, and the Abbreviated Trauma Score are other classification systems for TBI. Although all of these classification systems have limitations, they are still important to health care providers in understanding the clinical management and outcomes of TBI.

Treatment

It is important that anyone with signs of TBI receive medical attention as soon as possible. While the initial phase of injury is irreversible in nature, it is vital to stabilize the individual in an effort to prevent further injury. Priorities in early care include maintaining oxygen supply to the brain, maintaining adequate blood flow, and controlling blood pressure to prevent sudden fluctuations that might contribute to further damage.

Typically, patients with moderate to severe TBI will receive rehabilitation consisting of physical therapy, occupational therapy, speech language therapy, physical medicine, psychology, psychiatry, and social support. The extent a patient will require these clinical support services depend on the degree of initial injury and subsequent recovery.

Complications

Disabilities resulting from TBI depend on the severity and location of the injury, age of the patient, and coexisting medical conditions. Some of the more common disabilities resulting from TBI include issues with cognition (thinking and reasoning), sensory processing, communication, and behavior or mental health.

Some of the more common short- and long-term manifestations of TBI include problems with memory and reasoning, sensation (such as touch, taste, and smell), language (like communication, expression, and understanding), and emotion (including depression, anxiety, personality changes, aggression, acting out, and social inappropriateness). Given the variety of potential consequences of brain injury, it is easy to see how TBI can have a profound effect on family structure, creation of caregiver roles, and activities of daily living.

Caregiver Support

Stress and social isolation may result for close family members of the brain injured, particularly if they assume the role of primary caregiver. Peer and professional support groups exist to provide ongoing assistance in understanding the late and long-term effects of TBI, how to cope with the personality and lifestyle changes associated with TBI, and skills to maximize the individual's recovery from TBI. Peer support to deal with challenges of recovery is crucial, because oftentimes, the person with TBI appears quite normal physically, so outsiders expect him or her to operate at their normal (baseline) level of function.

Prevention and Current Research

Minimizing common sources of injury related to TBI is one way to reduce disease burden. Using the age-appropriate child-restraint device (car seat or booster) and adult seatbelts are two ways to prevent TBI caused by motor vehicle accidents. Wearing a well-fitted helmet properly while biking, playing contact sports, riding a horse, and other similar activities are also known to reduce the chance of TBI. In the elderly population, removal of tripping hazards such as throw rugs, installation of handrails, improving lighting, and remaining physically active can prevent injury.

Current TBI research includes developing and using animal models to test new therapies and treatments for severe TBI symptoms. For example, following brain injury, mitochondria (organelles used for cellular energy as well as apoptosis—programmed cell death) produce or initiate many of the primary and secondary pathologies seen in TBI such as cell death. To stop mitochondria from initiating unnecessary apoptosis, scientists are studying possible treatments for use in children with TBI. A preclinical trial is currently underway in examining how cyclosporine A (CsA) therapy can rescue the function of mitochondria so that there is less cell death at the injured site as well as reduced loss of neurological function.

Margaret Cook-Shimanek

See also: Apoptosis; Circle of Willis and Arterial Supply to the Brain—Building with Clay Activity; Optic Nerve; Seizures; Trauma

Further Reading

Brain Injury Association of America. (2012). *Brain Injury Association of America.* Retrieved from http://www.biausa.org/index.htm

Centers for Disease Control and Prevention. (2012). *Injury prevention and control: Traumatic brain injury.* Retrieved from http://www.cdc.gov/traumaticbraininjury/statistics .html

Ghajar, J. (2000). Traumatic brain injury. *The Lancet, 356,* 923–929.

National Institute of Neurological Disorders and Stroke. (2012). *NINDS traumatic brain injury information page.* Retrieved from http://www.ninds.nih.gov/disorders/tbi/tbi.htm

U.S. National Library of Medicine. (2012). *Traumatic brain injury.* Retrieved from http:// www.nlm.nih.gov/medlineplus/traumaticbraininjury.html#cat1

Tremor

Tremor is the most common, involuntary movement-based disorder and is characterized by rhythmic muscle oscillations (contractions and relaxations) of one or more parts of the body. Although the majority of tremor occurs in the hands, other body regions can be affected such as the arms, legs, trunk, head, face, and voice. Characteristics include shaking and trembling that may range from a very slight movement, to highly visible convulsions. Tremor may be brought on or further aggravated by strong emotion, stress, physical exhaustion, or during specific types of movement.

Tremor may also be a side effect of certain drugs, but most tremors manifest in an otherwise healthy population. The majority of afflicted patients are middle-aged and older. Men and women experience it equally and the tremor may be occasional, temporary, or chronic. Tremor itself is not directly life threatening, but many patients may feel embarrassment and/or frustration as a variety of everyday tasks are complicated. In some cases, tremor has directly resulted in accidents such as car crashes that range in severity from mild to fatal.

History

In the 19th century, Sirs Victor Horsley (1857–1916) and Edward Schäfer (1850–1935) were the first to conduct and publish an electrophysiological study of tremor. These authors may also have been the first to suggest that tremor may have a neurogenic basis. They found that the ongoing muscle activity, either organic or induced by motor tract stimulation, was universally characterized by superimposed 10-hertz twitches. Initially it was believed that the neurogenic mechanism responsible for tremor generation was an inevitable consequence of the nature of muscle organization with each motor unit producing a distinct contractile twitch. A second hypothesis stated that it was a peripherally arising phenomenon caused by the instability inherent in the reflex pathways. Still other scientists believed that tremor arose because of the mechanical tendency for body parts to oscillate at a certain frequencies.

Follow-up studies then showed that neural oscillations might represent binding or frequency coding of central nervous system activity. More recent studies suggest that physiological tremor may arise from rhythmic neural activity in the central nervous system, while pathological tremor results from a distortion or amplification of these central oscillations. Physiological tremor is the oscillation at approximately 10 cycles per second (or 10-hertz) accompanies the normal contraction of voluntary muscle. Pathological tremor is the abnormal, nonlinear oscillations that afflict those patients diagnosed with "tremor."

In terms of tremor generation, it is important to note that the individual motor units do not fire over a continuous frequency range. Instead they begin firing at a minimum frequency of about 8–10 hertz. It is hypothesized that this minimum frequency occurs through the influence of spinal mechanisms such as Renshaw inhibition, which is a form of collateral inhibition of motoneurons involving a special inhibitory interneuron. Studies conducted with EMG recordings of isometric contractions revealed an "interference pattern" that reflected the summation of activity of multiple motor units. Despite having a broad range of activity, the frequency spectra of these multi-unit recordings generally peaked in the 8–10 hertz frequency range.

Studies disagree, however, on the exact cause of tremor and its origin in the nervous system. A direct demonstration of corresponding central oscillation has yet to be performed. Nevertheless, there is a great deal of evidence to support the existence of central oscillations that produce certain types of tremor.

Types and Symptoms, Treatments, and Outcomes

There are two main types of tremor: resting tremor and action tremor. Resting or static tremor occurs when the affected muscle is relaxed such as when a patient's hands are resting in their lap. This type of tremor is frequently seen in patients with Parkinson's disease and it usually affects just the fingers or hands. As the disease progress, tremor can involve to other body parts like the head.

Action tremor occurs during movement of the affected muscle. These tremors are then categorized based on the different actions: intention, postural, and isometric tremor. Intention or kinetic tremor is witnessed during isolated muscle movement. Intention tremor results specifically when a patient performs a purposeful movement toward a target such as touching his or her nose during a medical examination or reaching for a glass or cup. Postural tremor is caused by a sustained position such as holding one's arm out against gravity. Finally, an isometric tremor occurs during a voluntary muscle contraction without accompanied movement, such as pushing against a wall. This tremor, however, is less common. There are other rare types of tremor such at task-specific tremor. A task-specific tremor affects the performance of highly skilled or dexterous tasks such as handwriting, playing the piano, or speech.

The cause of tremor is typically a problem in the regions of the brain controlling coordinated muscle movement. There are several neurological disorders and conditions that may result in tremor including but not limited to multiple sclerosis, stroke, traumatic brain injury, and neurodegenerative diseases that damage or destroy parts of the brainstem or the cerebellum (the part of the brain that regulates controlled movements). Tremor may also be caused by a variety of recreational drugs and prescriptive medications, brain tumors, excessive alcohol consumption or withdrawal, low blood sugar, overactive thyroid, stress, anxiety, fatigue, stroke, caffeine, mercury poisoning, liver failure, and normal aging. Several types of tremor may be inherited while others have no known cause.

During a physical examination and neurological assessment performed by a health care provider (doctor, physician assistant, or nurse practitioner), the patient may be subjected to physical and blood chemical tests in order to determine the cause of the tremor. Tremor may then be diagnosed as a certain type by its appearance, cause, or origin. Seven of the most well-known types include essential, Parkinsonian, dystonic, cerebellar, psychogenic, orthostatic, and physiologic tremors.

Essential tremor may be mild and nonprogressive in some individuals, and slowly progressive in others. Sometimes referred to as a benign essential tremor, these are the most common form of abnormal involuntary muscle movement. Tremor frequency may decrease with age, but the severity may increase over time, compromising the patient's ability to perform daily tasks or activities. Onset of this type of tremor is most common after the age of 40, although essential tremor may be witnessed in people of any age. Originally there was no known pathology linked to the existence of essential tremor; however, recent studies suggest that this tremor may be linked to mild degeneration in certain regions of the cerebellum.

Parkinsonian tremor occurs characteristically as resting tremor and is often the first symptom of Parkinson's disease. This tremor most commonly affects the hands but may be seen in the lips, chin, legs, and trunk and may be markedly increased by stress or strong emotion. Movement typically originates on one side of the body and progresses to include the other side over time.

Dystonic tremor is experienced by patients of all ages afflicted by dystonia, a movement disorder characterized by sustained involuntary muscle contractions. This type of tremor is quite rare and is found in less than 1 percent of the population. The associated muscle tremors are typically irregular and jerky, but certain hand positions may impede the movement. Dystonic tremor occurs irregularly and can often be relieved by rest or slight touch stimulation to the affected part of the body.

Cerebellar tremor is caused by damage to the cerebellum that may result from a tumor, stroke, or disease. Chronic alcoholism and the overuse of drugs or medication are also common causes of cerebellar tremors. This tremor is different to action tremors as it is a slow tremor of the extremities that occurs at the end of a purposeful movement. Directed movement typically worsens the tremor. Speech problems, rapid involuntary eye movements, gait (walking) problems, and postural tremor of the neck and trunk may also accompany cerebellar tremor.

Psychogenic tremor, also known as functional or hysterical tremor, may appear as any form of tremor and accompany any type of movement. Psychogenic tremor is frequently characterized by sudden onset and remission, and increase in incidence with stress. Change in the direction of the tremor or distraction frequently lessens or impedes the tremor's symptoms. Psychological disorders and psychiatric disease have been strongly linked to the presence of psychogenic tremor. When diagnosing psychogenic tremor, health care providers must first determine what is missing such as the absence of other neurologic signs and no evidence of disease by laboratory or radiologic investigations. Next they determine if there are changing tremor characteristics, clinical inconsistencies, multiple undiagnosed conditions, presence of psychiatric disease, and an unclassified tremor (complex tremors). Finally, if the patient's tremor is responsive to placebo (a substance with no medical effect) and/or unresponsive to antitremor medications, then a diagnosis of psychogenic tremor is made.

Orthostatic (relating to standing up) tremor occurs in the legs and trunk in the patient immediately after standing. This tremor is typically perceived as unsteadiness rather than an actual tremor due to the high frequency of the muscle contractions. No other clinical signs or symptoms have been reported and the feeling of unsteadiness ceases after the patient sits, begins walking, or is lifted from the ground.

Lastly, physiologic tremor occurs in every normal individual to an extent. This tremor is rarely visible to the eye and may be heightened by physical exhaustion or fatigue, a strong emotion such as fear, hypoglycemia (low blood sugar), hyperthyroidism (overactive thyroid which assists in regulating metabolism), and heavy metal poisoning. Stimulants such as caffeine, as well as alcohol or drug overconsumption or withdrawal may also heightened physiologic tremor. Once a tremor becomes visible, they are known as enhanced physiologic tremor. The condition is usually reversible once the cause has been appropriately corrected.

There is currently no known cure for most tremors, but treatment can be effective provided the tremor is diagnosed correctly. Such tremor responds to treatment of the underlying condition, like treating the psychological disorder as in the case of psychogenic tremor. Drug therapy is also an option for the management of conditions such as Parkinson's disease. Eliminating certain "triggers," such as caffeine or severe stress, has also shown to be effective. Physical therapy may be used to increase strength and coordination, thereby controlling the symptoms of tremor in some individuals. Appropriate muscle control, bracing, and functionality skills may be taught when physical therapy is an option.

Future

Lastly, surgical intervention such as thalamotomy and deep brain stimulation may be performed to ease certain extreme tremor that cannot be controlled with drugs. Thalamotomy, a procedure first introduced in the 1950s, refers to the precise destruction of a tiny area of the brain called the thalamus that controls some involuntary movements. Thalamotomy, however, has fallen out of recent favor with the advent of deep brain stimulation.

Deep brain stimulation occurs by implanting electrodes that are connected by wires under the skin of the chest, below the collarbone. The activated electrodes may then send continuous electrical pulses to target areas of the brain via a device similar to a pacemaker. These pulses effectively blocks the impulses that cause tremors and does so without actually destroying parts of the brain as in the case of thalamotomy.

Both treatments have been used fairly commonly to treat patients diagnosed is Parkinson's disease. Surgical intervention of any type, however, may have severe side effects including problems with motor control of speech, temporary or permanent cognitive impairment such as learning and visual difficulties, and problems with balance. Experts are still unsure of exactly what causes tremor and how deep brain stimulation works to combat the symptoms of tremor. Further research is currently being conducted to determine these mechanisms.

Sarah Chang Foster

See also: Brain Stimulators; Huntington's Disease; Multiple Sclerosis; Parkinson's Disease; Spasm; Traumatic Brain Injury (TBI)

Further Reading

Bhidayasiri, R. (2005). Differential diagnosis of common tremor syndromes. *Postgraduate Medical Journal, 81*(962), 756–762. Retrieved from http://www.ncbi.nlm.nih.gov/pmc/articles/PMC1743400/

Crawford, P. (2011). Differentiation and diagnosis of tremor. *American Family Physician, 83*(6), 697–702. Retrieved from http://www.aafp.org/afp/2011/0315/p697.html

Fasano, A., Daniele, A., & Albanese, A. (2012). Treatment of motor and non-motor features of Parkinson's disease with deep brain stimulation. *Lancet Neurology, 11*(5):429–442. Retrieved from http://www.ncbi.nlm.nih.gov/pubmed/22516078

McAuley, J. (2000). Physiological and pathological tremors and rhythmic central motor control. *Brain, 123*(8), 1545–1567. Retrieved from http://brain.oxfordjournals.org/content/123/8/1545.full

National Institute of Neurological Disorders and Stroke (NINDS). (2012). *NINDS tremor information page.* Retrieved from http://www.ninds.nih.gov/index.htm

University of Maryland Medical Center. (2011). *Tremors.* Retrieved from http://www.umm.edu/ency/index.htm

Trigeminal Nerve

The *trigeminal nerve* (V) is the 5th of 12 pairs of cranial nerves. It carries primarily somatosensory (temperature, pressure, and pain) information of the head and face, but also some motor information to the front third of the head. The nerve is named three (tri-) twins (-geminus) in Latin, after its three major branches. Because of these distinct branches, each division is named after the region they innervate. Specifically, the branches are named ophthalmic (V_1), maxillary (V_2), and mandibular (V_3). The trigeminal nerve is one of the three largest and thickest cranial nerves in mammals, the others being the optic (for vision) and vagus (for autonomic function for the gut, heart, and lungs).

The ophthalmic (V_1) branch is mostly composed of sensory fibers (axons, the output of a neuron) and innervates the top half of the face, the cornea (part of the eye), tear duct, and part of the nasal cavity. The maxillary (V_2) branch is also primarily composed of sensory fibers and innervates the nasal cavity and the upper jaw, including the roof of the mouth. The mandibular (V_3) branch contains both sensory and motor fibers. The sensory fibers of the mandibular branch innervate the lower jaw, lips, tongue, and cheeks. The motor fibers of the mandibular branch innervate the muscles of the jaw responsible for chewing. Sensory trigeminal fibers originate in the trigeminal (or Gasserian) ganglia, which is a collection of the cell bodies of trigeminal sensory neurons laying in a depression in the bottom of the cranial cavity (the space inside the skull).

Brain Nuclei and Central Projections

The trigeminal nerve root enters the brainstem at the level of the pons, and fibers from motor and sensory neurons project to different brain nuclei (groups of cell bodies). The motor fibers of the mandibular branch originate in the trigeminal motor nucleus, which is located in the mid-pons. The trigeminal motor nucleus is sometimes called the masticator nucleus because it controls the muscles responsible for mastication or chewing. The trigeminal sensory nucleus is the largest of the cranial nerve nuclei and stretches from the mesencephalon, through the pons (passing laterally to the trigeminal motor nucleus) and into the spinal cord ending at the level of second cervical vertebrate.

Sensory fibers from the trigeminal ganglia project to different areas of the trigeminal sensory nucleus depending on the type of sensation carried. Sensory neurons from the trigeminal ganglia, called first-order neurons because they are the initial neuron in the neural circuit, form synapse with second-order neurons, which are the second neuron in the circuit. Fibers sensitive to vibration and touch pass into the pons and form synapses with second-order sensory neurons in the pontine portion of the trigeminal nucleus. Pain and temperature sensitive fibers also enter the brain at the level of the pons but descended to form synapses in the spinal trigeminal nucleus. Second-order neurons in the trigeminal sensory nucleus all produce axons that cross the midline of the brain and ascend to the thalamus, where they form synapses with neurons that carry information to the primary somatic sensory cortex.

With one known exception, the cell bodies of all primary sensory neurons are found in ganglia outside the central nervous system. The one established exception is the sensory neurons found in the mesencephalic portion of the trigeminal sensory nucleus. The neurons of the mesencephalic trigeminal nucleus directly innervate the same muscles as the motor neurons originating in the motor trigeminal nucleus. These sensory neurons allow for proprioception (awareness of position in space) of the muscle involved in mastication. The sensory neurons of the mesencephalic trigeminal nucleus project centrally to the motor trigeminal nucleus and allow for reflexive control of chewing.

Chemesthesis

Chemesthesis is the stimulation of the somatosensory system by chemicals rather than by tactile stimulus. Most somatosensory nerves are protected from chemicals by a layer of keratinized skin. However, the trigeminal nerve innervates mucus membranes which are not so protected, allowing for the stimulation of trigeminal nerve fibers. Chemesthetic chemicals are commonly used in cooking as spices. For example, capsaicin, a chemical found in chili peppers, stimulates temperature sensitive pain fibers creating the sensation of heat. Other spices, which contain chemicals that stimulate the somatosensory system, are garlic, basil, and mint. In the nasal cavity, chemesthetic stimulation is generally considered painful and results in reflexive changes in respiration rate to protect the airway. It is common for the sensations of chemesthesis and taste or smell to be confused with each other but they are all distinct sensory modalities, mediated by entirely different cranial nerves.

Trigeminal Neuralgia

Trigeminal neuralgia is pathological condition typified by reoccurring facial pain. The pain can occur unilaterally or bilaterally and is typically described as burning or stabbing. The sensation usually reoccurs in the same region of the face but has been reported to spread from the original location as time with the condition passes. In some cases, trigeminal neuralgia is caused by compression of the nerve by tumor, cyst, or aneurism (an unusually large expansion in the wall of an artery that causes weakness and possibly tears in the arterial wall). In these cases, treatment of the underlying condition can provide relief. However, in many cases, the exact cause of trigeminal neuralgia can be idiopathic, meaning the exact cause of the condition cannot be determined.

Speculative causes of this disease have included tension placed on the trigeminal nerve at points where it exits the skull, compression of trigeminal ganglia due to anomalies in local circulation, and demyelination (damage to the myelin sheath) of the nerve root. The demyelination hypothesis is supported by the occurrence of trigeminal neuralgia in many individuals with multiple sclerosis. Initial treatments for trigeminal neuralgia usually focus on alleviating the pain with a combination of narcotics, anti-inflammatories, and steroids. Anticonvulsants have been successfully used to preventive bouts of pain but these treatments generally become less effective over time. Surgically relieving the vasculature pressure on the trigeminal ganglia can relieve the pain in some situations. In extreme cases, cutting the trigeminal ganglion or nerve can bring relief but carries the risk of significant side effects, including permanent facial numbness or paralyzation (complete loss of muscle function) of the muscles of mastication. This means that patients with such complications may not be able to chew on the side of mouth where the cut was made.

Current Research

Historically, sensations of irritation mediated by chemicals were thought to be caused when the chemicals acted on free nerve endings in the epithelium. Many of these chemicals were later found to activate ion channels or receptors located in free nerve endings. Capsaicin, for example, acts on an ion channel in the transient receptor potential (TRP) channel superfamily. Other members of the TRP channels family have also been found on somatosensory nerve endings and are activated by temperature (either heat or cooling sensations as in mint), acids, or isothiocyanates (a class of chemicals found in mustard and wasabi). Compounds that activate these ion channels typically must be fat soluble to pass through the epithelial layer that protects the free nerve endings. That is why dairy products such as milk or sour cream will help ease the pain from spicy foods because they too are fat soluble.

Recent studies have identified sensory cells in respiratory epithelium that provide a mechanism by which the trigeminal nerve can detect water-soluble irritants. Solitary chemosensory cells (SCCs) are found scattered thought the respiratory epithelium of the nose and form synapse with trigeminal pain fibers. SCCs utilize receptors and signaling pathways similar to bitter sensitive cells found in taste buds. However, while SCCs respond to "bitter" substances, the sensation they produce when stimulated is not bitter but rather irritation. This is a result of the law of specific nerve energies, which states that the sensation produced when a particular nerve is stimulated is determined by the central projection of that nerve and not the means of stimulation.

While SCCs respond to many classically bitter compounds, they also respond to bacteria metabolites. Some gram-negative bacteria in the respiratory tract produce chemical signals to communicate with each other. One class of these chemicals, acyl-homoserine lactones, are called quorum-sensing signals because their concentration increases with the number of bacteria. Some bacteria undergo changes in gene expression to become more virulent when quorum-sensing signals reach high enough concentrations. SCCs are stimulated by acyl-homoserine lactones and in turn stimulate the trigeminal nerve causing irritation, inflammation, and protective changes to respiration. It has been suggested that this allows SCCs to detect a growing bacterial infection and mount protective respiratory reflexives and immune response before the bacteria become virulent.

C. J. Saunders

See also: Central Nervous System (CNS); Cranial Nerves; Multiple Sclerosis; Nerves; Somatosensory Cortex/Somatosensory System

Further Reading

Basbaum, A. I., Bautista, D. M., Scherrer, G. & Julius, D. (2009). Cellular and molecular mechanisms of pain. *Cell, 139*(2), 267–284.

Bryant, B. P., & Silver, W. (2000). Chemesthesis: The common chemical sense. In T. E. Finger, W. Silver, and D. Restrepo (Eds.), *Neurobiology of taste and smell* (pp. 73–100). New York: Wiley-Liss, Inc.

Finger, T. E., & Bottger, B., Hansen, A., Anderson, K. T., Alimohammadi, H., & Silver, W. L. (2003). Solitary chemoreceptor cells in the nasal cavity serve as sentinels of respiration. *Proceedings of the National Academy of Sciences USA, 100*, 8981–8986.

Prasad, S., & Galetta, S. (2009). Trigeminal neuralgia: Historical notes and current concepts. *Neurologist, 15*(2), 87–94.

Silver, W. L., & Finger, T. E. (2009). The anatomical and electrophysiological basis of peripheral nasal trigeminal chemoreception. *Annals of the New York Academy of Sciences, 1170*, 202–205.

Silver, W. L., Roe, P., & Saunders, C. J. (2010). Functional neuroanatomy of the upper airway in experimental animals. In J. B. Morris and D. Shusterman (Eds.), *Toxicology of the nose and upper airways* (pp. 45–64). New York, NY: Informa Healthcare.

Tizzano, M., Gulbransen, B. D., Vandenbeuch, A., Clapp, T. R., Herman, J. P., Sibhatu, H. M., . . . Finger, T. E.. (2010). Nasal chemosensory cells use bitter taste signaling to detect irritants and bacterial signals. *Proceedings of the National Academy of Sciences USA, 107*, 3210–3215.

Trochlear Nerve

The *trochlear nerve* is the smallest of 12 cranial nerves, which are part of the peripheral nervous system. It supplies motor (efferent) function only to the *superior oblique muscle* of the eye. All cranial nerves are paired, meaning one nerve supplies the right side and the other nerve supplies the left. The trochlear nerve is the 4th of 12 paired cranial nerves, and is also called *cranial nerve IV*. The trochlear nerves work in tandem with two other cranial nerves: *oculomotor* (*cranial nerve III*) and *abducens* (*cranial nerve VI*) nerves. Together, these three cranial nerves supply motor function to six extraocular muscles so that the eyes move with exact precision, fluidity, and grace.

Anatomy and Physiology

Within the *tegmentum* (roof) of the *midbrain* (part of the brainstem), the neurons that make up the trochlear nerve are located near the midline in the *trochlear nuclei* (a group of cell bodies). These nuclei (one on the left side and one on the right) are at the level of the *inferior colliculi* and ventral to the *cerebral aqueduct* (a natural opening containing cerebrospinal fluid). Inside the cranium, the fibers (axons) of the trochlear nerve travel the furthest of all the cranial nerves. The axons travel together around the cerebral aqueduct toward the back (dorsally). They cross over and exit the midbrain on the dorsal side. Because the trochlear nerve crosses within the brainstem, it innervates (terminates and activates) the muscle on the opposite side (contralateral). This means the neurons in the left trochlear nucleus innervate the superior oblique muscle for the right eye and vice versa.

The trochlear fibers continue to travel around to the ventral side (front), over the *cerebral peduncle,* to run next to the abducens nerve. Together, the nerves penetrate the *dura* (one of the brain coverings), enter the *cavernous sinus* through the *tentorium cerebelli,* and follow the lateral wall of the sinus until they enter the orbit via the *superior orbital fissure.* The trochlear nerve moves medially and travels diagonally over the *levator palpebrae* and *superior rectus* muscles. Finally, it branches into three or more parts to innervate the superior oblique muscle along its proximal edge.

Once the superior oblique muscle is innervated, activation of the trochlear nerve causes the muscle to contract. This results in the eye having an inward rotation with a downward and lateral movement. The superior oblique muscle is continually opposed by the *inferior oblique muscle,* which rotates the eye outward with an upward and medial movement. Together, the superior and inferior oblique muscles work against each other to allow the eye to move smoothly when focusing or tracking an object.

Clinical Symptoms, Diseases, and Treatment

If the trochlear nerve is damaged, the result is paralysis of the superior oblique muscle causing the eye to rotate outward (*extortion*). This occurs because the inferior oblique muscle no longer opposes the superior oblique muscle. Patients will have double vision (*diplopia*) as well as have difficulty keeping an object in focus while tracking a moving object. Damage to the trochlear nerve generally arises from inflammation within the orbit or blockage by an *aneurysm* (abnormal ballooning of an artery), particularly of the *posterior cerebral* or *superior cerebral artery*. Tumors within the orbit may also cause inflammation to cranial nerve IV.

Persons with damage to their trochlear nerve may also have weakness in gazing downward, which can affect walking particularly when going downstairs. This is most pronounced when attempting to gaze medially, such as focusing on stairs. The person may compensate by tilting his or her head. In normal conditions, tilting the head results in the eyes rotating in the opposite direction of the anteroposterior axis. This allows the image on the retina to stay on the vertical axis. When persons with cranial nerve IV palsy tilts their head to the unaffected eye, it causes the diplopia to resolve and binocular vision to be obtained. This is because the normal eye will rotate inwardly (*intortion*) to line up with the extorted eye. The main care for trochlear nerve palsy is to treat the inflammation or to remove the tumor causing the damage.

Jennifer L. Hellier

See also: Abducens Nerve; Aneurysm; Cranial Nerves; Nerves; Oculomotor Nerve; Visual System

Further Reading

Liang, B. (2012). *The 12 cranial nerves.* Retrieved from http://www.wisc-online.com /objects/ViewObject.aspx?ID=AP11504

Moore, K.L., Agur, A.M.R., & Dalley, A.F. (Eds.). (2010). *Essential clinical anatomy* (4th ed.). Baltimore, MD: Williams and Wilkins.

Yale University School of Medicine. (1998). *Cranial nerves.* Retrieved from http://www .yale.edu/cnerves/

Tuberous Sclerosis Complex

Tuberous sclerosis complex (TSC, Latin and Greek terms meaning "hard swelling") is a rare, autosomal dominant disorder affecting about 25,000 to 40,000 individuals in the United States (NINDS, 2013). It can occur in both men and women and in any race or ethnicity. TSC may present with benign tumors called *harmatomas* (Greek meaning "an error or defect in the body") growing in the brain, eye, kidney, lung, and skin. In many patients with TSC, harmatomas appear in their first year of life. However, tuberous sclerosis can also present in subtle ways and may not be recognized.

Signs and Symptoms

The signs and symptoms of TSC are variable between individuals as well as change as the person ages. The most common types of harmatomas and their side effects are listed in the following.

In the brain, TSC may present with three types of abnormalities: (1) *cortical tubers*—hard harmatomas growing deep in the brain; (2) *subependymal nodules*—located in the walls of the ventricles, the region where cerebrospinal fluid flows, and are generally asymptomatic (no side effects); and (3) *subependymal giant cell astrocytomas* (SEGAs)—large harmatomas found in the walls of the ventricles that may obstruct the flow of cerebrospinal fluid. Patients with brain harmatomas may present with seizures, developmental delays, and autism. The seizures may be of all types including *tonic clonic seizures, tonic seizures, akinetic seizures,* and *myoclonic seizures.* Infantile spasms are often associated with tuberous sclerosis. Patients with TSC frequently have seizures, which are difficult to control. Patients with TSC may also have developmental delays with a wide range from mild to severe mental retardation. Patients with TSC may have behavioral problems including aggression, rage, attention deficit hyperactivity disorder, obsessive-compulsive disorder, and potentially self-harming behavior.

In the eye, TSC may present with *retinal harmartomas* or *astrocytomas.* These benign tumors may resemble a white spot on the retina (the photosensitive lining on the back of the eye) and usually do not cause problems with vision. However, they are a noninvasive way to diagnose TSC.

In the heart, TSC may present with benign tumors called *rhabdomyomas* (Greek and Latin terms meaning "rod-shaped swellings in muscles"). These are typically found in infancy in patients with TSC. If rhabdomyomas are large, they can cause a blockage in blood circulation at birth. However, if these are not large at birth, they typically become smaller with time and do not cause medical problems.

In the lung, TSC may present with lesions called *lymphangioleiomyomatosis* (LAM). This condition is more common in women than men. LAM is a tumor-like disorder in which cells proliferate in the lungs. Lung destruction with cyst formation occurs. While many patients with LAM are asymptomatic, others suffer breathlessness than can worsen with time.

In the kidney, TSC may present with *cysts* and *angiomyolipomas* (*AMLs*). Cysts typically do not cause serious problems, but the AMLs (mixed muscle and fatty tissues) may grow large enough to cause kidney dysfunction including hypertension (high blood pressure), bleeding, and renal failure.

On the skin, TSC may present with (1) *ash leaf spots* (lighter patches of skin), (2) *facial angiofibromas* (mix of vascular and fibrous tissues) or *adenoma sebaceum,* (3) *shagreen patches* (located on the lower back), and (4) *subungual fibromas,* which grow under the nails and may cause bleeding.

Causes

TSC is caused by a defect also known as a mutation on two genes—*TSC1* and *TSC2*. The *TSC1* gene is located on chromosome 9 and *TSC2* gene is located on chromosome 16. *TSC1* codes for a protein called *harmartin,* and *TSC2* codes for a protein called *tuberin.* Both *TSC1* and *TSC2* are thought to control cell growth by inhibiting the activation of a protein kinase called mTOR. When mTOR is overactivated, cells are abnormally differentiated and abnormally large (particularly in TSC brain lesions). Only one of the two genes, *TSC1* or *TSC2,* needs to have a mutation for TSC to be present.

Treatment

There is active ongoing research for treatments of TSC, but there is currently no cure for the condition. Anticonvulsant medications are used to treat seizures related to TSC. However, these types of seizures are often difficult to control. Clinical trials with immunosuppressant drugs *rapamycin* and its analogue *everolimus* are ongoing for the SEGA tumors in the brain, Lung LAM, and kidney angiomyolipomas. Due to the potential for many organ systems involved in TSC, a multidisciplinary team approach is an ideal way to care for patients. Physicians involved in this team include neurologist, cardiologist, pulmonologist, neuropsychologist, and if needed, a neurosurgeon.

Audrey S. Yee

See also: Autism; Neurologist; Seizures

Further Reading

National Institutes of Neurological Disorders and Stroke (NINDS). (2013). *Tuberous sclerosis fact sheet.* Retrieved from http://www.ninds.nih.gov/disorders/tuberous_sclerosis/detail_tuberous_sclerosis.htm

Schwartz, R. A., Jozwiak, J., & Pedersen, R. (2013). *Genetics of tuberous sclerosis clinical presentation.* Retrieved from http://emedicine.medscape.com/article/951002-clinical

Tunnel Vision

Vision occurs when light from all angles of the visual fields hit the *retina,* the photosensitive lining of the back of the eye. However, in some cases the light from the periphery (the sides) is not seen, resulting in *tunnel vision.* Specifically, tunnel vision is a visual field defect where peripheral (side) vision is lost while keeping visual acuity in the central regions. If the peripheral vision is slowly lost over a period of time, a person may not realize that they have tunnel vision. That is why it is important to have your vision checked every year by an optometrist or ophthalmologist. Glaucoma is one of the many causes of tunnel vision, which becomes more prevalent in persons over the age of 40. Glaucoma is a severe condition that can lead to blindness if left untreated.

Causes, Signs, and Symptoms

Tunnel vision can be a result of damage to the *optic nerve* (cranial nerve II, which is the primary nerve used for sight and connects the eye to the brain), the *retina,* or the *occipital lobe* (part of the brain that processes visual input). When the damage is to the optic nerve, it is called *optic neuropathy.* A specific type of optic neuropathy is *optic neuritis,* which is the inflammation of the optic nerve. It can occur any where along the length of the optic nerve and its cause is unknown. Scientists have suggested that optic neuritis may be a type of autoimmune disorder, where the body's immune system abnormally attacks itself.

Other noninflammatory causes of optic neuropathy may include glaucoma, which is associated with increased pressure within the eye; reduced blood flow to the eye; neurological diseases such as diabetes; tumors along the optic nerve; deficiencies in nutrition; and excessive tobacco or alcohol use, just to list a few. Since there are several causes of tunnel vision, this entry will only discuss the most common causes: *cataracts, glaucoma,* and *retinitis pigmentosa* (a degenerative eye disease that damages the retina).

Cataracts are a clouding of the lens within the eye. This clouding decreases normal vision as if a film is over the eye. Cataracts increase in probability as a person ages but some infants can be born with cataracts (congenital cataracts). Cataracts are the most common cause of blindness and can be surgically corrected.

The term glaucoma refers to several conditions that cause damage to the optic nerve. It is a slow but steady loss of peripheral vision and can lead to blindness if not treated. The most common type of glaucoma is an abnormal increase in eye pressure, called intraocular pressure. This may happen when too much fluid is produced within the eye or if the natural drainage (outflow channels called trabecular meshwork) of this fluid is blocked. Glaucoma may also occur with normal eye pressure but there is reduced blood flow to the optic nerve. Glaucoma must be treated as soon as possible to reduce the chances of permanent blindness.

Finally, retinitis pigmentosa is a rare degenerative disease that is first identified when a person complains of night blindness. This tends to be followed by several years or even decades later of peripheral tunnel vision loss. Retinitis pigmentosa is an inherited disease that affects both eyes and often leads to blindness.

Treatment

It is very important to see a doctor as soon as possible if a person is experiencing tunnel vision. As in most cases, treatment for tunnel vision depends on the underlying cause. If glaucoma is detected in the early stages, medical intervention can stop the loss of peripheral vision all together. Glaucoma is usually treated with eye drops, lasers, and/or surgery to prevent further loss of vision. Additionally, vitamin A derivatives may be beneficial in improving retinal degenerative diseases such as retinitis pigmentosa.

Patricia A. Bloomquist

See also: Congenital Defects (Abnormalities); Optic Nerve; Visual Fields; Visual Perception (Visual Processing); Visual System

Further Reading

Dalferth, M. (1989). How and what do autistic children see? Emotional, perceptive and social peculiarities reflected in more recent examinations of the visual perception and the process of observation in autistic children. *Acta Paedopsychiatrica, 52*(2), 121–133.

Davis, J. C., McNeill, H., Wasdell, M., Chunick, S., & Bryan, S. (2012). Focusing both eyes on health outcomes: Revisiting cataract surgery. *BMC Geriatrics, 12,* 50.

Perusek, L., & Maeda, T. (2013). Vitamin A derivatives as treatment options for retinal degenerative diseases. *Nutrients, 5*(7), 2646–2666.

Vagus Nerve

Cranial nerves are part of the peripheral nervous system and are paired, meaning one nerve supplies the right side and the other nerve supplies the left. They are the specific motor (efferent) and/or sensory (afferent) nerves that deliver neuronal signaling to the head, face, and neck. Roman numerals starting from the rostral end of the brain (near the nose) number the cranial nerves. The *vagus nerve* is the 10th of 12 paired cranial nerves. Thus, it is numbered as *cranial nerve X*.

The vagus nerve is a mixed nerve, meaning that it contains both sensory and motor components. Specifically, it has an extensive motor and sensory distribution to thoracic and abdominal viscera, as well as to structures in the pharynx and larynx. It emerges from the brainstem, particularly from the posterior region called the *medulla oblongata,* as a bundle of small rootlets. From there, it wanders inferiorly below the head and neck to enter the chest and abdomen. This is how it received its Latin term, *vagus,* which means, "wandering." There are two major roles of the vagus nerve. First, it functions as the parasympathetic motor output of the autonomic nervous system; and secondly, it functions to relay information about the viscera (organs) to the brain via sensory neurons. These sensory neurons are called primary visceral sensory neurons. In fact, most of the nerve fibers in the vagus nerve are sensory in nature.

Anatomy and Physiology

The vagus nerve originates in the medulla oblongata from four main nuclei (groups of neuronal cell bodies in the central nervous system): *nucleus solitarius, nucleus ambiguus, dorsal nucleus of the vagus nerve,* and the *spinal trigeminal nucleus.* The fibers from the nucleus solitarius receive sensory taste information along with sensory input from organs. The nucleus ambiguus fibers send parasympathetic output to the heart, which is used to lower heart rate. Fibers from the dorsal nucleus of the vagus nerve send parasympathetic output to abdominal organs, which results in increased secretory activity of glands and increased rates of peristalsis (used in the process of digestion). Finally, the spinal trigeminal nucleus receives sensory information from the outer ear and the mucus layer of the larynx. It travels a long distance from its point of origin in the brainstem to the various organs of the neck, thorax, and abdomen that it innervates.

In its journey, cranial nerve X exits the skull through the jugular foramen (a hole at the base of the skull) along with cranial nerves IX (glossopharyngeal) and XI (accessory). The vagus nerve then descends in a covering (called the carotid sheath) with the internal jugular vein and internal carotid artery, inferiorly through the neck and eventually into the chest and abdomen. Along the way, the vagus nerve gives off several branches on both sides of the body to innervate various organs and/or skeletal muscles. It has two enlargements: *the superior ganglion*—which is near the opening of the foramen that receives general sensory information and connects with neurons from cranial nerves IX and XI—and *the inferior ganglion*—which receives sensory input from various organs. Because the vagus nerve carries so many different afferent fibers from so many different visceral organs, it is a very large and thick nerve that is easily identified within the neck, thorax (chest cavity), and abdominal cavity.

In the thorax, the right and left vagus nerves take different paths on their way to the abdomen. The left vagus nerve is closely aligned with the arch of the aorta (the largest artery in the body as it is the main artery that exits the heart) and gives off a branch, the *left recurrent laryngeal nerve.* This branch then hooks around a ligament under the arch before ascending up into the neck to supply motor function and sensory sensation to the larynx (voice box). On the right side, the *right recurrent laryngeal nerve* comes off of the right vagus nerve much higher up, hooking around the right subclavian artery before ascending up the neck.

The recurrent laryngeal nerves will innervate (terminate on and stimulate) the intrinsic muscles of the larynx, such as the *thyroarytenoid, posterior and lateral cricoarytenoid,* and *arytenoid muscles.*

Because the left recurrent laryngeal nerve passes under the aortic arch, it is longer than the right recurrent laryngeal nerve. Along the way, both recurrent branches give off smaller branches to the heart, esophagus, trachea, and pharyngeal constrictor muscles before reaching their destination, the larynx.

The vagus nerves enter the abdomen through a natural hole in the diaphragm called the *esophageal hiatus,* which allows the esophagus, vagus nerve, and a few vessels to pass through the diaphragm. This section of cranial nerve X supplies motor parasympathetic fibers to all organs (except the adrenal glands) from the neck down to the latter third of the transverse colon. It also will innervate some muscles in the larynx that are involved in speech, the throat, and palate (the roof of the mouth). Based on the location of the vagus nerves branches, cranial nerve X is responsible for a variety of tasks that include the control of heart rate and blood pressure, gut peristalsis, speech, and breathing.

Clinical Symptoms and Diseases

Isolated lesions of the vagus nerve are uncommon, but damage to the recurrent nerves can occur. Cancers of the larynx or thyroid glands or during thyroid surgery can injury these nerves. The result is decreased movement of the vocal fold on the damaged side, causing hoarseness. Bilateral damage to the recurrent branch can result in difficulty in swallowing, reduced gag reflexes, and dysarthria (problems with speaking due to the lack of muscle control). To test which vagus nerve is damaged, an easy clinical diagnostic assessment is to see if the patient's uvula deviates to one side. If it does, the uvula will move away from the side of the lesion. In addition, patients will not be able to elevate their palate.

Disorders of cranial nerve X can occur from other disease states that may induce inflammation or infection. When the vagus nerve is affected, it can either produce overstimulation or inactivity of the nerve. Overstimulation results in excessive neurotransmitter release, while inactivity results in the lack of neurotransmitter release. Symptoms may include pain, organ dysfunction—like abnormal heart rate, difficulty in urinating, or a change in a person's voice, peptic ulcers, gastroperesis—decreased ability to digest food, and fainting. Peptic ulcers, which are painful and serious, are caused by an overproduction of peptic acid and may lead to gastroesophageal reflex disease (GERD). Thus, cutting the vagus nerve (vagotomy) was historically used to control acid release in the stomach in patients with peptic ulcers. This procedure is no longer used now that more effective and less invasive treatments are available, such as proton pump inhibitors that decrease the production of gastric acid by medication.

Using the Vagus Nerve as a Medical Intervention

Today, stimulating or blocking cranial nerve X has been shown useful for different medical therapies, including seizure management, clinical depression, some heart rate irregularities, and weight loss. To stimulate the vagus nerve, a pacemaker-like device is implanted in a patient's chest. When the stimulator is activated, it can control certain types of seizures. This same vagal nerve stimulation therapy has also been shown to improve patients with drug-resistant clinical depression. Currently, neuroscientists are testing the stimulator device to reduce tinnitus (a constant ringing sound in the ear), as a small branch of the vagus nerve supplies the outer ear.

Since the vagus nerve controls heart rate, patients with supraventricular tachycardia or atrial fibrillation may use vagal nerve stimulation manually. Patients with such heart conditions are taught to hold their breath for a few seconds, cool their face down with cold water, cough, or tighten their stomach muscles to mimic a bowel movement. If these treatments do not help, surgical and/or pharmacological intervention(s) may be required.

Lastly, blocking cranial nerve X output has shown to help obese patients to lose weight. In a recent study in rabbits where their vagus nerve was blocked, scientists saw a reduction in the animal's weight by 14 percent and in food intake by 40 percent within one month (Mizrahi et al., 2012). Although vagotomy is no longer used to treat peptic ulcers, it is currently being studied to reduce weight in morbidly obese patients. This procedure would be an alternative to gastric bypass surgery. The result is the patient feels less hungry. However, patients with vagotomy need to take a daily supplement of vitamin B12 for the rest of their lives to prevent a deficiency that can lead to nerve damage, if untreated.

Robin Michaels and
Jennifer L. Hellier

See also: Autonomic Nervous System; Cranial Nerves; Epilepsy; Nerves; Peripheral Nervous System; Seizures

Further Reading

Liang, B. (2012). *The 12 cranial nerves.* Retrieved from http://www.wisc-online.com/ob jects/ViewObject.aspx?ID=AP11504

Mizrahi, M., Ben Ya'acov, A., & Ilan, Y. (2012). Gastric stimulation for weight loss. *World Journal of Gastroenterology, 18*(19), 2309–2319.

Moore, K. L., Agur, A. M. R., & Dalley, A. F. (Eds.). (2010). *Essential clinical anatomy* (4th ed.). Baltimore, MD: Williams and Wilkins.

Yale University School of Medicine. (1998). *Cranial nerves.* Retrieved from http://www .yale.edu/cnerves/

Ventricles

Ventricles are the spaces or cavities deep within the brain that are filled with a clear, watery liquid called cerebrospinal fluid (CSF). There are four ventricles in the human brain: the two lateral ventricles in the right and left cerebral hemispheres; the third ventricle within the diencephalon (the caudal portion of the forebrain); and the fourth ventricle between the pons and the cerebellum. The four ventricles communicate with each other through the right and left *interventricular foramina* (opening between the ventricles) that run between the lateral ventricles and the third ventricle, and the *cerebral aqueduct,* which connects the third and the fourth ventricles. The fourth ventricle opens into the protective coverings of the brain called the meninges. Specifically, it opens into the space below the arachnoid mater called the *subarachnoid space* via the lateral and median apertures. This allows passage of CSF from the ventricles to the surface of the brain and spinal cord.

Ventricles house specialized tissue structures called *choroid plexus,* which is responsible for the production of CSF. CSF circulates not only throughout the ventricles but also bathes the outside of the brain and spinal cord. The ventricles provide a mechanism by which metabolic waste of the neural tissues can be easily removed from the deep regions of the brain by the CSF. The fluid is then filtered at the *arachnoid villi* or *granulations* within the meninges that eventually drains into the venous system (veins). CSF in the ventricles as well as in the subarachnoid space provides buoyancy that allows the brain and spinal cord to float rather than directly rest on its hard boney casing. Thus, CSF protects the delicate neural tissues from compression or traumatic contusion against the skull or backbone with every jolt and movement that everyday normal activities produce.

History and Function

With limited knowledge of cellular and molecular organization of the body, early philosophers believed that it was the ventricles in the brain that possessed the animal spirit (also known as psychic pneuma), which they believed was responsible for carrying out all functions of the brain. This notion of brain and body regulation by the ventricles was termed the "ventricular-pneumatic doctrine." Between the fourth and fifth century AD, the "three-cell theory" evolved in which each brain ventricle was thought to provide a specific function. The lateral ventricles were grouped together and were believed to receive all sensory information. The third ventricle was considered to be responsible for logical thought processes, and the fourth ventricle was deemed as the storage of memory. The idea that the empty spaces in the brain was the "seat of the soul" and responsible for brain function, rather than the actual brain tissue itself, was developed from the early religious leaders' beliefs that souls are not physical structures. Hence, it must occupy an empty space of the head.

In the 16th century, Andreas Vesalius (1514–1564) and Leonardo da Vinci (1452–1519) contributed more accurate depictions and understanding of brain anatomy through their thorough dissection and study of the brain. But it was not until the 1600s that anatomists started arguing that the ventricles were nothing more than spaces passively formed within the brain and that it could not be the seat of the soul.

The current understanding of ventricles being chambers filled with CSF is quite the contrary to the first theories proposed by ancient anatomists. Scientists have now shown that ventricles provide a network of chambers within the brain to house

CSF, which provides buoyancy to the brain, removes metabolic waste, and delivers hormones and other signaling peptides to the deep portions of the brain.

Anatomy and Physiology

It is useful to understand the anatomy of the brain to appreciate the shape and location of each ventricle. The brain is composed of the cerebrum, which is the large, paired hemispherical bulk of the brain. It is separated into right and left sides by a deep groove along the midline called the *longitudinal fissure*. The right and left cerebral hemispheres are connected to each other by a thick band of white matter called the *corpus callosum*. Two lateral ventricles, each in the shape of the letter "C," lie in the deep center of each cerebral hemisphere, running in the direction from the front to the back of the cerebrum. Deep inside the cerebrum and below the corpus callosum lies the diencephalon, which is composed of distinct structures called the epithalamus, thalamus, and hypothalamus. Within the small globular neural tissue of diencephalon lies the third ventricle. Each lateral ventricle communicates with the third ventricle and also with each other via a paired opening called the interventricular foramina, also known as the foramina of Monroe. The midbrain is the short segment of the brainstem just below the diencephalon that contains the cerebral aqueduct. The cerebral aqueduct is a single and narrow channel that allows passage of CSF from the third ventricle into the fourth ventricle. The fourth ventricle is located in between the pons and cerebellum of the brain. This roughly diamond-shaped space receives CSF from the higher ventricles through the cerebral aqueduct and channels it to the outside of the brain into the subarachnoid space through the two openings on either side called the lateral apertures and one midline opening called the median aperture.

The complex shape and network of chambers that comprise the ventricles of the brain also serve as the sites of CSF production. The structure responsible for producing CSF is the choroid plexus, which is found on the floor of each lateral ventricle, the roof of the third ventricle, and the lower portion of the fourth ventricle. The choroid plexus is made of numerous folds of vascular connective tissue that is covered with *ependymal cells,* a special type of neural cells that line all the ventricles of the brain and central canal of the spinal cord. The highly folded nature of choroid plexus makes them resemble cauliflower in appearance. Here, the blood-brain barrier does not exist and plasma from the blood vessels is filtered and modified by the ependymal cells. The newly filtered fluid is released into the ventricular spaces. Commonly, CSF travels through the ventricles in one direction: from the lateral ventricles, to the third, through the cerebral aqueduct, to the fourth ventricle, then to the subarachnoid space outside of the brain and spinal cord. The one-directional flow of CSF is hypothesized to be induced by intracranial pressure, arterial blood pressure, and the current created by the ependymal cells' cilia that beat in one direction. Once the CSF leaves the brain through the lateral and median apertures, the fluid travels through the subarachnoid space surrounding the surface of the brain and spinal cord. Arachnoid granulations are dilated swellings of arachnoid mater that protrude into the dural sinus of the protective brain coverings, where excess amounts of CSF and metabolic waste are filtered and returned to blood circulation.

Diseases

The main clinical condition associated with the ventricles is hydrocephalus. The direct translation of hydrocephalus is "water on the brain." In this condition, CSF accumulates in the ventricles of the brain and in turn increases intracranial pressure. The rising amount of CSF and the increasing pressure it creates are dangerous because they can make the brain to swell and be pushed against the rigid bone (skull) encasing the brain. In a severe or prolonged case of hydrocephalus, brain damage and even death may result.

The most common cause of hydrocephalus is an obstruction of the normal flow of the CSF throughout the ventricles and outside of the brain. The obstruction may be inside the brain (intraventricular) or outside of the brain (extraventricular). The most common site of intraventricular obstruction is at the cerebral aqueduct, the narrow channel between the third and the fourth ventricles. Extraventricular obstruction may result from diverse causes such as infection, inflammation, intracranial hemorrhage (bleeding), and poor return of CSF into the circulatory system at the arachnoid villi. In rare cases, hydrocephalus can result from an over production of CSF without any obstruction of the flow.

Hydrocephalus affects mostly children and is frequently present in children with myelomeningocele, a form of neural tube defects in which the spinal cord and its bony casing (vertebrae or spine) formation is abnormal. At the affected area, the spinal cord is tethered to the spine and as the infant grows, the rapidly growing backbone pulls down on the spinal cord, eventually leading to a herniation of the brain through the *foramen magnum* (large hole) of the skull. The narrowed foramen magnum reduces the amount of CSF draining out of the brain and into the subarachnoid space surrounding the spinal cord. This eventually results in hydrocephalus and increased intracranial pressure.

Common symptoms of hydrocephalus include headache, vomiting, and uncoordinated movements as well as visual impairment. In some cases, large intracranial pressure and expansion of the brain may enlarge or alter the shape of the babies' heads since the bones of the skull have not yet fused in infants and young children. Current treatments for hydrocephalus focus on draining the excess CSF via *lumbar puncture,* placements of shunts in the ventricles, or placement of stents at obstructed regions. In severe cases, surgery may be required to remove the obstructing tissues.

Lisa M. J. Lee

See also: Cerebrospinal Fluid; Hydrocephalus; Meninges

Further Reading

A history of the brain. (n.d.). Retrieved from http://www.stanford.edu/class/history13/earlysciencelab/body/brainpages/brain.html

Moore, K. L., Agur, A. R., & Dalley, A. F. (2011). *Essential clinical anatomy* (4th ed.). Philadelphia, PA: Lippincott Williams & Wilkins.

National Institute of Neurological Disorders and Stroke. (2013). *NINDS hydrocephalus information page.* Retrieved from http://www.ninds.nih.gov/disorders/hydrocephalus/hydrocephalus.htm

The medieval cell doctrine of brain function. (n.d.). Retrieved from http://www.princeton.edu/~cggross/BVM_Imhotep3.pdf

Vertebra

The human body is composed of 206 bones that have five distinct functions: movement, support, protection, storage of ions, and blood cell production. The skeleton can be divided into two broad regions, the *axial skeleton*—all of the bones along the axis, including the skull, ribs, vertebral column, and the sternum—and the *appendicular skeleton*—the bones in the appendages, including the pectoral girdle, the pelvic girdle, the arms, and the legs. Both the skull and the *vertebral column* play an integral role in protecting the central nervous system (CNS) from damage. Human bodies have, on average, 33 vertebra—7 cervical (upper portion in the neck), 12 thoracic (middle portion), 5 lumbar (lower back), 3 to 5 fused together to form the sacrum, and 3 to 5 fused together to form the coccyx (tailbone). Each vertebra is separated by an intervertebral disk that forms a fibrocartilaginous (made of connective tissue that is fibrous) joint that is capable of slight movement of the spine. Intervertebral disks also act to adhere the vertebrae together so that there is no slippage.

Structure and Surfaces

Each vertebra has a similar structure with minor variations. The vertebrae are made up mostly by the body, which is the most anterior or front structure when it sits in the vertebral column. Intervertebral disks sit in between each vertebral body. The posterior aspects of the vertebrae are formed by the vertebral arch, which is made up of a pair of pedicles (connect the arch to the body) and a pair of lamina (come together posteriorly to form the vertebral spinous process). Within the vertebral arch is the vertebral foramen (opening within each vertebra), which houses the spinal cord.

Each vertebra has seven processes, four articulating processes (or articulating facets) that connect vertebra to vertebra, two transverse processes, and one spinous process. Not only do the processes act as a surface to connect bone to bone, but they also form a location for muscle attachments. These processes and facets act to inhibit movement of the spine in order to protect the fragile spinal cord running the length of the vertebral column (ending approximately at the level of the second lumbar vertebra, L2).

Regions

The five regions of the vertebral column are, from superior to inferior, cervical, thoracic, lumbar, sacral, and coccygeal. The cervical region encapsulates the first seven vertebrae and these vertebrae are named as C1, C2, and so on. C1 and C2 are specialized vertebrae named the atlas and the axis, respectively, and make up the atlanto-occipital joint and the atlanto-axial joint, which connects the skull to the rest of the vertebral column allowing for movement up and down and rotation from side to side. There is no intervertebral disk between the skull and the atlas or the atlas and the axis. The rest of the cervical region has short spinous processes and are smaller in general. In between the pedicles of each vertebra, the eight cervical spinal nerves exit the spinal cord and travel to the rest of the body. Cervical vertebrae also have small transverse foramina, which allow the vertebral arteries to pass into the skull to supply the brain with blood and nutrients.

The thoracic region contains the next 12 vertebrae and is the location where the ribs connect to the vertebral column. The thoracic vertebrae are named T1 through T12. There are specialized divots or facets on each thoracic vertebra that provide a surface for the articulation of the ribs to the vertebrae. The thoracic vertebrae are slightly larger than the cervical vertebrae with more pronounced spinous processes. They allow for slight rotation but not a lot due to the articulation with the rib cage.

The lumbar region of the vertebral column is made up of the next five vertebrae labeled L1 through L5. These vertebrae are much larger than the cervical and thoracic as they support the most weight. The lumbar region allows for the most flexion and extension (bending forward and backward) and some lateral flexion or side-to-side bending. The lumbar vertebrae are curved inward creating a lumbar lordosis or a natural "sway" in the lower back. This is created by the way the vertebrae and intervertebral discs interact.

The sacrum is three to five fused vertebrae that are labeled S1 to S5. These vertebrae do not have any intervertebral discs between them and act as one bone. They do not allow for any movement between them. The coccyx is also three to five fused vertebrae (most commonly four) that are labeled Co1 through Co5 and also has no intervertebral discs allowing for no movement. The coccyx is also considered the tailbone and in many creatures can contain more than five vertebrae.

Abnormalities

One of the most common abnormalities of the vertebral column is a slipped intervertebral disc resulting in a pinched nerve. The spinal nerves that run between the two vertebrae and the slipped disc becomes pinched by the vertebrae. This results in back pain and, sometimes, pain radiating outward from that spot. Another abnormality of the vertebral column is spina bifida, a developmental disorder where the vertebrae do not fully form, resulting in a space where the meninges (protective covering of the spinal cord) and spinal cord can protrude. This most commonly occurs in the lumbosacral region. Spina bifida can be surgically repaired but results in permanent damage of the spinal cord where it protruded from the vertebral column.

Laminectomy

The spine is made up of 33 bones called *vertebrae* (plural, *vertebra* is singular). This makes the spinal column rigid to protect the soft tissues that run through the opening of each vertebra. The soft tissues are the spinal cord, spinal nerves, and spinal rootlets. A *laminectomy* is the removal of part of a vertebral bone. Specifically, it is a surgical cut of the lamina between the spinous process, the lateral pedicles, and the transverse processes of the vertebra. The surgery is performed by a neurosurgeon as a last resort to treat severe back pain from a herniated disk(s), spinal injury, spinal stenosis (narrowing of the canal), or tumors. Each of these can cause compression of the spinal cord or the nerve roots resulting in severe back and leg pain. In 1887, Sir Victor Alexander Haden Horsley (1857–1916) was the first person to successfully perform a laminectomy. During this surgery he removed a spinal tumor. For developing this and several other surgical techniques, Dr. Horsley is considered one of the fathers of neurosurgery.

The term laminectomy means to cut the lamina; however, a conventional laminectomy includes cutting the *posterior spinal ligament* and some or all of the spinous process. It also includes detaching many of the small back muscles that are attached to the vertebra. By opening and removing these structures, the spinal cord, spinal nerves, and the rootlets have a larger space to expand and are no longer being compressed. Recovery from a laminectomy is generally faster compared to more complex spinal surgeries, such as spinal fusions or placing spinal rods. It can take a few weeks or months for the patient to have pain relief and they can have a good prognosis that may last for several years.

Jennifer L. Hellier

See also: Spinal Cord

Further Reading

Johns Hopkins Medicine. (n.d.). *Laminectomy.* Retrieved from http://www.hopkins medicine.org/healthlibrary/test_procedures/orthopaedic/laminectomy_92, P07681/

The vertebral column can also have abnormal curvatures in some individuals. Scoliosis is the most common abnormal curvature and results in a lateral curvature of the vertebral column (curves to the left or right). Scoliosis results from unequal development of each side of the vertebrae. Another abnormal curvature is Kyphosis, which is an exaggerated posterior curvature of the spine producing a "humpback." Lordosis is an exaggerated inward curvature of the cervical and lumbar region resulting in "swayback." Oftentimes, pregnant women develop a temporary lordosis due to the extra weight being carried.

Riannon C. Atwater

See also: Herniated Discs; Lumbar Puncture; Pinched Nerve—Building with Clay Activity; Skull; Spina Bifida; Spinal Cord

Further Reading

Unknown. (n.d.). *The vertebral column and spinal cord.* Retrieved from http://www.emory .edu/ANATOMY/AnatomyManual/back.html

Hines, T. (2013). *Anatomy of the spine.* Retrieved from http://www.mayfieldclinic.com /pe-anatspine.htm#.Uv_-aIV36Gw

Jones, O. (2014). *Osteology of the vertebral column.* Retrieve from http://teachmeanatomy .info/back/vertebral-column/

Ullrich, P. F. (2009). *Vertebrae in the vertebral column.* Retrieved from http://www.spine health.com/conditions/spine-anatomy/vertebrae-vertebral-column

Vestibular System

The *vestibular system* is a sensory system that detects the position and movement of the head. By monitoring the position and movement of the head, the vestibular system contributes to the sense of balance and equilibrium. The main organs of the vestibular system are located within the inner ear on both sides of the head, just posterior to the cochlea of the auditory system. There are two components in the vestibular system: the semicircular canal system and the otoliths. Each component is responsible for detecting different types of movement. The semicircular canals detect rotational movement, and the otoliths detect gravity and linear acceleration. The vestibular system is closely tied to the visual centers of the brain that control eye muscle movement as well as areas of the autonomic nervous system within the cerebellum that maintain subconscious muscle tension. When the vestibular system is malfunctioning and the subconscious muscle tension is abnormal, it may cause symptoms like motion sickness, vertigo, or uncontrolled eye movements.

History

Early anatomist mistook the vestibular system as a part of the auditory system; it was postulated to be an entry to the auditory system. This is why it was called the vestibular system, vestibule meaning a channel that leads to or is an entrance to another cavity. It turned out that the small canals had their own sensory function that is independent of the auditory system. The vestibular system is an organic mechanism for detecting the force of gravity or the location of "down." The vestibular system and auditory system are not directly related; however, they do use the same mechanism of signal transduction, hair cells. Hair cells contain tiny hair like projections on their top surface called cilia. Bending the specialized cilia creates receptor potentials that trigger action potentials in their corresponding nerve. In the vestibular system, the hair cells transduce mechanical movement in response to head orientation into neuronal signals. Both the vestibular and auditory systems evolved from the lateral line organs, which are found in aquatic vertebrates. Lateral line organs use hair cells to detect vibrations and pressure changes in the surrounding water. As reptiles evolved onto land, the lateral line organs disappeared, but the hair cells remained and evolved into the inner ear systems found in humans today.

Anatomy and Physiology

The vestibular system has two portions: the otolith organs and the semicircular canals. The otolith organs are two, fluid-filled, round structures that detect the force of gravity, tilts of the head, and linear acceleration (sensation of speeding up in a car). The semicircular canals, on the other hand, are made up of three, half-circle, fluid-filled tubes that detect rotational and head tilt movements. Both of these organs are found in the inner ear just posterior to the cochlea. The otolith organs are found centrally between the cochlea and the semicircular canals, and the semicircular canals loop out posteriorly from the otolith. There is a set of vestibular organs located on each side of the head within the temporal bone.

The three semicircular canals detect head rotations such as nodding vertically, shaking horizontally, or movement from shoulder to shoulder. The semicircular canals also detect angular acceleration that is created by a sudden rotation, like spinning in a circle. Each canal is located in a plane that is 90 degrees to the other two semicircular canals. The hair cells are located within an enlargement at the base of each canal called the ampulla. The hair cells within the ampulla are attached to the crista, which is analogous to the organ of Corti in the cochlea. The cilia of the hair cells extend into a membrane called the cupula. When there is a head rotation, the wall of the canal and the cupula move, but the fluid movement lags behind due to inertia. The opposing movement between the fluid and the cupula bends the cilia of the hair cells in the opposite direction of the head movement. The bending motion in one direction causes an excitation of the hair cells and a release of neurotransmitters, which are chemicals used to activate neurons. Moving in the opposite direction inhibits neurotransmitter release. The released neurotransmitters stimulate action potentials within the vestibular nerve. The on/off arrangement of the hair cells allows the brain to detect the orientation of the head at all times. The function of the semicircular canals is easily demonstrated by spinning rapidly in a circle for 15 to 30 seconds and then stopping. The sustained motion within the semicircular canals eventually stops bending the cupula and the sensation of spinning subsides. However, once the spinning motion ceases the fluid causes the cupula to bend in the opposite direction, which gives the sensation of motion in the opposite direction.

The otolith organs are located between the semicircular canals and the cochlea; it contains a pair of large chambers called the saccule and the utricle. These two structures within the otolith detect changes in the angle of the head and linear acceleration, which are all responses to gravity. The utricle and saccule have a sensory epithelium called the macula that is vertical in the saccule and horizontal in the utricle when the head is upright. The vestibular macula contains hair cells with their cilia projecting into a gelatinous membrane called the otolith membrane. Otolith means ear stone in Greek, and within the otolith membrane are many tiny calcium carbonate stones (1–5 micrometers in diameter), the otoliths. These stones are heavier than the surrounding fluid and membrane, so gravity pulls them down. The weight of the otoliths being pulled down by gravity also causes the membrane to be pulled down and thus bends the cilia of the hair cells. Bending in one direction stimulates an action potential in the vestibular nerves and bending in the opposite direction inhibits an action potential. The hair cells within the macula can detect head movement in any direction due to their respective orientation within the utricle and saccule. In addition, the otolith organs on each side of the head are mirror images of one another. This means that a head tilt will result in the activation of hair cells on one side of the head, while the corresponding location on the opposite side of the head will be inactivated. Any head tilt or acceleration will result in the activation of certain hair cells and the inactivation of others. Collectively the brain can interpret these activation/inactivation patterns for all forms of head orientations unambiguously. A great example of the otolith organs at work is being on a moving sidewalk. A person will experience a sudden acceleration stepping onto the walkway and then feel a deceleration stepping off.

The vestibular axons extending from the hair cells form the vestibular portion of cranial nerve VIII (the vestibulocochlear nerve). The vestibular portions of this nerve make connections to several areas of the brain including the vestibular nucleus within the brainstem and the cerebellum. The visual system, somatic sensory system, and the cerebellum, all send inputs to the vestibular nucleus in order to regulate different aspects of equilibrium and balance. The cerebellar pathways help to regulate balance by adjusting muscle tension and posture in response to stimuli within the vestibular system. The vestibular system in conjunction with the visual system makes up the vestibulo-ocular reflex (VOR). The VOR senses rotations in the head and triggers a reflex in the muscles that control eye movements. This allows an animal's vision to remain fixed on a target as its head moves. The VOR is regulated entirely by vestibular system input, so it continues to work even if a person closes their eyes.

Diseases

The most common disease associated with the vestibular system is vertigo. *Vertigo* is Latin for a "spinning movement." Individuals who suffer from vertigo often experience the feeling of moving despite remaining still. In addition to the sensation of movement, affected individuals often suffer from nausea and balance issues that make it difficult to stand or walk straight. Vertigo can be classified into two categories: peripheral or central. Peripheral vertigo is the result of vestibular system dysfunction within the semicircular canals or the otolith organs. The most common cause of this type of vertigo is benign paroxysmal position vertigo, which is defined as a rotational vertigo that has a short duration and is induced by changing head position. This type of vertigo is often accompanied by an uncontrolled eye movement called nystagmus where the eye moves back and forth like a twitch for a few minutes during the episode. Other causes of peripheral vertigo include motion sickness, Meniere's disease, and infection or inflammation of the inner ear. Central vertigo is caused by direct damage to the vestibular centers within the brain. Most often the damage is in the vestibular nucleus of the brainstem or in the cerebellum. Central vertigo generally causes balance issues and not the perception of movement, like in peripheral vertigo. Causes of central vertigo are often stroke, brain tumor, hemorrhage, or epilepsy.

Treatment of peripheral vertigo depends on the underlying cause. For infections and inflammation, antibiotics and steroids can be used to treat the issue and the vertigo will subside. Other pharmacological treatments, like benzodiazepines, can be used to suppress the vestibular system and reduce the sensation of movement. Central vertigo treatment depends on the disorder that is causing the vertigo. A tumor that affects the vestibular areas of the brain could be excised or treated with chemotherapy.

Lynelle Smith

See also: Auditory System; Autonomic Nervous System; Cochlea; Epilepsy; Meniere's Disease; Nystagmus; Vestibulocochlear Nerve

Further Reading

Bear, M. F., Connors, B. W., & Paradiso, M. A. (2007). *Neuroscience exploring the brain* (3rd ed.). Baltimore, MD: Lippincott Williams & Wilkins.

Gray, L. (2013). *Vestibular system: Structure and function* (Chap. 10). Retrieved from http://neuroscience.uth.tmc.edu/s2/chapter10.html

Watson, M. A., & Black, F. O. (2013). *The human balance system.* Retrieved from http://vestibular.org/understanding-vestibular-disorder/human-balance-system

Vestibulocochlear Nerve

The *vestibulocochlear nerve* is a cranial nerve that is part of the peripheral nervous system and supplies motor (efferent) and/or sensory (afferent) function to the head, face, and neck. All cranial nerves are paired, meaning one nerve supplies the right side and the other nerve supplies the left. The cranial nerves are numbered starting from the nose (rostral end of the brain) and moving caudally (toward the back of the head) as Roman numerals. The vestibulocochlear nerve is the 8 of 12 paired cranial nerves. Thus, it is also called *cranial nerve VIII.* The vestibulocochlear nerves are purely sensory and have two divisions: vestibular and cochlear. The vestibular portion deals with the sensation of balance, while the cochlear division is used for hearing (auditory information).

Anatomy and Physiology

Within the skull and deep to the external ear, the vestibulocochlear nerve's sensory receptors are located in the *membranous labyrinth*. This is a very delicate small structure that is tubular, filled with *endolymph* (a special fluid), and connected to a series of tunnels within the *petrous portion* (meaning the hard or stony section) of the temporal bone. The tunnel walls are called the *bony labyrinth*. The bony labyrinth is connected to the inner ear by two openings, the oval window with the *stapes* bone and the round window with a flexible membrane called the *round window membrane*. The stapes vibrates when a sound wave hits it, resulting in a pressure wave into both the bony and membranous labyrinths. This pressure wave travels through the channels and make the round window membrane vibrate. In turn, the endolymph moves resulting in the sound wave being propagated.

Semicircular Canals

The *semicircular canals* are found within the vestibular apparatus in the inner ear. There are two sets of semicircular canals, one in the left inner ear and one in the right. Their function is to sense head rotations in the X-, Y-, and Z-axes, which are called the yaw, pitch, and roll axes in flight. There are three semicircular canals one for each axis and each are tiny fluid-filled tubes attached to a larger, bony region containing the *utricle* and *saccula*. They are named for their orientation within the vestibular apparatus: horizontal, superior, and posterior semicircular canals. Together, these canals help animals maintain their balance by detecting acceleration in three perpendicular planes. The hair cells in the semicircular canals are similar to those in the *organ of Corti* (used for hearing); however, they detect movements of the fluid in the canals due to angular acceleration. The semicircular canals are connected to the *vestibulocochlear nerve* (the 8th of 12 paired cranial nerves) in the inner ear.

The horizontal semicircular canal senses movement on a vertical basis—rotating the head up and down on the neck. The posterior semicircular canal detects rotations on a sagittal plane—rotating the head left and right. The superior semicircular canal detects head rotations on the anterior-posterior axis—moving the head forward and backward. Damage to the semicircular canals could be twofold. If any part of the canal does not work, then a person may seem like they have lost their sense of balance. Damage to the vestibulocochlear nerve could also make a person lose their sense of balance and/or the diminished ability to hear. Injuries related to damage of the semicircular canals include, but are not limited to: the sensation of spinning or the feel the room is spinning around (*vertigo*), the sensation of being off balance (*disequilibrium*), or the feeling of lightheadedness or feeling faint (*presyncope*).

Renee Johnson

See also: Dizziness and Vertigo

Further Reading

Purves, D., Augustine, G. J., Fitzpatrick, D., Hall, W. C., LaMantia, A.-S., McNamara, J. O., & Williams, S. M. (Eds.). (2004). *Neuroscience* (3rd ed.). Sunderland, MA: Sinauer Associates.

The sensory receptors in the cochlea (called hair cells) and vestibular structures (called the macula, which consist of hair cells covered in a gelatinous mass) are small and can be easily damaged. The outputs (axons) of these sensory receptors travel a short distance to their receiving neurons, which are located in the cochlea and the *semicircular canals*. The cells in the cochlea make up the *spinal ganglion* (a group of cell bodies), while the neurons in the base of the semicircular canals make up the *vestibular ganglion*. These neurons' axons bundle and travel together making up cranial nerve VIII. The nerve travels through the *internal auditory meatus* with the facial nerve (cranial nerve VII). Both the vestibulocochlear and facial nerves then enter the brainstem at the junction of the pons and medulla. This is where the two divisions of the vestibulocochlear nerve begin to diverge from each other.

Vestibular Component of the Nerve

The fibers from the vestibular division terminate in the *vestibular nuclear complex* within the floor of the fourth ventricle. This makes up the vestibulocerebellar tract. The axons from the vestibular nuclear complex will terminate in several nuclei within the brainstem and spinal cord to affect the muscles used for maintaining balance. The *lateral vestibulospinal tract* is made of ipsilateral (same side) fibers from the lateral vestibular nucleus to terminate down the spinal cord onto neurons that control extensor muscles (antigravity muscles). The medial and inferior vestibular nuclei have shared connections to the cerebellum to control and coordinate balance while the body is moving. This is called the *vestibulocerebellar tract.* Finally, all vestibular complex nuclei project to the three cranial nerve nuclei used to control the muscles of the eyes. This makes up the *medial longitudinal fasciculus,* which is critical to maintaining the body's orientation in space as well as maintaining fixation of an object during head movement. These fibers terminate onto both the left and right nuclei of cranial nerves III (oculomotor), IV (trochlear), and VII (abducens). These interconnections show how the vestibular division is highly integrated with vision.

Cochlear Component of the Nerve

The fibers from the cochlear division terminate in the *dorsal* and *ventral cochlear nuclei.* The dorsal cochlear nucleus receives high frequency information, while the ventral cochlear nucleus receives information about low frequencies. The pathway to the cerebral cortex from here is not well understood. However, a few synapses have been studied in patients with cortical deafness, which are described in the following. The outputs of the dorsal and ventral cochlear nuclei cross to the other side (contralateral) of the brainstem and ascend toward the brain. This forms the *lateral lemniscus,* a tract of ascending axons to the cerebral cortex. Some axons cross over and synapse in the contralateral *trapezoid body* or the contralateral *superior olivary nucleus* before joining the lateral lemniscus. There are few fibers that do not cross over and terminate in the ipsilateral *superior olivary nucleus* and ascend in the ipsilateral lateral lemniscus. From here, axons of both the left and right lateral lemnisci terminate in the *inferior colliculus.* The inferior colliculus axons terminate into the thalamus, which sends its axons to the *transverse temporal gyrus.* It is here where sound is interpreted in the brain.

Clinical Symptoms, Diseases, and Treatment

Vestibular Component of the Nerve

If the vestibulocochlear nerve is damaged, the result is reduction or complete loss of balance. In particular, patients will feel dizzy, may fall more often, and have abnormal eye movements. The person may also have nausea causing them to vomit. The most common lesion to the vestibulocochlear nerve is a tumor of the Schwann cells surrounding the nerve. Removal of the tumor may be necessary for balance function to return. Finally, patients may be trained to overcome their balance deficit by using their eyes more effectively as vision can override vestibular issues. This is because the eyes can see the horizon and realize that it is stable and not truly moving.

Cochlear Component of the Nerve

If the vestibulocochlear nerve is damaged, the result is reduction or complete loss of hearing. This usually occurs from skull fractures or ear infections. Tumors can occur in the internal auditory meatus, which can damage both divisions of the vestibulocochlear nerve as well as the facial nerve. Finally, lesions to the lateral leminscus typically result in a characteristically partial deafness on the contralateral side. This is because the small amount of ipsilateral fibers is spared on the affected side and can carry the auditory information to the brain. Treatment may include antibiotics to heal the infection or hearing aids.

Jennifer L. Hellier

See also: Auditory System; Cranial Nerves; Dizziness and Vertigo; Nerves; Vestibular System

Further Reading

Liang, B. (2012). *The 12 cranial nerves.* Retrieved from http://www.wisc-online.com/objects/ViewObject.aspx?ID=AP11504

Moore, K. L., Agur, A. M. R., & Dalley, A. F. (Eds.). (2010). *Essential clinical anatomy* (4th ed.). Baltimore, MD: Williams and Wilkins.

Yale University School of Medicine. (1998). *Cranial nerves.* Retrieved from http://www.yale.edu/cnerves/

Visual Fields

Of the five senses (hear, smell, sight, taste, and touch) that humans depend upon, the visual system is the one that is utilized the most. The visual system is a complex assortment of neurons (brain cells that communicate motor and sensory information between each other) that allows animals and humans to see the world around them. This system is made of a series of different tracts (a long group of fibers that transmits information electrically) and nuclei (groups of cell bodies) much like the "tracks" and "ports or stations" on a railroad system. Each part of the track is important and when there is damage to any one part, it ultimately affects the *visual field*.

History

More than 2,000 years ago, Hippocrates (460–377 BC) was one of the first to recognize the visual field. The first documented testing, in fact, was performed by asking the patient to cover one eye while watching a fixed point. The tester would

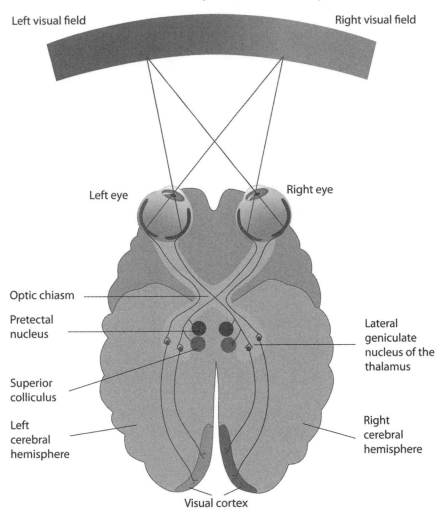

The Visual Projection Pathway

Left visual field

Right visual field

Left eye

Right eye

Optic chiasm

Pretectal nucleus

Lateral geniculate nucleus of the thalamus

Superior colliculus

Left cerebral hemisphere

Right cerebral hemisphere

Visual cortex

Diagram explaining how visual signals are received by the brain. (Dreamstime.com)

then ask the patient to identify objects held in the sides and outer edges of the visual field usually at four points. This type of testing is called *confrontation visual field evaluation.* This testing was expanded by British ophthalmologist Jannik Bjerrum (1851–1920) in the 19th century. Bjerrum mapped visual fields by holding a white object in front of a black screen known as the *tangent screen.*

Over time, additional tests were developed, such as the Amsler grid. This grid measures a person's central visual field. The patient is asked to fix his gaze on a small black dot in the center of a grid of black horizontal and vertical lines. The patient will note areas that are blurry or distorted.

Hans Goldmann (1899–1991), a Swiss ophthalmologist, developed a method of visual field testing using bright lights as targets on a white background on a bowl-shaped perimeter. These targets have different colors, sizes, and brightness. This perimetry is known as a kinetic perimetry in which a stimulus is first seen as marks on the outer edge or perimeter of the visual field.

In 1970s, a computer became an automated aid in testing. The Humphrey visual field analyzer, Goldmann field testing, and matrix as well as the octopus perimeter made testing more accurate in locating defects or loss in the visual field. Many of these tests are still used today during a routine eye exam. Because vision is so critical to humans, it is important for everyone to have an annual eye exam to maintain a healthy visual system.

Anatomy and Physiology

In the simplest of terms, when light enters the eye, it strikes the optic nerve. This information is then transported to the primary visual cortex (or striate cortex of the occipital lobe) where an image is produced. This system can be broken down into simpler parts, so a better understanding of the system may be obtained. When a human looks at an object, the total amount of area that can be seen is known as the *visual field*. Health care providers test the visual field by having a person focus on an object directly in front of them without moving their eyes or their head. Because the eye is a sphere, the resulting visual field is divided into the size of the angle seen both vertically and horizontally from a single eye. Thus, the typical dimensions for a human's visual field is 60 degrees superiorly (above eye level), 75 degrees inferiorly (below eye level), 60 degrees nasally (toward the nose), and 100 degrees temporally (toward the ear or temporal bone).

The visual field is broken into two halves: the nasal and temporal fields. The nasal visual field is on the medial or side toward the nose. The temporal field is on the lateral or outside toward the ear. Both of these fields are then broken down further into superior and inferior sections, thus giving the visual field four distinct quadrants. Because animals have two eyes, there are two visual fields.

When looking out at the target object, it is important to understand that as light enters the eye though its lens, the image is then rotated 180 degrees (meaning the image is turned upside down when projected onto the retina—the back of the eye). Thus, the light that is coming from the nasal visual field crosses the lens and strikes the lateral or outside portion of the inner eye. Similarly, this means that the temporal field crosses the eye and strikes the medial or inside portion of the inner eye. This tract will then go down the optic nerve and cross at the optic chiasm.

There are different ways to test an individual's visual field ranging from very simple tests that are done in a doctor's office using only hand movements to very complex computer-generated exams.

Visual Field Test

Humans, like most animals, are highly visual beings. When there is a deficit in vision, a health care provider may have the patient undergo a series of tests to examine the extent of their visual field. This is called a *visual field test,* which determines the entire range of vision for each individual eye. A visual field test assesses both the central and peripheral visions for each visual field quadrant. Generally, one eye is completely covered and the patient is asked to push a button when an object is seen within the visual field of the uncovered eye. The pushed button results in a "click" to the computer that is recording and "mapping" the visual field. The number of incorrect or missed clicks in each quadrant will tell the health care provider where the deficit exists, such as in the central vision, peripheral vision, or a specific quadrant. Thus, it is imperative that the person understands the tests and cooperates fully (meaning the patient pushes the button when they see an object) for the results to be reliable.

If the person is generally healthy, the visual field test is usually short from one to eight minutes long. If the patient is suspected of having glaucoma, then the tests are more complex and take about 15 to 25 minutes to complete. However, these longer tests can be tiresome to the eyes particularly in older patients. For all visual field tests, the person is asked to focus on a central object and to not move their eye. Then a light or a moving line at different intensities (bright versus dim, fast versus slow) appears. The next light or moving line will then appear randomly in a different location and/or quadrant. Each time the light or moving line is seen the patient pushes the button, which makes a computerized map of the visual field.

Jennifer L. Hellier

See also: Hubel, David H.; Optic Nerve; Visual Motor System; Visual Perception (Visual Processing); Visual System

Further Reading

Sheppard, J. (2007). Visual field test. Retrieved from http://www.medicinenet.com /visual_field_test/article.htm

Problems and Location of Injury

Humans are dependent on their sight for almost all aspects of everyday life. When problems arise in the visual system, they can be detrimental to our daily lives. Fortunately, scientists have a good understanding of the visual system and its pathway from the eye to the visual cortex. When damage occurs to the optic pathway, an individual's ability to see the world around him changes. The location in which their visual field is affected determines what portion of their vision or visual field is compromised. This may manifest as blind spots in their vision, blurred or hazy vision, or even total blindness. Injury to the visual tract can be caused by a variety of different things including infections, tumors, diabetes, strokes, high blood pressure, congenital defects (the abnormal anatomy a person is born with), blunt trauma (something hitting the head or entering an individual's eye), or following surgery.

To date, health care providers have found five basic areas where a lesion can cause problems in a person's visual fields: (1) optic nerve, (2) optic chiasm, (3) optic tract, (4) optic radiation, and (5) striate cortex. Starting at the optic nerve (the output of the retina), if an injury occurs before the optic chiasm (where the optic nerves meet and some fibers cross), it causes a break in the visual pathway. This break stops all the information from being sent to the visual cortex. When an injury of the optic never occurs, it will often result in total loss of vision on the side of injury. This is known as *monocular (one eye) blindness.*

The optic chiasm is where the information from both eyes meets before proceeding down the optic tract. Only the information from the nasal or medial visual field crosses here; the temporal or lateral tract just proceeds to the optic tract. The optic chiasm is positioned just anterior or in front of the pituitary gland. The pituitary gland is sometimes called the master gland and is about the size of a pea, but it produces a variety of different hormones that the body requires. Tumors on the pituitary gland can press on the optic chiasm causing injury. So when an injury is sustained here, it results in loss of both temporal fields. This condition is called *bitemporal hemianopsia.* The term "hemianopsia" means blindness or partial blindness. The optic chiasm splits and becomes two optic tracts. Damage to the optic tract will manifest as a condition called *homonymous hemianopsia.* This is due to the damage of nasal visual field on the ipsilateral or same side, and damage to the contralateral or opposite side temporal visual field.

The optic radiation is a network of neurons that take visual information from the lateral geniculate nucleus (part of the thalamus) to the primary visual cortex. This network is called Meyer's loop. When this structure is damaged, it results in a condition called *quadrantanopsia.* When a visual field test is conducted after injury to the optic radiation, the results will show decreased visual sensation in the same side nasal field and opposite side temporal field. Depending on where Meyer's loop is damaged, it can manifest in the superior or inferior portion of the visual field.

Finally, the striate cortex or Brodmann's area 17 is the end point for the visual tract. The striate cortex is in the occipital lobe, which is the most posterior portion of the brain. When there is damage to this area of the brain, it can result in a condition called *homonymous hemianopsia* with macular sparing. This means that all vision is lost in the ipsilateral nasal visual field and the contralateral temporal visual field, except for a small portion in the center of both visual fields that project to the macula (the center of the retina).

Adam K. Mills

See also: Blind Spot; Color Blindness; Occipital Lobe; Optic Nerve; Retina; Sensory Receptors; Tunnel Vision; Visual Perception (Visual Processing); Visual System

Further Reading

Carroll, J. N., & Johnson, C. A. (2013). *Visual field testing: From one medical student to another.* University of Iowa Health Care Ophthalmology & Visual Sciences. Retrieved from http://EyeRounds.org/tutorials/VF-testing/

Purves, D., Augustine, G. J., Fitzpatrick, D., Katz, L. C., LaMantia, A.-S., McNamara, J. O., & Williams, S. M. (Eds.). (2001). Visual field deficits. In *Neuroscience* (2nd ed.). Sunderland, MA: Sinauer Associates. Retrieved from http://www.ncbi.nlm.nih.gov/books/NBK10912/

Spector, R. H. (1990). Visual fields. In Walker, H. K., Hall, W. D., & Hurst, J. W. (Eds.). *Clinical methods: The history, physical, and laboratory examinations* (3rd ed., Chap. 116). Boston, MA: Butterworths. Retrieved from http://www.ncbi.nlm.nih.gov/books/NBK220/

Visual Perception (Visual Processing)

The *visual system* is a sensory system that is responsible for the sense of sight or vision. *Visual perception,* however, consists of the psychological process of how an animal or person sees a visual image. Specifically, visual perception is how the brain interprets the external environment and surroundings that are contained by visible light, and that interpretation can vary from person to person based on their previous experiences. Because of this difference, the visual system is a separate entry in this encyclopedia. Furthermore, this entry will focus on mammalian and human visual perception and processing. Animals are highly visual beings, particularly mammals and humans, as this sensory system along with the ability to process the information helps them see their prey, see their food, and see their surroundings. However, visual perception is more than translating what is projected onto the *retina,* the photosensitive lining of the eye. It is internalizing the image and its surroundings and how it pertains to the subject. Thus, sight is the combination of the visual system, visual processing, and visual perception.

History

For thousands of years, man has realized that the eye and brain are intimately interconnected. The visual pathway, from the eyes to the brain, was first documented and described by Galen of Pergamon (AD 130–200). For the technology at the time, scientists are still amazed at Galen's accuracy in many of his anatomical drawings and physiological understandings of the visual system. However, he did make a few mistakes that are now better understood with modern scientific tools. In Galen's drawing of the visual pathway he misinterpreted that the optic chiasm (meaning "cross") has a true decussation (cross over) of the optic nerve. Instead, he thought that the output of the neurons within the retina would come together and then continue on the same side that they originated. He also missed the fibers that connect to the *dorsal lateral geniculate nucleus* of the thalamus. He thought these fibers were connected to the natural spaces within the brain, the lateral ventricles. This is because the belief at the time was that nerves were hollow conduits that carried the "spirits" to the different parts of the brain and for vision, this would be the "visual spirit."

Modern understanding and particularly the neurophysiology of the visual system are attributed to Canadian neurophysiologist David H. Hubel (1926–2013) and Swedish neurophysiologist Torsten N. Wiesel (1924–). Together, Hubel and Wiesel won the 1981 Nobel Prize in Physiology or Medicine for their contributions to neuroscience about vision and are considered the fathers of the visual system.

Anatomy and Physiology

The visual system is made up of several anatomical structures including the *eye*—and its *retina; optic nerves*—the output of the retina and the second pair of cranial nerves (which are nerves that supply motor and sensory function to the head, neck, and face); *optic chiasm; optic tract; lateral geniculate nucleus; optic radiation; visual cortex;* and *visual association cortex.* Since mammals have two eyes, all of the aforementioned structures are found in both the left and right sides of the brain, except for the optic chiasm. There is only one optic chiasm as this is where the left and right optic nerves come together and cross some of their fibers.

Visual Processing

Once an object's image hits the retina, the neuronal signals for that image are carried through the aforementioned structures and terminate in the visual cortex. It is here where the signal is processed and then passed on to visual association cortices to be translated into visual perception. The visual cortex is found at the posterior (back) part of the brain called the occipital lobe. There are two occipital lobes, one on each brain hemisphere and they each receive information from the opposite *visual fields*. Each eye has its own visual field, what the eye sees when it is fixed and looking straight ahead. The visual field is artificially divided into four quadrants with the vertical and horizontal axes crossing in the middle. The visual field signals are projected to the occipital lobe with specifically the left visual fields signals from each eye are processed in the right occipital lobe and vice versa.

The signals are then relayed to the *V1 region* of the visual cortex. This is the first of the hierarchy for visual processing. The V1 region is also called the *primary visual cortex, Brodmann's area 17,* and the *striate cortex*. The striate cortex is named as such due its striped nature of white matter within the cortex. This white matter consists of highly myelinated fibers from layer IV of the lateral geniculate nucleus that terminate in V1. The visual cortex is responsible for the initial processing of image information. In humans, it makes up the largest of all sensory systems that are represented in the brain. The neurons located in V1 send their axons to three main brain regions: (1) the *extrastriate visual cortices (Brodmann's area 18* or regions *V2, V3, V3a,* and *V4)* for additional processing of the visual signal; (2) the superior colliculus to modulate eye movements; and (3) the lateral geniculate nucleus to have central control of the sensory input.

Neurons in the extrastriate cortex will then project to: the *medial temporal cortex (Brodmann's area 19*), the *inferotemporal cortex (Brodmann's areas 20* and *21*), and the *posterior parietal cortex (Brodmann's area 7*). From the output cells of the retina—the ganglion cells—a represented map is found not only in the lateral geniculate nuclei but also in the striate and the extrastriate cortices. In fact, there are six retinotopic maps in the occipital lobe with one each in: V1, V2, V3, V3a, V4, and in the *middle temporal area* that borders the temporal and occipital lobes (called V5, which is important for the perception of movement). In addition, the retinal representations are found in the inferotemporal cortex and in the posterior parietal cortex (Brodmann's area 7a). The posterior parietal cortex is responsible for integrating both somatic and visual sensations together. These topographical maps of the retina throughout the visual system show how the visual signals are conserved and organized so that the object's information is preserved in the brain.

The flow of neuronal connections within the visual cortex is different depending upon the animal species. In humans, neurons in the striate and extrastriate cortices process the most basic information, such as light intensity, colors, lines and edges making "bars," and orientation. For examples, neurons in V1 and V2 are activated when specific orientations of bars or combinations of bars are seen in a specific region of the visual field. It is thought that this helps with identifying corners and edges of the image, which are important for visual perception. As visual information passes through the hierarchy of the visual cortex, the processing becomes more and more complex, making the image more realistic.

As the object's visual signal reaches the visual association cortices (Brodmann's areas 7, 19, 20, and 21), the neurons will respond to complete objects that were seen in the visual field. This means that cells in the visual association cortex will be activated when a specific type of bird, like an adult bald eagle, is seen. This information is then moved into two different pathways of the brain, called the *ventral* and *dorsal streams,* to identify "what" the object is and "where" it is in space compared to the person. The ventral stream sends signals toward the temporal lobe while the dorsal stream sends signals toward the parietal lobe. The ventral stream is used in recognizing that the object is a "bird," then identifying the object as "an adult eagle," and then applying it to a specific category "an adult bald eagle." The dorsal stream will take the surrounding environment of the adult bald eagle to help place its location in reference to the person. This is called spatial attention.

Visual Perception

Visual perception takes the information from visual processing and attempts to "make sense" of the object. Additionally, visual perception is important for the *perception of movement,* the *perception of depth,* and *figure-ground perception.* These three types of visual perception are based in *Gestalt psychology,* which tries to understand how the human eye sees objects first as a whole and then as a sum of its individual parts. It also looks at how the entire object is anticipated even when the parts are not integrated, such as filling in the "blind spots" of the visual field to complete the entire image.

Dominant Eye Test

Humans do not only have a dominant hand (right or left), but also have a *dominant eye.* This develops during childhood and has a critical period for development. The medical term for dominant eye is *ocular dominance.* It means that one eye is preferred for visual input over the other eye. Ocular dominance may not be on the same side as the person's dominant hand. This is because both the left and right hemispheres of the brain control vision as well as control different halves of the visual field and of each retina (the back of the eye where objects are visually formed). Just like most humans are right handed, most are also right-eye dominant.

There are two easy ways to determine a person's dominant eye. Both tests start with having the person hold their arms out at eye level. Next have the person make the letter "L" with each hand. Specifically, have their palms outward, fingers up, and thumbs out—making the L-shape. Have the person bring their hands together and cross one over the other. This makes a triangle space: one thumb over the other and one set of fingers over the other. Now have the person look through the triangle at an object with both eyes. It is preferable to have the entire object almost completely fill the space. Now the two tests alter. Test one: keeping the hands together, have the person bring their hands back to their face toward one eye. If the image stays within the open space, that is the person's dominant eye. Now have the person start over and bring their hands back to the other eye. The object should completely disappear from the opening. Test two: keeping the hands together, have the person close one eye and then the other. If the image stays within the open space, that is the person's dominant eye. The object will look to "jump" sideways when the dominant eye is closed.

To perceive movement, the neurons located in region V5 are activated when the speed and direction of an object are seen. In humans, the vestibular system is also necessary for understanding motion perception. This is because it compares the speed of the person against the speed of the object to determine the motion. There are some people who cannot perceive movement. This rare condition is called *akinetopsia*. Persons with akinetopsia see the world in several "still" pictures instead of fluid actions. Research has shown that these individuals have a lesion in V5, thus confirming the location of motion perception.

Seeing the world in three dimensions (3D) and how far an object is from a person is called depth perception. This perception is best with binocular vision as well as utilizing depth cues such *stereopsis, parallax,* and *convergence of the eyes.* Stereopsis is the impression of depth by viewing a 3D scene (or external environment) with both eyes. The different locations of each eye on the head present a disparity in what is seen, which is then processed by the brain to perceive depth. Parallax is used to determine distance by looking at an object at two different lines of sight and measuring it against the angle made by the two lines. Closer objects have a larger parallax compared to far objects. Using parallax is how ancient astronomers determined the distance of the moon, sun, and stars. Finally, the inward movement of both eyes (looking toward the center) is called convergence. This helps in focusing the object onto the retina and producing binocular vision and stereopsis.

In figure-ground perception, it is the process of determining a "figure" from the "background." For example, it is how you are reading this entry and seeing each letter and word as its own figure and not part of the white background (or white paper). Specifically, figure-ground perception looks at edges (or borders) of the figure as well as its shape, so that it can be perceived in the brain as a singular object. One of the most famous figure-ground perception examples comes from Danish psychologist Edgar Rubin (1886–1951). It is a vase-face drawing that is also considered an optical illusion. The vase is white and in the middle of a black background. However, the black looks like two faces looking at each other with a white space between them. This drawing—called the Rubin vase—focuses on the edges of the vase, which are also the edges of the two faces. Depending if the person focuses on the white side of the border, the brain will see a white vase. But, if the person focuses on the black sides of the edges, the brain will interpret the image as two faces. The visual system will go back and forth between the two images and the two interpretations.

For the brain to determine which to look at as the "figure" and the "ground," it uses other cues that are based on the size, the shape, the color, and the movement of the object. Generally, the object is smaller than the background, the shape tends to be curved—particularly convex, the color is more distinct and varied for an object compared to the "monotone" color of the background, and the movement of the object is faster than the "static" background.

Jennifer L. Hellier

See also: Blind Spot; Color Blindness; Hubel, David H.; Occipital Lobe; Optic Nerve; Retina; Sensory Receptors; Tunnel Vision; Visual Fields; Visual System; Wiesel, Torsten N.

Further Reading

Bear, M. F., Connors, B. W., & Paradiso, M. A. (2007). *Neuroscience exploring the brain* (3rd ed.). Baltimore, MD: Lippincott Williams & Wilkins.

Dragoi, V., & Tsuchitani, C. (1997). Visual processing: Cortical pathways. In *Neuroscience Online, an electronic textbook for the neurosciences* (Chap. 15). Open-access educational resource provided by the Department of Neurobiology and Anatomy at the University of Texas Medical School at Houston. Retrieved from http://neuroscience.uth.tmc.edu/s2/chapter15.html

Kandel, E. R., Schwartz, J. H., Jessell, T. M., Siegelbaum, S. A., & Hudspeth, A. J. (Eds.). (2012). *Principles of neural science* (5th ed.). New York, NY: McGraw-Hill.

Purves, D., Augustine, G. J., Fitzpatrick, D., Hall, W. C., LaMantia, A. S., McNamara, J. O., & Williams, S. M. (Eds.). (2004). *Neuroscience* (3rd ed.). Sunderland, MA: Sinauer Associates.

Visual System

The *visual system* is a sensory system that is responsible for the sense of sight or vision. This vision can be monocular (one eye without depth perception) or binocular (two eyes with depth perception). Animals are highly visual, particularly mammals and humans, as this sensory system helps them see their prey, see their food, and see their surroundings. The visual system is one of the most well-studied central nervous system processes as vision is extremely important to humans. The visual system is comprised of several structures, all of which collect and concentrate light and images from the eye to the brain, so that these stimuli can be interpreted in the brain. *Visual perception,* however, consists of the psychological process of how a person sees a visual image. Because of this difference, visual perception is a separate entry in this encyclopedia. Furthermore, this entry will focus on mammalian and human visual systems.

History

Between the years of 600–400 BC, the ancient Greeks were the first to name the anatomical structures associated with vision. However, it took more than half a century for humans to understand the visual pathway to the brain, which was discovered by Galen of Pergamon (AD 130–200). Galen, who is officially named Claudius Galenus, is considered the most accomplished Roman physician for his dissection techniques and drawings and was the first person to diagram the visual pathway from the eyes to the brain. Scientists today are still amazed at his precision in many anatomical and physiological understandings of the human body for his time. Nonetheless, he made some anatomical mistakes that are now better understood with more modern scientific tools and techniques. For example, Galen's anatomical depiction of the optic chiasm (meaning "cross") did not have a true decussation (cross over) of the optic nerve. We know today that some of these fibers do cross while others continue on the same side that they originated, as shown by Galen. Other errors in anatomy were driven by the beliefs in the second century. At the time, nerves were considered to be hollow conduits that carried an individual's "spirits" within the brain. Thus, Galen drew some of the optic nerve fibers to the lateral ventricles to show the "visual spirit." It is now known that these fibers actually terminate in the lateral geniculate nucleus, which is part of the thalamus and helps form the walls of the lateral ventricles.

Today, modern understanding and particularly the neurophysiology of the visual system are attributed to Canadian neurophysiologist David H. Hubel (1926–2013) and Swedish neurophysiologist Torsten N. Wiesel (1924–). Together, Hubel and Wiesel won the 1981 Nobel Prize in Physiology or Medicine for their contributions to neuroscience about vision and are considered the fathers of the visual system.

Anatomy and Physiology

The visual system is made up of several anatomical structures. This entry will focus on the main and primary anatomical structures including: the *eye*—and its *retina; optic nerves*—the output of the retina and are the second pair of cranial nerves (which are nerves that supply motor and sensory function to just the head, neck, and face); *optic chiasm; optic tract; lateral geniculate nucleus; optic radiation; visual cortex;* and *visual association cortex.* Since mammals have two eyes, all of the aforementioned structures are found in both the left and right sides of the brain, except for the optic chiasm. There is only one optic chiasm, as this is where the left and right optic nerves come together and cross some of their fibers.

Eye

The eye is a complex organ that acts like a camera as it uses the laws of optics, which are based in physics. The eye uses light from an external object to focus an image onto its photoreceptors (specialized proteins that respond to light). These photoreceptors are found at the posterior portion (back) of the eye in the retina. To help focus the light and project the image, the eye will refract the incoming light first through the cornea—a transparent structure at the anterior portion (front) of the eye that covers the iris (the color of an eye that controls the size of the pupil), pupil (a natural hole in the center of the iris), and anterior chamber. It then passes through the pupil and is refracted again via the lens (a transparent, biconvex structure). Together, the cornea and the lens act like a compound lens to project the image upside down on the retina.

Retina

The retina is made up of 10 distinct layers of neurons (specialized cells that transmit nerve impulses) that will modulate the light stimulus. The neural processing of the retina is very complex but can be reduced to four main stages: photoreception, transmission to bipolar cells, transmission to ganglion cells, and transmission to the optic nerve. Of all the different neurons within the retina, there are only two types of photoreceptor cells that respond to light (photoreception): the *rods* and the *cones.* The rods respond to dim light (such as moonlight) and produce black-and-white vision; while the cones respond to bright light (such as daylight) and produce color vision. Surrounding neurons within the other layers of the retina modulate the output signals from the rods and cones and then transfer this information to the bipolar cells. Further modulation of the signals is performed and the bipolar cells transmit this information to the ganglion cells, the outmost layer of the retina. Finally, the ganglion cells' axons produce action potentials that travel along the optic nerve into the brain.

Optic Nerves

The optic nerves are a pair of cranial nerves that transmit information about an image from the eye to the brain. The output of the retina consists of ganglion cells and their axons, which make up the optic nerves. The optic nerves travel along the underside (ventral portion) of the brain. The representation of the visual world within the fields of vision (either from the nasal half of the visual field or the temporal half) travels within the optic nerves all the way to the back of the brain. These brain regions are called the occipital lobes. But before the signals reach their final destinations, they must be processed by relaying the information to other brain structures. The majority of the axons travels to the thalamus (a deep brain structure) and terminates within the lateral geniculate nucleus (a group of cell bodies). The remaining axons travel to the superior colliculus in the midbrain (part of the brainstem), which is important for moving the head when something "catches the eye" and for controlling eye movements called saccades.

Optic Chiasm

As previously stated, the optic chiasm is where the optic nerves from both eyes meet and cross. However, not all of the fibers will cross. The optic chiasm can be found at the base of the hypothalamus. It looks like a large white "X" because of the large number of myelinated (a protective covering that helps transmit nerve impulses faster) axons. This crossing of information is important because it takes specific halves of the visual fields and projects them to specific halves of the brain. This means that the left halves of the visual fields of both eyes are crossed over and projected to the right cerebral hemisphere, while the right halves of the visual field of both eyes are sent to the left cerebral hemisphere. Small portions of the optic nerve axons that arrive from the centers of both visual fields are projected to both hemispheres for redundancy purposes.

Optic Tract

The optic tract begins immediately after the optic chiasm and eventually splits into two divisions: the left and right optic tracts. The information carried within these tracts is exclusive to the same side as its visual field. This means that images seen in the left half of the visual field will flow into the left optic tract and the right visual field halves enter the right optic tract. These tracts follow the posterior (behind) portion of the thalamus and end in the lateral geniculate nucleus.

Lateral Geniculate Nucleus

The term geniculate means to bend as this nucleus wraps to the lateral side of the posterior part of the thalamus and is ellipsoid in shape. The lateral geniculate nucleus is separated into six distinct layers with each layer receiving certain visual information. These layers have either parvocellular or magnocellular neurons, which are the target neurons for specific axons within the optic tract. Both of these neurons are relatively large and have specific functions. Parvocellular neurons are commonly called P cells and are necessary for processing color and edges of an image; while magnocellular neurons or M cells are important for depth perception and motion. Additionally, K cells (neurons within the retina that help with color vision) terminate on small neurons lying between the six layers. Layers one, four, and six receive information from the contralateral (opposite side) temporal visual field, while layers two, three, and five receive information from the ipsilateral (same side) nasal visual field. The output of the P, M, and K cells will make the optic radiation and end in the primary visual cortex.

Optic Radiation

From the left and right lateral geniculate nuclei, visual information is sent to the V1 region of the occipital lobe via the left and right optic radiations. V1 of the occipital lobe is also called the primary visual cortex and has six layers of neurons. The optic radiations move posteriorly and medially (toward the middle) to the most posterior portion of the occipital lobe. The axons of the P cells of the lateral geniculate nucleus will terminate in layer 4Cβ, while the M cells will end in layer 4Cα. Finally, the K cells will connect to blobs (large neurons) located in layers two and three of V1. Up to now, visual signals have been processed relatively straightforward. This will change once the signal enters the visual cortex.

Visual Cortex

The visual cortex is responsible for processing image information. In humans, it makes up the largest of the sensory systems that are represented in the brain. The visual cortex has a hierarchy of regions starting with V1, which is the primary visual cortex and is also called the striate cortex for its striped look. This region's input comes directly from the lateral geniculate nucleus. The extrastriate visual cortices are regions V2, V3, V4, and V5. The flow of connections is different depending upon the animal species. These secondary visual areas are necessary for processing the most basic information, such as light intensity, colors, lines and edges making "bars," and orientation. For examples, neurons in V1 and V2 are activated when specific orientations of bars or combinations of bars are seen in a specific region of the visual field. It is thought that this helps with identifying corners and edges of the image. As visual information passes through the hierarchy of the visual cortex, the processing becomes more and more complex making the image more realistic.

Ocular Dominance Columns

The visual system is the most well-studied sensory system of animals. From these studies it is known that processing vision within the brain is extremely complex. Part of this processing occurs within *ocular dominance columns*. Ocular dominance columns are groups of neurons that span several layers of the primary visual cortex. They are anatomical structures that make up the striate cortex, which is a portion of the primary visual cortex. Ocular dominance columns are found as a striped pattern on the surface of the striate cortex. They are perpendicular to another set of cells that make up the orientation columns. Drs. David H. Hubel (1926–2013) and Torsten N. Wiesel (1924–) discovered ocular dominance columns during their research in the primary visual cortices of cats. Since these experiments, ocular dominance columns have been found in many mammals, including humans.

These columns are activated primarily from the input of one eye and not the other. They develop before birth but can degrade during the critical period required for developing vision. Hubel and Wiesel found that blocking vision in one eye during the critical period resulted in the unaffected eye developing ocular columns in regions of the striate cortex that would normally be developed by the blocked eye. Originally, ocular dominance columns were hypothesized to be important for binocular vision. However, these columns are not as distinct or well developed in all animals with binocular vision, such as rats and squirrel monkeys. Now, scientists are wondering if ocular dominance columns are more a result of development particularly from synaptic plasticity or Hebbian learning. These functions can occur from the spontaneous activity of the retina of the developing fetus or from the lateral geniculate nucleus that projects to the striate cortex.

Jennifer L. Hellier

See also: Hubel, David H.; Wiesel, Torsten N.

Further Reading

Rice, M. L., Leske, D. A., Smestad, C. E., & Holmes, J. M. (2008). Results of ocular dominance testing depend on assessment method. *Journal of American Association of Pediatric Ophthalmology and Strabismus, 12*(4), 365–9.

Visual Association Cortex

Finally, the visual association cortex receives information from the hierarchy of the visual cortex. Here, the neurons will respond to complete objects that were seen in the visual field. For example, cells in the visual association cortex will be activated when a specific type of car, like a red Toyota Prius, is seen. This information is then moved into two different pathways of the brain, called the ventral and dorsal streams, to identify "what" the object is and "where" it is in space. The ventral stream moves toward the temporal lobe, while the dorsal stream moves to toward the parietal lobe. The ventral stream is used in first recognizing that the object is a "vehicle," then identifying the object as a "red car," and then applying it to a specific category "a red Toyota Prius." The dorsal stream will take the surrounding environment of the red Toyota Prius to help place its location in reference to the person. This is called spatial attention.

Jennifer L. Hellier

See also: Blind Spot; Color Blindness; Hubel, David H.; Occipital Lobe; Optic Nerve; Retina; Sensory Receptors; Tunnel Vision; Visual Fields; Visual Perception (Visual Processing); Wiesel, Torsten N.

Further Reading

Bear, M. F., Connors, B. W., & Paradiso, M. A. (2007). *Neuroscience exploring the brain* (3rd ed.). Baltimore, MD: Lippincott Williams & Wilkins.

Kandel, E. R., Schwartz, J. H., Jessell, T. M., Siegelbaum, S. A., & Hudspeth, A. J. (Eds.). (2012). *Principles of neural science* (5th ed.). New York, NY: McGraw-Hill.

Martins Rosa, A., Silva, M. F., Ferreira, S., Murta, J., & Castelo-Branco, M. (2013). Plasticity in the human visual cortex: An ophthalmology-based perspective. *BioMed Research International*, 2013, 568354. doi:10.1155/2013/568354. Retrieved from http://www.ncbi.nlm.nih.gov/pubmed/24205505

Von Hippel-Lindau Syndrome

Von Hippel-Lindau syndrome (VHL) is a rare autosomal-dominant (non-sex chromosome-dominant) condition, which predisposes carriers to grow both malignant and benign cysts and tumors. Although this disorder occurs throughout the body in multiple systems in the central nervous system (CNS), tumors preferentially grow near the cerebellum. *Hemangioblastomas*, which are highly vascularized benign tumors found in the brain, spinal cord, and retina (part of the eye) are the most common type of tumor generally seen in patients with VHL. Patients with VHL experience dizziness, headaches, vision problems, high blood pressure, difficulties with balance and walking, and weakness in the limbs. This syndrome affects both sexes equally and occurs in all ethnic groups. Approximately one out of every 32,000 people has VHL. Eighty percent of these cases are inherited, whereas the remaining 20 percent are considered new mutations. Most individuals affected by VHL do not present any clinical symptoms until after they are 80 years or older. Treatment for VHL varies based on the size and location of the tumor, and the standard of practice involves surgical removal of the mass. A more modern but not necessarily more ideal approach is the use of stereotactic radiosurgery. Prognosis also varies depending upon the size and location of the tumor, and early detection followed by total removal of the tumor is essential. Unfortunately, individuals affected by VHL generally have multiple tumors and multisystem complications are common causes of death.

History

Two individuals first discovered Von Hippel-Lindau disease in the early 1900s independently. Dr. Eugen von Hippel (1867–1938) was a German physician who was fascinated with disorders in the development of the eye. In 1904 he wrote "about a very rare disease of the retina" and several years later in 1911, he commented on the anatomical origin of the disease; he termed the disease angiomatosis retinae. In 1929, Dr. Arvid Lindau (1892–1958) also wrote about a similar condition. Lindau, a Swedish physician, began to link a condition of hemangiomas of the CNS to the retinal disorder that had been previously described by Dr. von Hippel. Lindau's findings earned him the prestigious Lennmalm's Prize (1929) from the Swedish Medical Society. Lindau's close relationship with Dr. Harvey Cushing (1869–1939), who is revered as the father of modern neurosurgery, allowed for Dr. Cushing to make Lindau's findings known in the United States. Although doctors von Hippel and Lindau published their findings in the early part of the 20th century, it took until 1969 for VHL syndrome to receive its current name.

Types, Treatments, and Outcomes

VHL in the central CNS involves the growth of hemangioblastoma tumors found near the cerebellum, retina, or cerebrum. While these tumors are benign, they provide the environment that lends to the growth of cysts (fluid-filled sacs) as well as benign or malignant tumors around the hemangioblastoma. These secondary growths often apply pressure on surrounding nervous tissue leading to the general symptoms of VHL. Within VHL, there exist four distinct subtypes based on the individual's genetics.

VHL syndrome is a genetically inherited autosomal-dominant disorder that is related to the tumor-suppressor gene *VHL*. It is hypothesized that the normal function of this gene is to prevent the growth of tumors; however, patients with VHL syndrome suffer from a loss-of-function mutation resulting in the *VHL* gene to be muted. Thus, patients with VHL have a higher occurrence of tumors than the general population. The four subtypes of VHL are based on the symptoms that are derived from different VHL mutations; the subtypes are Type 1, Type 2A, Type 2B, and Type 2C. However, scientists are debating whether Type 2C actually exists.

Type 1 results from a deletion of the *VHL* gene and has a strong chance of tumor occurrence in the CNS, low risk of adrenal gland tumors, and a high risk of renal (kidney) and pancreatic tumors. Type 2A results from the *VHL* gene being substituted by an amino acid. It carries a strong chance of CNS tumor occurrence as well as adrenal tumors, but a low risk of renal and pancreatic tumors. Type 2B results from a deletion of the *VHL* gene and carries a high risk for all tumor types. Type 2C results from an amino acid substitution of the *VHL* gene. It statistically has a high risk for adrenal tumors but low risk for CNS, renal, and pancreatic tumors.

Treatment for VHL tumors is dependent upon the location and size of the growth. Additionally, it is imperative that health care providers correctly diagnose the patient with VHL, as it is a complex multisystem affective genetic disorder and a tumor of the cerebellum can be directly related to a tumor of the kidneys; if these are treated as separate instances, the prognosis becomes less optimistic. Typical treatment involves a neurosurgeon to resect the tumor in an aggressive manner while still leaving adjacent tissue intact. In the event that the location and/or size of the tumor does not allow a safe approach for the surgeon, an experimental procedure such as stereotactic radiosurgery may be used.

VHL is currently not curable, and the prognosis for patients with this disorder varies depending on the size and location of the mass. It is important to note that this is a genetic disorder, meaning that even if a tumor is fully removed from the patient, there is a high probability of tumor recurrence. With early detection and treatment, prognosis is greatly improved and, in some cases, complications can be completely avoided.

Future

VHL research is being conducted to help with earlier detection, improving prognosis, and even working toward a cure. Scientists can now perform genetic screening for the presence of the *VHL* gene, allowing the ability to rule-out individuals from having the disorder as well as creating a precedent for screening families known to have the genetic abnormality. The research of Marston Linehan, currently at the National Cancer Institute, focuses on the metabolic properties of these tumors. Linehan performs studies on interrupting glycolysis for these tumors as an effective approach to treatment. Specifically for CNS-related VHL, scientists are developing new multimodal drug and gene therapies.

Eric W. Prince

See also: Cerebellum; Cerebral Cortex; Dizziness and Vertigo; Retina

Further Reading

Genetic and Rare Diseases Information Center (GARD). (n.d.). *Hemangioblastoma.* Retrieved from http://rarediseases.info.nih.gov/GARD/Condition/8232/Hemangioblastoma.aspx

National Institute of Neurological Disorders and Stroke. (2010). *NINDS Von Hippel-Lindau disease (VHL) information page.* Retrieved from http://www.ninds.nih.gov/disorders/von_hippel_lindau/von_hippel_lindau.htm

The VHL Family Alliance. (2013). *VHL Family Alliance.* Retrieved from http://www.vhl.org/

W

Waldeyer-Hartz, Heinrich W. G., von (1836–1921)

Heinrich Wilhelm Gottfried von Waldeyer-Hartz (commonly referred to as "Waldeyer") was an anatomist from Germany. He is most famous for consolidating the neuron theory—which is used to describe the organization of the nervous system—and developing the term "neuron" to describe the basic structural unit of the nervous system. With his expertise in anatomy, Waldeyer coined the term *chromosome* and has two large anatomical structures named after him: the *Waldeyer's tonsillar ring* and *Waldeyer's gland.* Waldeyer's tonsillar ring is the lymphoid tissue ring of the naso- and oro-pharynx, while the glands of the eyelid are called the Waldeyer's glands. In addition, the sheath that encircles the terminal ureter is commonly named the Waldeyer sheath.

Waldeyer's work was based on other discoveries made by neuroanatomists Camillo Golgi (1843–1926) and Santiago Ramon y Cajal (1852–1934). Golgi and Cajal designed and used a silver nitrate method of staining nervous tissue. This stain allowed Golgi and Cajal to study the branching processes of nerve cells (axons and dendrites). The observed interconnections of the nerve cells appear to form chains and neural networks which helped to explain the transfer of information between neurons. At the time Golgi and Cajal were developing a theory to describe the structures and functions of the central nervous system; however, they had opposing ideas. Golgi was in favor of the *syncytium theory,* while Cajal was in favor of the *neuron doctrine.* This was an ongoing discussion between several top neuroscientists during the late 1800s and early 1900s. Waldeyer was interested in the topic and learned Spanish to be able to discuss his viewpoints with Cajal. Waldeyer's friendship and mentee relationship with Cajal helped to develop additional recognition of Cajal's work to the Germans, who were the dominant experts in microscopy at the time. With Waldeyer's influence, he introduced Cajal's theories by publishing them as a series of articles in the *Deutsche Medizinische Wochenschrift,* which is the main medical journal of Germany. Thus, Cajal's work was recognized by many more scientists, which helped his neuron doctrine (or neuron theory) to be the most accepted. The neuron doctrine is still used today by neuroscientists.

Waldeyer was born in Braunschweig, Germany, and attended school at Paderborn, which started his interest in math and science. In 1856, Waldeyer was accepted to the University of Gottingen. While at the university, he met the famous anatomist Friedrich Gustav Jacob Henle (1809–1885) and instantly became interested in anatomy and changed his major from mathematics to natural sciences. He continued his studies in medicine under the influence of Henle until 1859 when he transferred to the University of Greifswald and studied under Julius Ludwig Budge (1811–1888) at the anatomy institute. Waldeyer eventually moved to Berlin and became a professor at the University of Berlin for more than 33 years.

Jennifer M. Sorgatz

See also: Central Nervous System (CNS); Introduction: Neuroscience Overview; Neuron

Further Reading

von Waldeyer, W. (1891). Ueber einige neuere Forschungen im Gebiete der Anatomie des central nerven systems. *Deutsche Medicinische Wochenschrift, 17,* 1213–1218, 1244–1246, 1287–1289, 1331–1332, 1350–1356. (His most famous statement and summary of the neuron theory).

Who Named It. (2013). *Heinrich Wilhelm Gottfried von Waldeyer-Hartz.* Retrieved from http://www.whonamedit.com/doctor.cfm/1846.html

Wernicke's Area

Wernicke's area is a region of the human brain that is thought to mediate the interpretation and comprehension of spoken and written language. When Wernicke's area is injured, most commonly following a stroke, the result is a form of *aphasia*. An aphasia occurs when a person is unable to communicate, both verbally and written. When a person has aphasia resulting from injury to Wernicke's area, a condition known as Wernicke's aphasia, the words spoken by the patient flow freely but they are nonsensical and difficult to interpret.

History

Wernicke's area was originally described by a 26-year-old German physician named Karl Wernicke (1848–1905). His paper, published in 1874, discussed two patients he had seen that had profound deficits in their comprehension of the spoken language. Though they had no problems forming sounds, the sounds that they formed did not resemble any words in German or any other language. This has been described more recently as "cocktail chatter." Further, the patients did not appear to notice that anything had been disrupted with their speech patterns. Upon examination of one of the patient's brains at autopsy, Wernicke noticed a lesion in the left hemisphere, just posterior to, or behind, the primary auditory cortex. This portion of the brain has been shown to be responsible for sound processing and ultimately hearing. Wernicke's original description is what caused the region to later be known as Wernicke's area.

Prior to the discovery of Wernicke's area, a surgeon named Pierre Paul Broca (1824–1880) had defined and written about another region of the brain that seemed to control a distinct, and separate aspect of language from that controlled by Wernicke's area. This area is now known as Broca's area. The patient that Broca's descriptions were based on, in addition to having a right-sided hemiparesis or weakness, had difficulty forming words. Unlike Wernicke's patients that were able to form words that did not make any sense, Broca's patient had the ability to utter just a single, albeit recognizable syllable. Also unlike Wernicke's patients, Broca's patient seemed to understand what he was being told; however, he just was not able to articulate his thoughts through words. Broca's patient died several days later, and upon autopsy Broca noticed a lesion in the frontal lobe on the third gyrus, or ridge of the brain, which is now known as Broca's area.

Anatomy and Physiology

The exact location of Wernicke's area has been the subject of debate since its original description in 1874. In other words, the precise region that needs to be lesioned to produce the symptoms of the resultant affliction known as Wernicke's aphasia is not rigidly defined. One commonly used method for describing locations in the human brain is using the "Brodmann's Area" numerical system. Similar to the Dewey Decimal System commonly employed in libraries to make book finding easier, Brodmann's Areas are named for regions in which the cells are thought to participate in a similar function as those surrounding it. They were originally numbered solely for structural similarities, but this has changed over the years. Wernicke's area is also known as Brodmann Area 22, which corresponds to a location that is above and slightly behind the left ear. The function of the brain regions surrounding Wernicke's area, as well as some of the regions that Wernicke's area communicates with from afar, provide insight into the function of Wernicke's area. The best way to determine the function of a brain region is to see what happens when that area is injured or damaged. Specifically for Brodmann area 22, when it is injured, it produces particular defects in the comprehension of language.

The general region of the brain that Wernicke's area is located in is known as the temporal lobe. The temporal lobe has many functions in addition to those performed by Wernicke's area, including memory storage and the processing of sensory information. The particular portion of the temporal lobe that contains Wernicke's area is known as the *posterior superior temporal lobe,* which simply means the upper rear part of the temporal lobe. One of the main functions of the neurons contained within this area is to allow the person to understand sounds that he or she has heard, whether that be another voice, his or her own voice, or various inputs from the environment. There are also neurons in or near Wernicke's area that are responsible for the comprehension of written communication or visual information.

However, Wernicke's area is not the first stop for this type of auditory information. After being sensed by specialized cells within a person's ear, the sound information travels to several regions, such as the primary auditory cortex (Brodmann area 41). The information continues on to the higher-order auditory cortex (Brodmann area 42). Here, preliminary processing of the sound input occurs. Not long afterward, this information is sent to Wernicke's area so that it is interpreted as sound or as language. Wernicke's area helps a person make sense of the sounds that he or she has heard, and allows them to comprehend words that are heard in everyday interactions. After Wernicke's area comes Broca's area. The sound information, having now been processed by Wernicke's area, is sent to Broca's area (Brodmann area 45) via projections known as the *arcuate fasiculus.* In Broca's area, the sounds are processed into a certain structure, such as that of a sentence or of a phrase.

Disease, Symptoms, and Treatment

Disease and injury help neuroscientists understand where language is processed in the brain and specifically what functions these regions perform in the auditory processing pathway. Similar to Karl Wernicke's initial studies, much of this anatomical information has been determined during autopsies of patients with particular conditions. If it was observed frequently enough that people with particular symptoms had lesions in specific regions of their brains, scientists could then study those regions. This process allows neuroscientists to (1) assign specific functions to the brain region, (2) understand how the central nervous system interpret signals from the outside world, and (3) determine how the damaged area communicates with other regions of the brain to perform complex functions. Understanding the function and dysfunction of different brain regions is an important first step toward ultimately treating and curing diseases associated with those areas.

While correlations between symptoms and brain regions can be informative from a scientific perspective, these same symptoms can be tragic and life changing for the individual patient experiencing them. Symptoms associated with lesions to Wernicke's area can be catastrophic for the patient and unfortunately this is a brain region that is commonly affected in certain disease states, particularly *stroke*.

Though there are several mechanisms in which Wernicke's area can be injured, by far the most common is stroke. Stroke comes in multiple forms, including bleeding or hemorrhaging into particular regions in the brain, or from blockage of arteries supplying blood to the brain. Like all cells in an organism's body, the *neurons* in the brain require a continual supply of oxygen. This allows the neurons to make the energy they need to perform their functions. When the supply of oxygen is disrupted, as it is in stroke, cells can be damaged. If neurons in the brain are damaged, it may lead to cell death and the functions that they perform will be lost. Using MRI (magnetic resonance imaging) technology, a physician will be able to (1) visualize the particular regions of the brain that have been damaged by the loss of oxygen, (2) begin to understand the symptoms the patients will experience, (3) determine what functions a patient may be able to recover, and (4) realize possible options for therapy and treatment.

One of the most common arteries to be affected in stroke is the middle cerebral artery (MCA). This is a large artery that supplies blood to many regions of the brain. The temporal lobe, which contains Wernicke's area, receives a large portion of its blood supply from the MCA. When the MCA is blocked, for instance by a blood clot, the temporal lobe and Wernicke's area can be permanently damaged. When brain regions that are responsible for understanding or formulating spoken language are damaged, the result is a condition known as an *aphasia*. In fact, one of the earliest warning signs of a stroke can be disruption of normal speaking patterns. Recognizing the typical signs of stroke may facilitate timely intervention, resulting in increased survival rates and a better quality of life following the event.

Many different forms of aphasia have been identified. The function that is lost as a result of the brain injury determines the type of aphasia that the patient will experience. When Wernicke's area is injured, the kind of aphasia that occurs has been termed *receptive aphasia*. It is also commonly referred to as Wernicke's aphasia. Other types of aphasia include (1) Broca's aphasia, (2) conduction aphasia, and (3) global aphasia. Because the neurons contained within Wernicke's area are involved in comprehension of language, both spoken and visual, Wernicke's or receptive aphasia displays deficits in these fields. Specifically, the patient will have no trouble formulating sounds, but will be unable to comprehend both the words he or she is speaking, and the words being spoken to them. The result is a situation that is often described as "cocktail chatter," otherwise known as *logorrhea* or *press of speech.* The words flow freely and in a generally normal cadence and rhythm, but are nonsensical and confused. For example, if a patient with Wernicke's aphasia is asked what time it is, they may respond with, "A car and a candy bar are both worth one hundred dollars and both are very tasty and move faster than the speed of light." If portions of Wernicke's area that are responsible for comprehension of visual language are impaired, the patient may also be unable to understand written language, which can affect both reading and writing.

Once damage to the brain occurs and a patient is stricken with aphasia, options for treatment and regeneration are limited. If the cause of the patient's aphasia is a stroke, timely intervention can result in spared tissue (meaning decreased cell death) and function. Specifically, health care providers may try to break the blood clot that is causing the stroke by administering a substance known as tissue plasminogen activator (tPA). tPA is a naturally produced chemical that breaks up clots, and when introduced at higher concentrations into the patient's system, it can dissolve the stroke-causing clot and hopefully restore blood flow to the damaged tissue. Sometimes, physicians are able to physically break up a stroke-causing clot by using advanced imaging techniques to probe the clot with a catheter that is threaded from an artery somewhere in the body.

To date, the options for curing aphasia are very limited. As stem cells and potential stem cell therapeutics are being increasingly well understood, it is possible that in the future, stem cells could be introduced to damaged regions to repopulate areas that have had extensive cell death. Patients with aphasia are prescribed speech therapy and have shown encouraging results. Because speech and language are both complex entities, it is likely that each case of aphasia is unique, and thus will respond uniquely to different treatment options.

Conclusion

Wernicke's area is a region in the brain of both historical and medical significance. The work performed by Karl Wernicke and others in describing it and the symptoms associated with damage to Brodmann area 22 are a prime example of this type of anatomical and clinical harmony. Because stroke is so commonplace in today's society, understanding the various symptoms that can result from them are important. As scientists become better at understanding the causes of stroke and aphasia, options for treatments and cures are anticipated to improve.

Christopher Knoeckel

See also: Aphasia; Broca's Area; Brodmann Areas; Language; Magnetic Resonance Imaging (MRI); Stroke

Further Reading

The Aphasia Center. (2012). *What is Wernicke's aphasia?* Retrieved from http://www.the aphasiacenter.com/2012/01/what-is-wernickes-aphasia/

Chulder, E. H. (n.d.). *"Oh say can you say" the brain and language.* Retrieved from http:// faculty.washington.edu/chudler/lang.html

Krestel, H., Annoni, J. M., & Jagella, C. (2013). White matter in aphasia: A historical review of the Dejerines' studies. *Brain Language.* S0093–934X(13)00117-X. doi:10.1016/j .bandl.2013.05.019.

Mayo Clinic Staff. (2012). *Aphasia.* Retrieved from http://www.mayoclinic.com/health /aphasia/DS00685

National Institute on Deafness and Other Communication Disorders (NIDCD). (2010). *Aphasia.* Retrieved from http://www.nidcd.nih.gov/health/voice/pages/aphasia.aspx

Scott, S. K. (2012). The neurobiology of speech perception and production—can functional imaging tell us anything we did not already know? *Journal of Communication Disorders, 45*(6), 419–425.

Whipple's Disease

Whipple's disease is caused by an infection from the bacterium *Tropheryma whipplei*. This bacterium affects all systems of the body but first attacks the gastrointestinal tract. Thus, it was originally thought to only affect the digestive system. Whipple's disease interferes with the body's ability to metabolize fats. The infection is long lasting and requires more than a year of antibiotics for treatment. Whipple's disease is seen more often in men than in women, and often infections can recur throughout a person's lifetime. In general, Whipple's disease is common in farmers as the bacteria are found in affected soils and animals. American pathologist George Hoyt Whipple (1878–1976) was the first to describe the clinical findings and researched the disorder, which he termed *lipodystrophia intestinalis*. Whipple also identified the bacteria that caused the injection. Thus, Whipple's disease and the bacterium were named after their founder.

The symptoms of Whipple's disease may include many of the following: (1) severe diarrhea, (2) weight loss, (3) fatigue, (4) general weakness, (5) gastrointestinal pain, (6) abnormal muscle movement of the face and eyes, (7) seizures, (8) confusion, (9) uncoordinated movements (ataxia), (10) memory loss, and (11) impaired vision. Other symptoms that may manifest are fever, joint pain, and coughing.

It is imperative to treat and cure Whipple's disease as soon as possible. This is because if left untreated, the infection is fatal. The main treatment is to use a class of antibiotics to kill the *Tropheryma whipplei* bacteria by subscribing a type of penicillin, tetracycline, or sulfonamide. The antibiotic must be taken for one to two years to be effective. Sulfonamides have been shown to treat the neurological symptoms of Whipple's disease. Recently, pairing doxycycline from the tetracycline class of antibiotics with hydroxychloroquine (an antimalarial drug) for about 18 months has shown to be most effective for curing Whipple's disease.

Jennifer L. Hellier

See also: Ataxia; Learning and Memory; Seizures

Further Reading

Mayo Clinic Staff. (2012). *Diseases and conditions: Whipple's disease.* Retrieved from http://www.mayoclinic.org/diseases-conditions/whipples-disease/basics/definition/CON-20025442

White Matter

White matter are specific areas of tissue within the central nervous system (CNS) which contain heavily bundled, myelinated, axonal fibers and glial cells. The myelin, which provides a fatty insulation to the axons, gives a whitish hue and is how it received the term "white matter." The major cellular components of white matter are axons, both myelinated and unmyelinated, glial cells such as astrocytes and oligodendrocytes, and blood vessels. The other area of the CNS which is rich in neuronal cell bodies is known as the gray matter. The function of white matter is to connect different areas of the brain and spinal cord to form a complex and intricate network in which cognitive and motor functions are tightly regulated. White matter is critical to transfer information processed by the neurons in the surrounding gray matter. Diseases of white matter can cause mild to severe changes in emotion, cognition, and motor functions. Differences in white matter volume have also been linked to behavioral diseases such as autism and psychiatric disorders such as schizophrenia.

History and Function

In 1543, in his seventh book entitled *De Humani Corporis Fabrica,* the Renaissance anatomist Andreas Vesalius (1514–1564) was the first to distinguish between white and gray matter in the cortex. He identified the corpus callosum, or largest white matter tract in the brain, and described it in great detail. In 1664, Marcello Malpighi (1628–1694) used a primitive method to show that white matter was composed of fibers. Throughout the next few centuries, scientists began discovering that there were many fiber tracts in the white matter, which connected different areas of the brain. In the late 1800s, breakthroughs using the Golgi staining method of potassium bichromate and silver nitrate staining to identify axons, and the development of methylene blue staining by Paul Ehrlich (1854–1915), allowed researchers to clearly distinguish all of the myelinated fibers of the CNS. Some of these staining techniques are still used today in neuroscience research.

The white matter of the brain consists of an abundance of myelinated axons. Myelin is a lipid-rich substance that ensheaths the axons in a process known as myelination. Myelin acts as an electrical insulator. Its function is to facilitate the speedy conduction of electrical impulses down a nerve fiber or axon. In the cerebral cortex, the outer layer consists of the gray matter containing neurons, while the white matter is located deep within. It is quite the opposite in the spinal cord, where the gray matter is centralized, and the white matter surrounds the gray matter. White matter development, or myelination, is quite a different process than the formation of gray matter. The neuronal population, which constitutes the majority of gray matter, contains a maximal number of neurons at birth. Humans are born with many more neurons than what are actually needed and after birth, neurons that do not form proper connections with other cells in the CNS will die. The process of myelination, which constitutes the areas of white matter, does not begin until after birth and progresses until young adulthood. During infancy, myelination begins around three months of age and moves in a head to toe direction, enabling motor skills to develop. The myelin sheath is critical for the rapid and synchronization of coordinated movements and higher order cognitive abilities, which correlates with the amount of myelin in the mammalian CNS. The prefrontal cortex, part of the brain involved in higher learning, is not completely myelinated until about 10 to 12 years of age. As humans get older, and experience cognitive decline, there is also a decrease in total white matter volume.

White matter consists of three different types of fibers: projection, association, and commissural. Each fiber type has specific functions and locations within the CNS. Projection fibers form the main descending tracts out of the brain to the muscles and the ascending tracts to the brain from the sensory receptors. Association fibers link one area of the cerebral cortex to another within the same hemisphere. These fibers do not cross to the other cortex. Lastly, commissural fibers carry information between the left and right hemispheres allowing them to communicate. These fibers make up the corpus callosum as well as the anterior and posterior commissures.

Areas of White Matter

Within the cerebrum, or largest part of the brain, the largest commissural fiber tract resides, known as the corpus callosum. This tract predominantly contains cortico-cortical axonal projections, connecting the left and right hemispheres of the brain. This allows the frontal lobes of the brain to have the highest degree of conductivity. Within the corpus callosum, specialized glial cells, known as oligodendrocytes, reside. Oligodendrocytes are the glial cells in the CNS, which make myelin. However, in the peripheral nervous system (PNS), Schwann cells produce myelin to the axons exiting the brain and spinal cord. Two smaller commissural tracts within the cerebrum are the anterior and posterior commissures, which connect the temporal lobes of the two hemispheres.

The second largest part of the brain is the cerebellum. The cerebellum is located below the cerebral cortex and participates in the integration of signals to fine-tune motor activity such as coordination and precision. It is also critical for maintaining equilibrium and regulating muscle tone involved in postural control. The cerebellum is composed of outer layers of gray matter surrounding an inner layer of centralized white matter. The different cell types in the cerebellum work together to reinforce accurate movements. Below the cerebellum is a white matter–enriched structure, the brainstem. The brainstem connects the cerebrum to the spinal cord and it is responsible for vital functions, such as breathing, heartbeat, and blood pressure.

Within the spinal cord, the white matter is composed of six ascending and descending tracts arranged in columns, known as funiculi. The ascending tracts regulate the signal transduction of sensory information from cutaneous receptors (receptors that are found in the skin—dermis and epidermis), proprioreceptors (receptors located in muscles and joints), and visceral receptors (receptors found in the internal organs or viscera). The descending tracts are responsible for relaying information from the motor cortex in the brain to the muscles in the body.

Disease of White Matter

Abnormalities of white matter can have other implications. Such abnormalities are classically known as demyelinating or dysmyelinating diseases. White matter is quite vulnerable, and can be damaged by toxins. White matter is also affected and damaged following a stroke, traumatic brain injury, or neurodegenerative disease. White matter may play a very important role in controlling our emotions and behavior. Abnormalities in cerebral white matter are associated with a spectrum of emotional disturbances. Psychiatric patients with known white matter disorders can suffer from depression, mania (an abnormally elevated mood), psychosis (a loss of understanding the difference between reality and not reality), and euphoria (intense happiness). Implications for white matter and its role in schizophrenia patients have been identified by brain imaging studies. These studies were able to detect microscopic abnormalities in white matter structures as well as widespread myelin and oligodendrocyte dysfunction that were linked with altered cerebral contact (Davis et al., 2003). Correlations have also been made between children with attention deficit/hyperactivity disorder and a diminished volume of right frontal lobe matter resulting in impaired sustained attention. In autism, it has been observed that there is an increase in volume of hemispheric white matter in all lobes.

The more classically known diseases of white matter can be classified into two groups. Dysmyelinating diseases are abnormalities in myelin protein production or the process of myelination during development, while demyelinating diseases include damage or loss of healthy myelin. Dysmyelinating diseases, otherwise known as leukodystrophies, are usually genetically inherited and can cover a broad spectrum of neurodegenerative disorders that affect the integrity of myelin throughout the body. A commonly occurring dysmyelinating disease in the PNS is Charcot-Marie-Tooth (CMT), which affects one in 2,500 people in the United States. CMT is a hereditary disease that can result from mutations in different genes. Other leukodystrophies include Krabbe disease, childhood ataxia with central nervous system hypomyelination or CACH (vanishing white matter disease), Alexander disease, Refsum disease, and Pelizaeus-Merzbacher disease. Symptoms can occur in infancy and early adolescence and can include movement and speech disorders as well as stunting in physical and mental health. While there are currently no cures for these disorders, preferred treatment is speech, physical, and occupational therapy including moderate strength training and aerobic exercise. Bone marrow transplantation may be available as a possible treatment in the future.

In the CNS, multiple sclerosis (MS) is the most common demyelinating disease. Worldwide, MS affects about 2.1 million people. MS is an immune-mediated disease such that the body's own immune system attacks itself, resulting in damage to the myelin and surrounding nerves. There are two forms of MS: relapse, which is characterized by acute episodic periods, and chronic MS, which is progressive deterioration. There are other known demyelinating diseases such as optic myelitis (damage to the optic nerve tract), transverse myelitis (inflammation of the spinal cord), acute disseminating encephalomyelitis (an immune-mediated disease that usually occurs after a viral infection), and adrenomyeloneuropathy (a group of inherited disorders that disrupts the breakdown of fats). For all demyelinating diseases, symptoms usually include vision deficits or loss, hearing loss, headaches, seizures, muscle spasms, weakness, loss of coordination, paralysis, and loss of sensation.

Currently, there is no cure for MS but there are therapeutic strategies to treat exacerbations and manage the symptoms. The National MS Society recommends that persons consider the Food and Drug Administration (FDA)-approved "disease-modifying" drugs to decrease the severity of episodic attacks and try to prevent further deterioration of the brain. With the available drugs to help manage the symptoms of the disease, rehabilitation and sustaining motor and cognitive function are possible.

Clinical diagnoses for most diseases of myelin include a neurological exam and imaging scans. Diagnosis of white matter diseases has rapidly progressed due to the advancements in neuro-imaging. Magnetic resonance imaging (MRI) is commonly used to assess white matter deficits in the brain. It is possible to distinguish white matter tracts using diffusion-weighted imaging (DWI) as an MRI method. DWI measures the dispersion of water in white matter tracts. In healthy white matter, water diffuses in the direction of the specific tract being imaged. In damaged white matter, water diffusion is isotrophic, less directional, and chaotic. This method of imaging is now a standard for diagnosing white matter diseases. It is also being used as a method to study the development of myelination throughout childhood.

Future

Diseases of white matter are an intense field of research with the high prevalence of MS. The PNS has a much greater capacity of regenerating white matter, or the myelin sheath around nerves when damaged. Schwann cells, the cells responsible for myelination, have different conditions than oligodendrocytes in the CNS, which allow them to recapitulate the production of myelin during development when a nerve sheath faces insult or injury. It is still not fully understood why Schwann cells have this capacity of remyelination. Because of the complexity of the white matter in the CNS, in organization and its necessity for higher order behavior, researchers are trying to discover the key cellular regulators within the brain and spinal cord which could aid in the efficacy of remyelination of damaged areas. Different animals models exist which try and mimic MS, leukodystrophies, and even psychiatric disorders. Currently, with the advancement in imaging techniques coupled with the funding and research initiatives, scientists and physicians are working to find therapeutic treatments to enhance remyelination of white matter in the CNS.

Kathryn K. Bercury

See also: Attention Deficit Disorder/Attention Deficit Hyperactivity Disorder; Glia; Multiple Sclerosis; Myelin; Optic Nerve; Schizophrenia

Further Reading

Davis, K. L., Stewart, D. G., Friedman, J. I., Buchsbaum, M., Harvey, P. D., Hof, P. R., . . . Haroutunian, V. (2003). White matter changes in schizophrenia. Evidence for myelin-related dysfunction. *Archives of General Psychiatry, 60,* 443–456.

National Institute of Neurological Disorders and Stroke (NINDS). (2011). *Charcot-Marie-Tooth disease fact sheet.* Retrieved from http://www.ninds.nih.gov/disorders/charcot_marie_tooth/charcot_marie_tooth.htm

National MS Society. (n.d.). *Frequently asked questions about multiple sclerosis.* Retrieved from http://www.nationalmssociety.org/about-multiple-sclerosis/what-we-know-about-ms/faqs-about-ms/index.aspx

Schmahmann, J. D., & Pandya, D. N. (2007). Cerebral white matter—Historical evolution of facts and notions concerning the organization of the fiber pathway. *Journal of the History of the Neurosciences: Basic and Clinical Perspectives, 15,* 237–267.

Wiesel, Torsten N. (1924–)

Torsten N. Wiesel (1924–) is a Nobel laureate who earned this award for his pioneering work in the visual system. In 1981, Dr. Wiesel shared the Nobel Prize in Physiology or Medicine with David Hubel for their work investigating how visual information is transmitted to and processed in the brain's visual cortex. Their investigations studied specialized functions and mapping of the functional architecture of individual cells within the visual cortex. Their efforts further examined the development of the visual cortex and the role of innate and experiential factors. This work analyzed the flow of nerve impulses from the eye to the visual cortex and described structural and functional details of that part of the brain. Wiesel and Hubel's work led strong support to the view that prompt surgery is imperative in correcting certain eye defects that are detectable in newborn children, such as congenital cataracts (cloudiness in the lens of the eye).

Dr. Wiesel was born in Uppsala, Sweden, in 1924, and received his medical degree from Karolinska Institute in 1954. His academic career spans the Karolinska Institute, The John Hopkins University Medical School, and a 24-year position at Harvard Medical School where he did much of his neurophysiological research work within the department of neurobiology. After earning his medical degree, Dr. Wiesel became a postdoctoral fellow at the Wilmer Institute, Johns Hopkins Medical School where he met his colleague, Dr. David Hubel. This began their 20-year scientific collaboration and leading to their Nobel Prize. In addition, Drs. Wiesel and Hubel have written a book together describing their research and collaborative work titled *Brain and Visual Perception: The Story of a 25-Year Collaboration* (2004).

Torsten Wiesel has received numerous awards for his work in neuropsychological research to include most recently, the 1996 Helen Keller Prize for Vision Research, the 1998 Society for Neuroscience, Presidential Award, the 2005 Institute of Medicine, David Rall Medal, the 2005 National Medal of Science Award (USA), the

2006 Spanish National Research Council Gold Medal, and the 2007 Marshall M. Parks, MD Medal of Excellence, Children's Eye Foundation Award which he shared with colleague David Hubbel.

Dr. Wiesel's work includes serving on the Committee of Human Rights of the National Academies of Science (USA) and the International Human Rights Network of Academies and Scholarly Societies. He is a founding member of the Israeli-Palestinian Science Organization (IPSO). Furthermore, Dr. Wiesel has served as chair of the board of the Aaron Diamond AIDS Research Center (1995–2001), president of the International Brain Research Organization, IBRO, (1998–2004), chair of the Board of Governors of the New York Academy of Sciences (2001–2006), and on the board of directors of the Population Council (1999–2008).

In 2007, Wiesel's efforts to support research on eye diseases were recognized when the Torsten Wiesel Research Institute was established as part of the World Eye Organization, based in Chengdu, China. This institute allows scientists to engage in basic and clinical research on eye diseases prevalent in Asian populations.

Karen Savoie

See also: Visual System

Further Reading

Hubel, D.H., &Wiesel, T.N. (2004). *Brain and visual perception: The story of a 25-year collaboration.* New York, NY: Oxford University Press.

Wilson Disease

Wilson disease is a rare genetic disorder that is a result of copper accumulating in tissues of the affected person. Specifically, it is a mutation to the *ATP7B* gene, which is called the *Wilson disease protein.* If a person has one mutated gene, they are called a carrier. To have Wilson disease, a person must have two copies of the mutated gene, which occurs in about 1 in 100,000 persons (Ala et al., 2007). British neurologist Samuel Alexander Kinnier Wilson (1878–1937) was the first to describe the clinical findings and researched the disorder. Thus, Wilson disease was named after its founder.

Abnormal copper accumulation causes (1) severe liver damage that may require a liver transplant later in life, (2) brain damage that may lead to difficulty in swallowing (dysphagia), slurred speech (dysarthria) and excessive drooling, and (3) damage to the eyes that results in a rusty-brown ring around the cornea. Other symptoms may include tremor of the head and limbs, abnormal posture caused by impaired muscle tone, and uncoordinated movements (ataxia).

The two main treatments for Wilson disease are first to remove current amounts of copper in the body and second to stop the accumulation of copper. Zinc has been shown to block copper absorption in the stomach and is the primary treatment of choice. To remove copper, patients need to excrete the excess metal and are given copper chelators such as penicillamine. Finally, patients must have a low-copper diet, that is, they should not eat mushrooms, chocolate, nuts, dried fruit, and shellfish. If a person is diagnosed and treated early, they can live a normal life. Nonetheless, treatment is required for lifetime as this is a genetic disease.

Jennifer L. Hellier

See also: Dysarthria; Tremors

Further Reading

Ala, A., Walker, A. P., Ashkan, K., Dooley, J. S., & Schilsky, M. L. (2007). Wilson's disease. *Lancet, 369*(9559), 397–408.

Wundt, Wilhelm Maximilian (1832–1920)

Wilhelm Maximilian Wundt was the first person in history to be called a "psychologist," as he examined the mental and behavioral characteristics of an individual or group. Dr. Wundt studied medicine in his native country, Germany, at the Universität Heidelberg, and received his medical degree in 1856. His work led to the establishment of psychology as a unique branch of science and in 1874, he identified physiological psychology as a "new method of science."

While Wundt is known as the father of experimental psychology; he is remembered for his influence on the true development of psychology as a discipline. He was the first person to teach a course in physiological psychology at Universität Heidelberg in 1862, and in 1874, his work was published in *Principles of Physiological Psychology.* This led to the establishment of the first psychology laboratory in 1879 at Germany's University of Leipzig. Wundt's research took psychology from a subdiscipline of philosophy and biology to a unique scientific discipline. Early in his career, Wundt investigated immediate experiences of consciousness, emotions, ideas, and feelings through an internal perception or self-examination of conscious experience by objective observation. Wundt was a significant influence on early psychology and his students included James McKeen Cattell (1860–1944) and G. Stanley Hall (1844–1924). In 1883, G. Stanley Hall created the first experimental

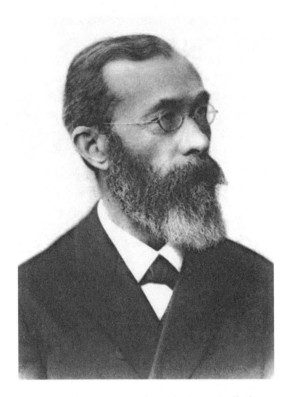

German philosopher and psychologist Wilhelm Wundt. (König, Edmund. *W. Wundt: Seine Philosophie und Psychologie*. Stuttgart: Fr. Frommanns Verlag, 1901)

psychology lab in the United States at Johns Hopkins University.

According to Wundt's work, the sciences are divided into two families: the formal sciences (e.g., mathematics) and the real sciences (the natural and spiritual aspects of reality). Furthermore, Wundt recognized philosophy as the means of taking psychological results and abstracting normative rules that govern the organization of human and natural sciences. Thus, he defined psychology as the foundation of all human sciences and the doctrine of spiritual processes. He believed that psychology mediated between the sciences and philosophy.

In Wundt's 10-volume work, *Volker Psychologie,* he addressed issues of truth and methodology in the social and human sciences, and referred to it as "folk psychology." According to Wundt, folk psychology "traces the lawful development through cultural participation, or higher human processes." He believed that the movement of human societies followed historical stages and identified these stages as the Age of Primitive Man, the Totemic Age, the Age of Gods and Heroes, and the Present Age. These stages led to interpretation of diverse human cultures and understanding influences on individuals within communities. Wundt's theory of how people view the world from their perspective (perspectivism) is exemplified in his interpretation of apparent psychological motives in communal existence, which leads to an understanding of individuals.

Wundt is remembered as a challenging psychologist as his research was largely ignored and his efforts to define a culturally sensitive approach to psychology were rejected during his lifetime. He did not deter from his efforts to lead psychology to follow principles of the physical sciences while being paired with the social sciences. Instead, he developed another form of psychology termed "scientific metaphysics," which combines both lab research with other scientific findings. Wundt is remembered for redefining psychology as the study of the structure of experiences with his empirical methodologies that developed psychology as a distinct disciplinary entity, independent from philosophy.

Karen Savoie

See also: Behavior; Psychology/Psychiatry

Further Reading

Wade, N., Piccolino, M., & Simmons, A. (n.d.). *Portraits of European neuroscientists.* Retrieved from http://neuroportraits.eu/

Experiments and Activities

This section includes experiments and activities that will build understanding of certain neuroscience processes and anatomy. For example, there are many activities in this section for building parts of the brain and nervous system with clay. Other experiments show procedures that should be completed in a school laboratory setting. Each activity or experiment shows which entry in the encyclopedia it relates to; in some cases the activity or experiment relates to another experiment or activity, which is also noted.

Astrocyte—Building with Clay Activity

Activity Relates to Blood-Brain Barrier; Glia

Astrocytes are supportive neurons within the central nervous system (CNS). They are named after their star-shaped morphology. The main function of astrocytes is to transport nutrients and waste between neurons and the blood-brain barrier (BBB). These cells are essential to the structure and function of the BBB. The integrity of the BBB is essential because it keeps macromolecules, microorganisms, and other chemicals from entering the CNS. If such compounds were to enter, it could be deadly for the individual. As most biological cells, astrocytes contain, but not limited to, cell membrane, cytoplasm, nucleus, ribosomes, endoplasmic reticulum (ER), and mitochondria.

Materials: Four colors of clay (red, green, yellow, and blue), wax paper, tabletop, paper towels, and toothpick.

Methods:
Roll a walnut-sized ball of red clay; this will represent the cell membrane and cytoplasm together forming the cell body (soma). Flatten this into a quarter-inch thick, two-inch diameter "pancake." Pinch and pull the edges of the "pancake" to make multiple points of a star; these will be the vascular feet of the astrocyte, used to help form the BBB. The vascular feet thin out as they move away from the soma. Clean your hands each time you switch colors.

Using a pecan-sized ball of green clay, flatten it to be approximately one inch in diameter and an eighth of an inch thick. This will represent the ER. Place the clay on top of the soma, relatively in the center. With a toothpick, poke several small holes into the central section of the ER. These holes represent ribosomes, used to make proteins.

Take a peanut-sized ball of yellow clay and roll it into a ball. This will represent the nucleus of the astrocyte. The nucleus houses the genetic material. Slightly flatten one side and place on top of the ER; the nucleus is not always in the center of the cell.

Finally, make four to five tic-tac-sized ovals. These are the mitochondria, which generate energy for the cell. Place throughout the cytoplasm.

Riannon C. Atwater

See also: Blood-Brain Barrier; Glia; Glioma

Further Reading

Kandel, E. R., Schwartz, J. H., Jessell, T. M., Siegelbaum, S. A., & Hudspeth, A. J. (Eds.). (2012). *Principles of neural science* (5th ed.). New York, NY: McGraw-Hill.

Basket Cells—Building with Clay Activity

Activity Relates to Inhibition; Neuron

Basket cells (BCs), named for their appearance, are specialized interneurons that act to inhibit neural signals by using a neurotransmitter called GABA (γ-aminobutyric acid). These cells are found in three locations within the brain: the cerebellum, hippocampus, and cerebral cortex. BCs have branched axons (output), which are capable of acting on multiple neurons at once. Their dendrites (input) are also branched. As most biological cells, BCs contain, but are not limited to, cell membrane, cytoplasm, nucleus, ribosomes, endoplasmic reticulum (ER), and mitochondria.

Materials: Four colors of clay (red, green, yellow, and blue), wax paper, table-top, paper towels, and toothpick.

Methods:
Roll a walnut-sized ball of red clay; this represents the cell membrane and cytoplasm together forming the cell body (soma). Flatten this into a quarter-inch thick, two-inch diameter "pancake." Pinch and pull the edges of the "pancake" to make multiple branches; these represent dendrites of the BC. Pinch and pull each dendrite into further branches. Roll a pecan-sized ball into a worm. Attach the worm to one edge of the soma and create a few branches off of it. This represents the cell's axon, which propagates a signal by releasing GABA into the space between two neurons, the synapse. Clean your hands each time you switch colors.

Flatten a pecan-sized ball of green clay to one inch in diameter and an eighth of an inch thick. This represents the ER. Place the clay on top of the soma, relatively in the center. With a toothpick, poke several small holes into the central section of the ER. These holes represent ribosomes, used to make proteins.

Slightly flatten one side of a peanut-sized ball of yellow clay. This represents the nucleus of the BC. Nuclei house the genetic material. Place on top of the ER; the nucleus is not always in the center of the cell.

Finally, make four to five tic-tac-sized ovals. These are mitochondria, which generate energy for the cell. Place throughout the cytoplasm.

Riannon C. Atwater

See also: Inhibition; Neuron

Further Reading

Kandel, E. R., Schwartz, J. H., Jessell, T. M., Siegelbaum, S. A., & Hudspeth, A. J. (Eds.). (2012). *Principles of neural science* (5th ed.). New York, NY: McGraw-Hill.

Behavioral Experiments

Experiments Relate to Behavior; Behavioral Tests; Olfaction

Behavioral experiments are used to determine if an animal model for a neurological disease has similar behavioral actions or deficits as persons with the same neurological disease. Several behavioral experiments can be performed; however, each test must correlate with the associated behavior. For example, scientists will count and classify seizure-like activity in animal models of temporal lobe epilepsy. Furthermore, the seizures will be identified if they occur at a specific time of day or during a specific activity like memory testing, as observed in humans with epilepsy.

Simple behavioral tests are routinely used in other diseases. For example, the sense of smell, which is called olfaction, is a very important behavior that can be disrupted in Alzheimer's disease, aging, and schizophrenia. Neuroscientists have developed several behavioral experiments to test odor identification, odor discrimination, odor threshold, and early odor learning preference, to name a few. These tests can help identify normative and diseased responses in animal models.

Q1: How do behavioral experiments identify deficits or neurological diseases in animal models?

Materials:

Two different odorants (extracts)   Mineral oil
Pipettes and tips   Six bottles (cleaned)
Paper and pencil   Human volunteers—male and female

Procedure:

For this experiment, prepare odor mixtures to a known concentration (0.1 and 1.0% of an odorant in mineral oil to a final volume of 10 milliliters). Mineral oil will be the vehicle for the extract mixtures. Place the odor mixture in a clean bottle and label the bottle so that the experimenter knows the concentration and odorant name but the volunteer does not (e.g., odor A-1, odor A-2, odor B-1, and odor B-2). Have the volunteers sniff the odor while slowly shaking or swirling the mixture, so that the odorant volatilizes. Ask the volunteer the following: (1) What does the odorant smell like? and (2) Which bottle has a higher concentration of the same odor? (Which one smells stronger?). Record the answers from men and women and compare the number of correct responses between: (1) identifying odorants and (2) odor concentrations.

Make two graphs, answers from men in one graph and answers from women in the other.

> Q2: How often was each sex correct in identifying the odorant?
>
> Q3: Which group was right in identifying higher odor concentrations?

For the next experiment, mix the odors with the same concentration together, making a one to one mixture of odor A and odor B (0.1% odor A mixed with 0.1% of odor B). Have the volunteers sniff the new mixture while slowly shaking or swirling the bottle so that the odorants volatilize. Ask the volunteer: (1) What does the odorant smells like? and (2) How many odors do you smell? Record the answers from men and women and compare the number of correct responses between (1) identifying odorants and (2) the number of odorants. Make two similar graphs as described earlier.

> Q4: How often was each sex correct in identifying the odorants?
>
> Q5: Based on these results, is there a difference in olfaction between the sexes?

Jennifer L. Hellier

See also: Behavior; Behavioral Test; Olfaction

Further Reading

Bjorn, G. (2010). Olfaction differences between the sexes. *The Daily Smell.* Retrieved from http://dev.thedailysmell.com/2010/11/12/science-of-smell-olfaction-differences-between-the-sexes/

Fox, K. (n.d.). The smell report: An overview of facts and findings. Social Issues Research Centre. Retrieved from http://www.sirc.org/publik/smell.pdf

Brain Building with Clay Activity: Cerebellum, Cerebral Cortex

Activity Relates to Brain Anatomy; Cerebellum; Cerebral Cortex; Frontal Lobe; Occipital Lobe; Parietal Lobe; Temporal Lobe

The central nervous system (CNS) consists of the *brain, brainstem,* and the *spinal cord.* The brain serves as the control center for the CNS. The brain is responsible for coordinating responses to stimuli and exerts control over all the other organs in the body. The three main divisions of the surface of the brain are the *cerebrum*—responsible for higher order function; the *cerebellum*—responsible for modulation of brain signals; and the *brainstem*—responsible for regulation of the cardiovascular, respiratory systems, and for connecting the brain to the spinal cord. The cerebrum can be further divided into lobes that are named after the bones that overlie them. The lobes are the *frontal, temporal, occipital, and parietal lobes.* One additional region of the brain is the insula, which is found deep in the frontal, parietal, and temporal lobes. The following table shows the function for each major brain region.

Table EA1   Brain Lobes and Their Function

Lobe	Function
Frontal lobe	Houses the primary motor cortex, reward, attention, short-term memory, and motivation
Temporal lobe	Retention of visual memories, language, storage of memories (long-term memory), and emotions
Occipital lobe	Visual processing center
Parietal lobe	Integration of sensory information, houses the primary sensory cortex, and special awareness (particularly where the body position is in space)
Insula	Plays a role in consciousness, emotion, maintaining homeostasis, perception, and self-awareness

Materials: Five colors of clay (red, green, yellow, blue, and white), wax paper, tabletop, toothpick, and paper towels.

Methods:
On the wax paper to protect the tabletop, roll a gumball-size piece of yellow clay into a "worm," approximately one-eighth of an inch thick. Take this worm and slowly fold it into a loose ball in your hand. This will represent the

frontal lobe of the cerebrum. Set this aside for later and clean your hands with the paper towels. Do this between each color.

Next, roll a walnut-size piece of green clay into another worm one-eighth of an inch thick. This will represent the temporal lobe of the cerebrum. As earlier, fold this clay into a loosely shaped ball and set aside.

Take a walnut-size piece of blue clay and roll it into a worm approximately one-eighth of an inch thick. Fold this clay into a ball; this will represent the occipital lobe of the cerebrum.

Then take a walnut-size piece of red clay and roll it as previously. Fold the clay into a ball; this represents the parietal lobe of the cerebrum.

Next, use a gumball-size piece of white clay and flatten one side. Using a toothpick, carve several horizontal lines across the rounded side of the ball. Add a short tail; this represents the cerebellum and brainstem. Repeat the aforementioned steps to make the other half of the brain (do not repeat for the cerebellum).

Finally, arrange the balls of clay into a brain. The frontal lobes will sit in front followed by the parietal lobes, under which the temporal lobes will sit. In the back will sit the occipital lobes. Underneath the occipital lobes, place the cerebellum and brainstem so that the brainstem points down.

Riannon C. Atwater

See also: Brain Anatomy; Cerebellum; Cerebral Cortex; Frontal Lobe; Occipital Lobe; Parietal Lobe; Temporal Lobe

Further Reading

Kandel, E. R., Schwartz, J. H., Jessell, T. M., Siegelbaum, S. A., & Hudspeth, A. J. (Eds.). (2012). *Principles of neural science* (5th ed.). New York, NY: McGraw-Hill.

Brain Cut-Out Hat Activity

Activity Relates to Brain Anatomy; Language; Learning and Memory

The brain consists of the cerebral cortex and deep structures, such as the thalamus, hypothalamus, and the hippocampus. The main functions of the brain are to integrate and modulate both sensory and motor information as well as to produce cognition, higher reasoning, and thinking. The cerebral cortex is divided into two hemispheres with each containing the same lobes and deep structures. The four lobes and their general function are the frontal (higher reasoning, premotor cortex, and motor cortex), parietal (somatosensory cortex—senses from the body mainly touch, language processing, visual association cortices), occipital (visual processing center), and temporal (storage of memory and emotions, language comprehension). The function of the thalamus is to modulate all sensory and motor function except for olfaction (the sense of smell).

Materials: Scissors, white glue, tape, paperclips, card stock (preferably two different colors to represent the left and right hemispheres), and pencil or pen.

Methods:
Print out the left brain hemisphere hat pattern on one color of the card stock, and repeat with the right pattern on the other color of card stock. With a writing instrument, label the functions of each lobe and draw pictures pertaining to those functions. Note that the left hemisphere, for most humans, contains Broca's area (forming sentences) and Wernicke's area (understanding language), both necessary for language. When ready, cut out each hemisphere's pattern. Then cut all of the solid lines that form the Vs along the edges of the brain. Pull the cut edge to the backside of the paper, making a flap to the dashed line. Glue these in place using the paperclips to hold them together until they dry. Next, place one hemisphere about an eighth of an inch or less underneath the other and tape together. Place on head making sure the frontal lobe is in the front. Enjoy!

Riannon C. Atwater and
Jennifer L. Hellier

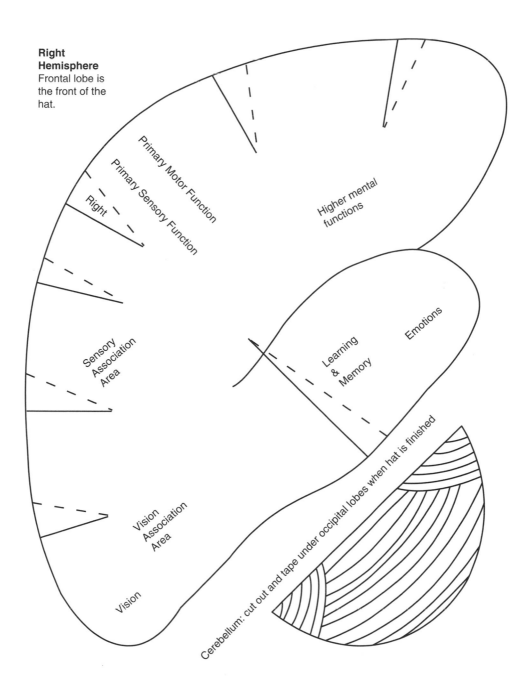

Right Hemisphere
Frontal lobe is the front of the hat.

Primary Motor Function

Primary Sensory Function

Right

Higher mental functions

Sensory Association Area

Learning & Memory

Emotions

Vision Association Area

Vision

Cerebellum: cut out and tape under occipital lobes when hat is finished

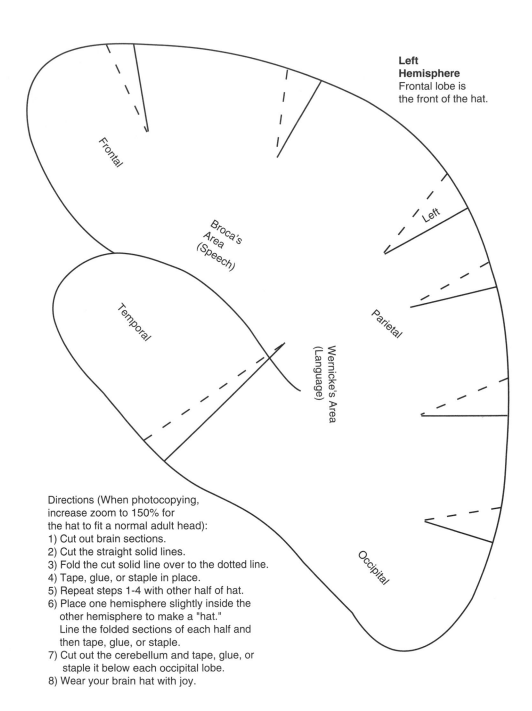

**Left
Hemisphere**
Frontal lobe is
the front of the hat.

Frontal

Broca's
Area
(Speech)

Left

Temporal

Parietal

Wernicke's Area
(Language)

Occipital

Directions (When photocopying,
increase zoom to 150% for
the hat to fit a normal adult head):
1) Cut out brain sections.
2) Cut the straight solid lines.
3) Fold the cut solid line over to the dotted line.
4) Tape, glue, or staple in place.
5) Repeat steps 1-4 with other half of hat.
6) Place one hemisphere slightly inside the
   other hemisphere to make a "hat."
   Line the folded sections of each half and
   then tape, glue, or staple.
7) Cut out the cerebellum and tape, glue, or
   staple it below each occipital lobe.
8) Wear your brain hat with joy.

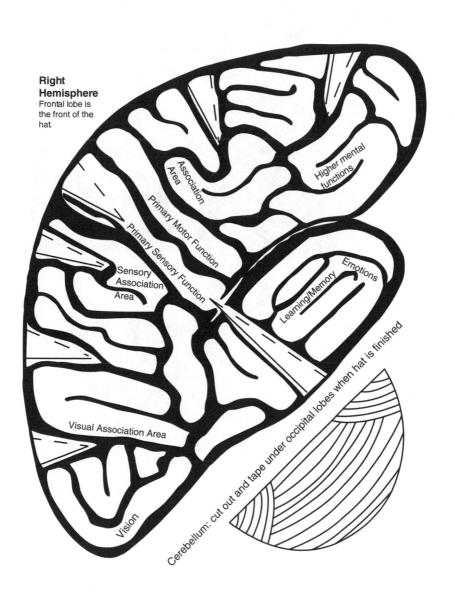

Right Hemisphere
Frontal lobe is the front of the hat.

Association Area

Higher mental functions

Primary Motor Function

Primary Sensory Function

Sensory Association Area

Emotions

Learning/Memory

Visual Association Area

Vision

Cerebellum: cut out and tape under occipital lobes when hat is finished

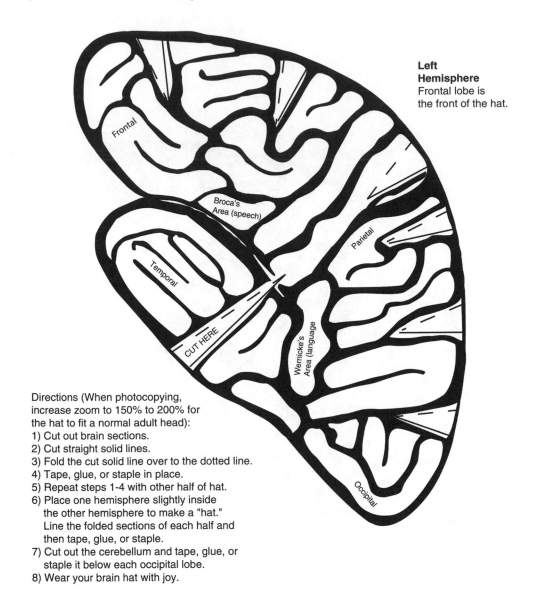

Left Hemisphere Frontal lobe is the front of the hat.

Frontal

Broca's Area (speech)

Parietal

Temporal

CUT HERE

Wernicke's Area (language

Occipital

Directions (When photocopying, increase zoom to 150% to 200% for the hat to fit a normal adult head):
1) Cut out brain sections.
2) Cut straight solid lines.
3) Fold the cut solid line over to the dotted line.
4) Tape, glue, or staple in place.
5) Repeat steps 1-4 with other half of hat.
6) Place one hemisphere slightly inside the other hemisphere to make a "hat." Line the folded sections of each half and then tape, glue, or staple.
7) Cut out the cerebellum and tape, glue, or staple it below each occipital lobe.
8) Wear your brain hat with joy.

See also: Brain Anatomy; Language; Learning and Memory

Further Reading

Purves, D., Augustine, G. J., Fitzpatrick, D., Hall, W. C., LaMantia, A.-S., McNamara, J. O., & Williams, S. M. (Eds.). (2004). *Neuroscience* (3rd ed.). Sunderland, MA: Sinauer Associates.

Cell Body (Soma)—Building with Clay Activity

Activity Relates to Glia; Neuron

The cell body or soma is the bulbous end of the neuron from which dendrites and the axon(s) protrude. Scaffolding proteins are essential in neural signals; they give the cell body its shape as well as carry organelles and proteins down the axon like train tracks. Housed in the soma are various organelles, which include, but are not limited to, cell membrane, cytoplasm, nucleus, cytoskeleton, ribosomes, endoplasmic reticulum (ER), Golgi apparatus, vesicles, and mitochondria.

Materials: Six colors of clay (red, green, yellow, blue, brown, and white), wax paper, tabletop, paper towels, and toothpick.

Methods:
Roll a walnut-sized ball of red clay; this represents the cell membrane and cytoplasm, together forming the soma. Flatten this into a quarter-inch thick, two-inch diameter "pancake." Clean your hands between each color.

Using a pecan-sized ball of green clay, flatten it to a one-inch diameter and an eighth of an inch thick pancake. This represents the ER. Place the clay centrally and on top of the soma. With a toothpick, poke several small holes into the central section of the ER. These holes represent ribosomes, used to make proteins.

Take a peanut-sized ball of yellow clay. This represents the nucleus of the soma, which houses the genetic material. Slightly flatten one side and place on top of the ER; the nucleus is not always in the center of the cell.

Make four to five tic-tac-sized ovals. These are mitochondria, which generate energy for the cell. Place throughout the cytoplasm.

Take a pea-sized ball of brown clay and form three to four small worms. Place these next to each other, between the ER and the edge of the cell body. These represent the Golgi apparatus, which packages nutrients, waste, and other chemicals into bundles to transport throughout the cell.

For the scaffolding proteins, make several thin long worms of white clay. Place throughout the cell. Connect the organelles to the nucleus and cell membrane with the white clay.

Riannon C. Atwater

See also: Glia; Neuron

Further Reading

Kandel, E. R., Schwartz, J. H., Jessell, T. M., Siegelbaum, S. A., & Hudspeth, A. J. (Eds.). (2012). *Principles of neural science* (5th ed.). New York, NY: McGraw-Hill.

Channel/Receptor—Building with Clay Activity

Activity Relates to Ion Channels

Channels are specialized proteins embedded within membranes of cells, particularly neurons. They act as gates through the membrane that selectively allow only certain molecules to travel through. The protein's conformation (shape) exists in the closed state for the majority of the time. When a neurotransmitter or other chemical binds to the receptors located on the channels, the protein's conformation changes to open, allowing molecules to pass through. This binding is crucial to ensuring the changes in membrane voltage so that neurons are able to transmit neural impulses. Without proper levels of neurotransmitters, neurons do not function properly.

Materials: Three colors of clay (brown, yellow, red), wax paper, tabletop, and paper towels.

Methods:
Take a walnut-sized piece of yellow clay and roll it on the wax paper to protect the tabletop. Form the clay into a worm, approximately a fourth of an inch in diameter. Cut this worm into three pieces, each an inch-and-a-quarter long. These pieces will represent one subunit of the channel. Clean your hands with the paper towels between each color of clay.

Repeat this process with brown clay, only cutting two pieces of clay. These pieces will represent the other subunit of the channel. Lay the subunits next to each other lengthwise, alternating colors. Gently push the pieces together so they will stick but not mix. Wrap the pieces into a hollow tube. This represents the channel.

Finally take two pea-sized pieces of the red clay and roll them into balls. These pieces will represent neurotransmitters that act as an agonist for the channel. Stick the pieces of red clay onto the channel gently. This is a receptor-bound channel that is open, allowing molecules to pass through the channel to the other side of the cell membrane. Remove the red clay from the receptor and gently twist the channel so that it is closed. When the channel is not bound by a neurotransmitter, molecules cannot pass through.

Riannon C. Atwater

See also: Acetylcholine and Its Receptors; AMPA and Its Receptors; Chloride Channels; Ion Channels; Potassium Channels

Further Reading

Hille, B. (2001). *Ion channels of excitable membranes* (3rd ed.). Sunderland, MA: Sinauer Associates, Inc.

Circle of Willis and Arterial Supply to the Brain—Building with Clay Activity

Activity Relates to Aneurysm; Stroke

Neurons within the brain have a very high metabolic rate and as such require a constant source of oxygen and glucose, which is provided by arterial supply. The *Circle of Willis* (also known as Loop of Willis and cerebral arterial circle) is a circular anastomosis (a reconnection of two streams that previously branched out) that connects various arteries within the brain. This anastomosis is vital because it creates collaterals, which allow the brain to continue to receive blood even in the event that one of the arteries becomes blocked. A blocked artery can occur during a stroke. Blood vessels can also be damaged when the wall of the vessel balloons resulting in an aneurysm and bleeding directly into the brain cavity.

The Circle of Willis was first identified by English physician Thomas Willis (1621–1675). It is found at the base of the brain, on the inferior surface surrounding the pituitary gland and optic chiasm. The Circle of Willis is composed of the following arteries: *the left and right anterior cerebral arteries, internal carotid arteries, posterior cerebral arteries, posterior communicating arteries,* and *the anterior communicating artery.* The basilar artery (lies on the pons and some of the medulla oblongata of the brainstem) and the left and right middle cerebral arteries (that wrap upward, around the cerebral cortex) are not considered part of the Circle of Willis, but also supply blood to the brain. The brain receives blood from two major arteries, the vertebral arteries and the internal carotid arteries. If blood supply is cut off from the brain, cell death and brain damage can result.

Materials: Red clay, wax paper, tabletop, and paper towels.

Methods:
Using the red clay, roll out a "worm" approximately one-quarter of an inch in diameter and four inches long on the wax paper, which is used to protect the table. Roll this worm into a circle; this will represent the anterior communicating artery and the left and right posterior communicating artery. Roll out seven additional worms that are approximately one-eighth of an inch in diameter all about two inches long. Take two of these worms and place them about an inch apart at the top of the circle; these represent the left and right anterior cerebral arteries. Place them so that they end in the circle. Using another two worms, place them in the middle of the circle on the left and right side so that they overlap the circle. These represent the right and left middle cerebral

artery (as they go away) and the internal carotid arteries (as they move to the center). With one of the remaining worms, place it at the bottom of the circle; this is the basilar artery. Finally, take the final two worms and place them on either side of the basilar artery. These are the posterior cerebral arteries.

Riannon C. Atwater

See also: Aneurysm; Stroke

Further Reading

Kandel, E. R., Schwartz, J. H., Jessell, T. M., Siegelbaum, S. A., & Hudspeth, A. J. (Eds.). (2012). *Principles of neural science* (5th ed.). New York, NY: McGraw-Hill.

Dendrites—Building with Clay Activity

Activity Relates to Neuron

The word *dendrite* is a term derived from Greek meaning, "tree" or "branched." They were named as such based on their morphology, meaning they look like branches of a tree. Thus, dendrites are the branched ends of the neuron (brain cells that send electrical impulses between other neurons or target cells) protruding from the cell body (soma). They are responsible for receiving neural signals and transmitting them through the soma to the axon to propagate the signal. Along with the axonal terminals, they form the synaptic cleft, the physical space between neurons or neurons and their target cell. Dendrites are the postsynaptic process in signal transmission and respond to various neurotransmitters (natural chemicals used to produce the electrical impulse) that are released by the axon terminals of other neurons. They are also responsible for determining which signals get propagated and how large the response will be. Dendrites branch extensively, forming a dendritic arbor. Generally, there is more than one dendritic branch from each soma.

Dendrites also determine the shape of a cell. For example, in pyramidal cells (which are found in the entorhinal cortex, hippocampus, and prefrontal cortex, to name a few brain regions), dendritic branches will come off of each "point" of the pyramid. Of these three branches, the one that extends from the apex of the pyramid is called an apical dendrite. These dendrites have been shown to integrate both inhibitory and excitatory signals that are used in specific functions such as learning and memory. Until recently, all dendrites were thought to propagate signals only toward the soma and then to the axon, however, studies have shown that some dendrites are able to support action potentials and release neurotransmitters themselves (e.g., Bergquist and Ludwig, 2008). These functions were thought to be specific to axons only.

Materials: Two colors of clay (red and yellow), wax paper (to protect the tabletop), tabletop, and paper towels.

Methods:
On the wax paper, roll a ping-pong-sized ball of red clay; this will represent the cell membrane and cytoplasm, together forming the cell body (soma). Flatten this into a quarter-inch thick, three-inch diameter "pancake." Pinch and pull the edges of the "pancake" to make multiple cell processes; pinch and pull each cell process into further branches. Continue to pinch each process until a vast arbor has been formed. This is the dendritic arbor of the neuron. Pinch a large portion of the clay and pull it into a long thick cell process.

This is the axon and axon hillock of the neuron. Clean your hands with the paper towels.

Next, take a peanut-sized ball of yellow clay and roll it into a ball. This will represent the nucleus of the neuron. The nucleus houses the genetic material. Slightly flatten one side and place on top of the soma; the nucleus is not always in the center of the cell.

Riannon C. Atwater

See also: Neuron

Further Reading

Bergquist, F., & Ludwig, M. (2008). Dendritic transmitter release: A comparison of two model systems. *Journal of Neuroendocrinology, 20*(6), 677–686.

Dendritic Spine—Building with Clay Activity

Activity Relates to Neuron

Neurons are made of a cell body (soma), dendrites (branches that receive synaptic input), and an axon (output of a neuron). The soma is the bulbous end of the neuron from which dendrites and the axon(s) protrude. When two neurons make a synapse, where chemical signaling occurs for the neurons to "talk" to each other, it *usually* consists of a dendrite from the presynaptic neuron and the axon bouton of the postsynaptic neuron. If the synapse is excitatory, a spine will protrude. This occurs because the spine serves as a storage site for extra glutamate receptors that are necessary for increasing synaptic strength during learning and memory. Dendritic spines have a bulbous head with a thin neck, which attaches to the dendrite. The head has an area called the postsynaptic density (PSD) where the collection of receptors and other scaffolding proteins is located. One dendrite can have hundreds to thousands of spines along its length, which increases its surface area and ability to connect to many more neurons.

Materials: Three colors of clay (red, yellow, and blue), tabletop, and paper towels.

Methods:

Roll a ball of red clay into a long snake (six inches long); this represents the cell membrane of the dendrite. Flatten this into a quarter-inch thick, two-inch diameter. On one horizontal side, pinch the clay to make a thin neck. The neck should be about one-inch long. Take a pecan-sized ball of red clay; flatten it to a one-inch diameter and an eighth of an inch thick pancake. Place on top of the neck, this represents the head. Clean your hands between each color.

Take a peanut-sized ball of yellow clay to represent the PSD. Slightly flatten one side and center it at the top of the head. Carve several short lines to represent extra receptors.

For the scaffolding proteins, make several thin long worms of blue clay. Place throughout the neck and dendrite. Connect the PSD with the blue clay.

Jennifer L. Hellier

See also: Learning and Memory; Neuron

Further Reading

Kandel, E. R., Schwartz, J. H., Jessell, T. M., Siegelbaum, S. A., & Hudspeth, A. J. (Eds.). (2012). *Principles of neural science* (5th ed.). New York, NY: McGraw-Hill.

Discriminative Touch Experiment

Experiment Relates to **Discriminative Touch; Sensory Receptors; Touch**

Touch is the most basic sense for animals. In mammals, and particularly humans, discriminative touch is essential for survival. For example, touch is necessary for infants to grow, feed, and bond with mothers, fathers, and other caregivers. It is the most basic form of communication (social touch), such as love through a kiss or a hug. Discriminative touch, or two-point discrimination, is important for animals to identify objects so they can use them as tools to access or pick up food. Discriminative touch employs small receptor fields (areas on the skin that receive external stimuli) to increase the intensity of the touch sense compared to crude touch, which uses large receptor fields. If a body region has an extensive number of small receptor fields, like in the fingertips, it will be more sensitive to external stimuli.

> Q1: What is two-point discrimination? What body region(s) do you think is(are) best at discriminative touch? Why?

Materials:

Ruler with metric measurements
Two toothpicks or similar items
Calculator, for calculating averages
Paper and pencil
Need a minimum of three different subjects (persons willing to be part of the experiment)

Procedure:

Select one person (a recorder) to record the results (write down the measurements), one person (a tester) to test the two-point discrimination of the different body parts, and a third person (a measurer) to measure distance in millimeters. The remaining people are the subjects. If you have a total of only three people, the recorder will also be the measurer. Rotate assignments so that everyone is a recorder/measurer, a tester, and a subject. For best results, you would like to have at least three measurements to average. However, more data points will produce a better mean.

1. To test two-point discrimination, the tester will take two toothpicks (or similar items) and simultaneously place them several inches apart onto

the *upper back* (between the neck and the shoulder) of the subject. The tester *does not* need to push hard to cause pain as this experiment is not testing pain. Instead the tester needs to exert enough pressure so that the subject can feel the two points. Start about eight inches (about 200 millimeters) apart, the length from the pinky finger to the thumb when the fingers are spread apart. Ask the subject, "How many points do you feel?" If the answer is, "one," then measure the distance in millimeters and record the distance between the two points. If it is, "two," then move the toothpicks closer together about one inch (about 25 millimeters) and simultaneously place them onto the back.

2. Repeat step 1 until the subject feels only one point; measure and record the distance in millimeters.

3. Repeat steps 1 and 2 on the *back of the hand* (the original distance will be about three inches—about 75 millimeters—apart) and ask the subject to close their eyes and turn their head. This is to ensure that the subject is only using their discriminative touch sense and not their visual sense to determine the number of points. Move the toothpicks closer together about 10 millimeters at a time.

4. Repeat steps 1 and 2 on the *fingertip* (the original distance will be about half inch—about 13 millimeters—apart) and ask the subject to close their eyes and turn their head. The finger is the most sensitive body part and if the points are too large, the tester will have a difficult time getting to "one point." Move the toothpicks closer together about 1–2 millimeters at a time.

5. Average the distances for each body part and graph the results.

Q2: Were the results significantly different in averaged lengths between the different body parts? If so, why did this happen?

Q3: How would this experiment change with older subjects (over the age of 50 years) compared to young subjects (under the age of 20 years)? Why?

Jennifer L. Hellier

See also: Discriminative Touch; Sensory Receptors; Touch

Further Reading

Purves, D., Augustine, G. J., Fitzpatrick, D., Hall, W. C., LaMantia, A.-S., McNamara, J. O., & Williams, S. M. (Eds.). (2004). *Neuroscience* (3rd ed.). Sunderland, MA: Sinauer Associates.

Electrophysiology Setup and Experiments

Experiment Relates to Cerebrospinal Fluid; Epilepsy; Frog Sciatic Nerve Experiment (in Experiments and Activities Section)

Electrophysiology is the study of electrical impulses and chemical signals that travel from neuron to neuron. Such recordings can identify how local circuits work in the "normal" brain, thus allowing scientists to compare "normal" and diseased network activity of the brain. For example, electrophysiology is used to study the cellular and molecular changes associated with temporal lobe epilepsy and other pathophysiological conditions (e.g., hypoxia and hypoglycemia). The trisynaptic circuit (three distinct synapses) of the hippocampus has been widely studied as it has inherent synaptic plasticity, which is necessary for learning and memory. Furthermore, the hippocampal slice is an optimal experimental preparation since the section retains most of its circuitry because of its laminar organization.

Scientists have recorded from both the dentate gyrus granule cells and CA3 pyramidal cells with either orthodromic (normal direction of neuronal impluses) or antidromic (reverse direction) stimulation. This results in recording local networks of neurons and their subsequent grouped firing of action potentials, which produce population spikes and field postsynaptic potentials (fPSP). Population spikes are synchronous action potentials from several neurons, and are analogous to the monophasic compound action potential of the frog sciatic nerve experiment.

Materials:

Extracellular preamplifier	Drip chamber
Slice chamber	Micromanipulators
Stimulator	Thermometer and external heater
Stimulus isolation unit (SIU)	O_2 and N_2 tanks
Oscilloscope	Fluid pump
Cables	Beaker
Artificial cerebrospinal fluid (ACSF)	Air table

Procedure:

The electrophysiological equipment setup is similar to the frog sciatic nerve setup. The hippocampal slice must be placed on the ramp of the slice chamber for about one to two hours with continual flow of ACSF and oxygen. This allows the hippocampal slice to equilibrate to its new environment. The relevant anatomy for this experiment is the hippocampal dentate gyrus, which contains the molecular layer, granule cell layer, hilus, and the beginning of the CA3 pyramidal cell layer. In the figure, identify the recording and stimulating electrodes and the respective regions in which they are placed.

1. *Field responses from orthodromic stimulation:* Set the stimulation to have a two-millisecond delay with 0.35 millisecond duration. At low stimulus intensities (less than 50 microamperes), a typical fPSP occurs with an amplitude of 1–2 mV. Slowly increasing the stimulating intensity will elicit a population spike. Eventually the amplitude of the population spike will stop increasing with stimulation intensity. Decrease the stimulation intensity to zero microamperes, and begin increasing the current until an initial response occurs. Record the threshold and amplitude of the fPSP, and then the population spike.

Q1: What is the utility of determining the threshold for the field PSP and/ or the population spike?

2. *Field responses from antidromic stimulation:* Move the stimulating electrode from the molecular layer to the hilus, such that the electrode is directly on the axons of the granule cells. The waveform will now look like the monophasic action potential. The population spike is the summation of action potentials from the group of granule cells near the recording electrode. Stimulate as before in step 1.

Q2: What is the difference between the observed orthodromic and antidromic responses?

Jennifer L. Hellier

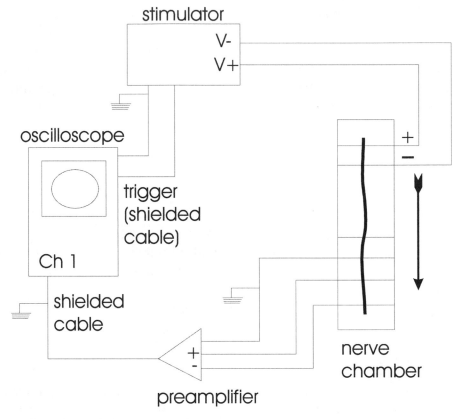

Figure EA.1   Frog sciatic nerve experiment.

See also: Cerebrospinal Fluid; Epilepsy; Frog Sciatic Nerve Experiment (in Experiments and Activities Section)

Further Reading

Sheperd, G. M. (Ed.). (2004). *The synaptic organization of the brain.* New York, NY: Oxford University Press.

Frog Sciatic Nerve Experiment

Experiment Relates to **Electrophysiology Setup and Experiments (in Experiments and Activities Section); Nerves**

Introduction:

Electrical stimulation can elicit simultaneous action potentials in a peripheral nerve containing thousands of axons. The collective response, called a compound action potential, can be recorded in a simple nerve chamber using standard extracellular recording techniques. The compound action potential elicited from the frog sciatic nerve is the classical preparation for the study of the action potential. Extracellular recording of peripheral and central axons is commonly used as a clinical diagnostic tool by neurologists, utilizing both threshold and nerve conduction velocity to define neurological diseases. This mode of recording is also used experimentally to study neurological diseases and nerve regeneration.

> Q1: What neurological diseases can be diagnosed by extracellular, physiological, recording techniques?

Materials:

Extracellular preamplifier	Stimulator
Nerve chamber	Oscilloscope
Amphibian physiological saline	Eight cables, two BNC cables must be shielded
Paper and pencil	
Frog sciatic nerve	

Procedure:

Connect the nerve chamber to the equipment as indicated in the figure. Arrange the electrodes so that the stimulator and recording electrodes are at opposite ends of the nerve and ground in the center. Connect the electrode cables to one end of the chamber and the other ends to the input of the preamplifier. Connect a third cable to one of the other electrodes about midway along the chamber and then to a ground terminal on the oscilloscope or stimulator. From the stimulator output, connect another pair of cables to the opposite end of the chamber with the negative electrode closest to the recording electrode. The trigger output of the stimulator should be connected to the trigger input of the oscilloscope, so that the oscilloscope sweep can be triggered by the stimulus.

Place saline in the bottom of the nerve chamber, making sure it does not contact the recording wires. The recording electrodes through capacitative coupling to the stimulating electrodes pick up the stimulus artifact, which is always the first deflection observed. Its amplitude and duration are a direct function of the stimulus parameters. To reduce the size of the stimulus artifact, set its duration to be as short as possible.

Place a frog sciatic nerve in the chamber so that the distal (thin) end is over the recording electrodes and the proximal (thick) end is over the stimu-lating electrodes. To study *biphasic action potentials,* set the stimulator to 0.1 volt, 0.4 millisecond with a 5.0-millisecond delay, and stimulate the nerve. Slowly increase the voltage until the compound action potential appears as a deflection in the baseline of the trace, following the stimulus artifact. Notice that the response is biphasic. As stronger voltages stimulate additional axons, the compound action potential will grow in amplitude. This reflects the dif-ferences in threshold that exist among the different sizes of fibers that make up the nerve. Eventually the compound action potential will stop increasing with voltage. Increase the stimulus duration to 2.0 milliseconds and decrease the voltage to 0.1 volt. Begin increasing the voltage until a response occurs. Record the threshold at several different stimulus durations, and plot thresh-old voltage versus stimulus duration.

Q2: What produces the biphasic waveform, and what is the basis for the positive and negative deflections?

Q3: How does stimulus duration affect threshold?

Jennifer L. Hellier

See also: Electrophysiology Setup and Experiments (in Experiments and Activities Section); Nerves

Further Reading

Junge, D. (1992). *Nerve and muscle excitation* (3rd ed.). Sunderland, MA: Sinauer Associates.

Membrane Potential Experiment—Understand Membrane Properties

Experiment Relates to **Action Potential; Electrophysiology Setup and Experiments (in Experiments and Activities Section); Ion Channel; Ion Pump; Membrane; Postsynaptic Potential**

The distinct feature of a neural cell (neuron or brain cell) is electrical excitability. It means the electric potential of the cell membrane (specifically the voltage across the cell membrane) can be dynamically changed and in certain conditions the cell can generate an *action potential,* the electrical output of a neuron. We can consider the cell membrane as an impermeable barrier separating the inside (intracellular or cytosol) and the outside (extracellular) of the cell. Because of this barrier, there are different concentrations of positive ions (sodium—Na^+, potassium—K^+, calcium—Ca^{2+}, and magnesium—Mg^{2+}) and negative ions (chloride—Cl^-, organic ions$^-$) inside and outside of the cell. The total difference between the intracellular and extracellular charge can be represented as an *electric potential* or *gradient.* However, there are openings in the membrane called *channels* that allow the flow of specific ions into and out of the cell, depending on their charge and direction of their electric gradient. The strength of the ionic flow depends on the channel's conductance and electric gradient. From physics, it is known that the flow of ions is an electric current, and according to Ohm's law, its value is proportional to the electric potential and membrane conductance:

$$I = U * G = \frac{U}{R}$$

where I is the current, U the potential, G the conductance, and R the resistance.

In addition to *resting channels* that stay open all the time, there are also (1) *ligand-gated channels* that open and close only in the presence of specific ligands, and (2) *voltage-gated channels* that open and close when the membrane potential is above and below certain levels, respectively. Another very important part of the cell membrane are *ionic pumps,* such as the Na^+/K^+pump, which uses adenosine triphosphate (ATP) energy to keep the electric gradient across the membrane by pumping three Na^+ out and two K^+ in. This system can reach balance when the total current flowing into the cell equals the flow out of the cell and is called the *resting membrane potential.* If not for the action of these pumps, the ions would flow freely across the membrane to balance the electric potential at 0 V (volts); however, for an average neuron, the resting membrane potential is negative and equals about −70 mV (millivolts).

Materials: 3 AA batteries, switch, 1 kΩ resistor, green LED, red LED, and 2000 µF capacitor.

Procedure:

1. To build the circuit, we will represent (1) the cell membrane as a capacitor (two vertical lines in the circuit), (2) the ionic pump as 3 AA batteries connected serially (the short and long dark lines), and (3) the ion channel conductance/resistance as a resistor (the rectangle). In order to see the direction of the current flow, we will use red and green LEDs, all connected as in the following diagram. The gray circle represents an imaginary cell and its dashed line is the cell membrane.

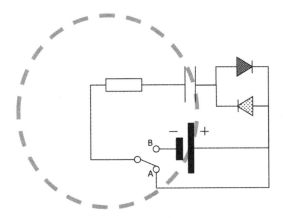

Diagram showing how to build a membrane potential circuit. Dashed line represents the imaginary cell membrane along with the resistor (rectangle) and capacitor (two vertical lines). The switch is the A-B toggle. Diodes (triangle with a line) represent the direction of electron flow. Ionic pumps are shown as 3 AA batteries connected serially (short and long vertical lines).

Questions:

1. What will happen when we turn the switch from A to B?
2. Which LED will light?
3. How long will the LED glow?
4. What is the value of the resting potential?
5. What will happen when we turn the switch back to A?

Waldemar B. Swiercz

See also: Action Potential; Electrophysiology Setup and Experiments (in Experiments and Activities Section); Ion Channel; Ion Pump; Membrane; Postsynaptic Potential

Further Reading

Kandel, E. R., Schwartz, J. H., & Jessell, T. M. (2005). *Essentials of neural science and behavior* (Chap. 8, p. 133). New York, NY: McGraw-Hill Medical.

Myelin Conduction Experiment

Experiment Relates to Axon; Multiple Sclerosis; Myelin; Nerves

Myelin is the protective covering or sheath that insulates the axons of neurons. This insulation makes the axon conduct action potentials (the output signal from a neuron) efficiently and rapidly. Some axons are unmyelinated and are less efficient in conducting action potentials compared to myelinated axons. Myelin is produced by glial cells, specifically *oligodendrocytes* in the central nervous system and by *Schwann cells* in the peripheral nervous system. These glial cells wrap their membranes around the axons several times. The more wrapping results in more insulation and faster conduction. There are a few diseases that cause the degeneration of myelin, such as multiple sclerosis (MS). When myelin is disrupted, it can cause symptoms of muscle weakness in humans.

Q1: What is the main function of myelin?

Materials:

A drinking straw
A single-hole puncher
Masking tape
Balloon
Rubber band
Timer
Paper and pencil

Procedure:

Place the balloon on one end of the straw and wrap the rubber band around the balloon and straw. This is to ensure that the balloon will remain on the straw when it is being blown up. Place your mouth on the other end of the straw to blow up the balloon. Using the timer, record the amount of time it takes for the experimenter to blow up the balloon. This is the baseline amount of time to blow up the balloon.

With the hole puncher, make several holes along the length of the straw, approximately four sets of holes. Now, time how long it takes to blow up the balloon without covering the holes. Record the time, *if* you are able to blow up the balloon.

Cover one set of holes with the masking tape. Only cover the holes with enough tape to wrap around the straw once. Blow up the balloon and record the time, if you can blow up the balloon. Cover the next set of holes with masking tape. Again only use enough tape to wrap around the straw once. Blow up the balloon and record the time. Continue to cover the next set of holes, following the same steps described previously. After covering all holes, blow up the balloon and record the time.

Next, cover each set of holes with another length of masking tape to wrap once around the straw. Blow up the balloon and record the time. Continue to wrap another length of masking tape to cover the holes. Blow up the balloon and record the time. Repeat these steps until you can blow the balloon up as quickly as the baseline time.

Q2: How many times did you need to wrap the straw to achieve the baseline time of blowing up the balloon?

Q3: How would this experiment change with different sized tubings? Or different sized holes?

Jennifer L. Hellier

See also: Axon; Multiple Sclerosis; Myelin; Nerves

Further Reading

Morell, P., & Quarles, R. H. (1999). The myelin sheath. In G. J. Siegel, B. W. Agranoff, R. W. Albers, et al. (Eds.). *Basic neurochemistry: Molecular, cellular and medical aspects* (6th ed.). Philadelphia, PA: Lippincott-Raven.

Neural Tube—Illustrating Activity

Activity Relates to Neural Tube

The *neural tube* is composed of the *neural plate* (a thickened region of the *ectoderm* that forms the *neuroectoderm*—this is, where the nervous system arises from), the *neural canal* (formed when the edges of the neural plate fold upward and meet), *neural crest cells* (highly motile cells that quickly divide to form the support cells of the nervous system, such as facial bones and the adrenal medulla), and the wall of the tube formed by *neuroectodermal cells* (which divide and specialize into neurons and into glial cells, which support the neurons by providing nutrients, etc.).

As the neural tube develops, around four weeks' gestation, the primary brain vesicles form. These are three swellings in the neural tube: *prosencephalon, mesencephalon,* and *rhombencephalon.* These primary vesicles give rise to secondary brain vesicles in the sixth week of development. The secondary vesicles consist of the *telencephalon,* the *diencephalon,* the *mesencephalon,* the *metencephalon,* and the *myelencephalon.* Each of these vesicles gives rise to a specialized region of the brain as diagrammed in the following (from anterior—toward the front, to posterior—toward the back).

Table EA.2 Development of the Central Nervous System from Neural Tube to Adult Brain

Primary Brain Vesicle (Week 4)	Secondary Brain Vesicle (Week 6)	Adult Brain Structure	Neural Canal Regions
Prosencephalon	Telencephalon	Cerebrum	Lateral ventricles
	Diencephalon	Thalamus, hypothalamus, epithalamus	Third ventricle
Mesencephalon	Mesencephalon	Midbrain, brainstem	Cerebral aqueduct
Rhombencephalon	Metencephalon	Brainstem, pons, cerebellum	Fourth ventricle
	Myelencephalon	Medulla oblongata	Central canal

Materials: Paper, colored pencils (red, orange, green, blue, and purple)

Methods:
Begin by drawing the primary brain vesicles, which form in the fourth week of embryogenesis. This illustration should be tube-like with three rounded swellings divided across the length of the tube. In this sketch, represent the prosencephalon with a red colored pencil. The prosencephalon is rounded at the most anterior surface. The mesencephalon will be illustrated with the green colored pencil. This is the middle section of the tube and is continuous with the other two primary vesicles. Finally, the rhombencephalon will be represented in purple colored pencil. This section should remain open at the most posterior end in this diagram. This is where the neural tube connects to the developing spinal cord.

For the secondary brain vesicles, begin by drawing Mickey Mouse ears and the top of his head in the red colored pencil. This represents the telencephalon. Continue the neural tube using the orange colored pencil by drawing to rounded projection from the next part of the neural tube; this represents the diencephalon. The mesencephalon should be drawn in green as a swelling in the tube. The metencephalon and myelencephalon, together, form the next swelling in the neural tube. In order to diagram this, draw the first half of the swelling on each side with the blue colored pencil; this represents the metencephalon. Finish the swelling in purple, leaving the posterior end open. This represents the myelencephalon connecting to the developing spinal cord.

Riannon C. Atwater

See also: Neural Tube

Further Reading

Kandel, E. R., Schwartz, J. H., Jessell, T. M., Siegelbaum, S. A., & Hudspeth, A. J. (Eds.). (2012). *Principles of neural science* (5th ed.). New York, NY: McGraw-Hill.
Purves, D., Augustine, G. J., Fitzpatrick, D., Hall, W. C., LaMantia, A.-S., McNamara, J. O., & Williams, S. M. (Eds.). (2004). *Neuroscience* (3rd ed.). Sunderland, MA: Sinauer Associates.

Oligodendrocytes—Building with Clay Activity

Activity Relates to Glia

Oligodendrocytes (derived from Greek meaning "cells with few branches") are supportive cells within the central nervous system (CNS). Their main function is to wrap axons within the CNS with a protective myelin sheath. Myelin sheaths are important as they help neurons transduce electrochemical signals much faster by allowing the impulse to jump from each *Node of Ranvier* (space between myelin sheaths on the axon) to the next node, a process called *salutatory conduction.* Speed of signal transduction is incredibly important, as it will allow the brain to react faster. As most biological cells, oligodendrocytes contain, but not limited to, cell membrane, cytoplasm, nucleus, ribosomes, endoplasmic reticulum (ER), and mitochondria.

Materials: Four colors of clay (red, green, yellow, and blue), wax paper, tabletop, paper towels, toothpick, and four pencils/sticks.

Methods:
Roll a walnut-sized ball of red clay; this will represent the cell membrane and cytoplasm together forming the cell body (soma). Flatten this into a quarter-inch thick, two-inch diameter "pancake." Pinch and pull the edges of the "pancake" to make four cell processes. These processes form the myelin sheaths that wrap around each axon. One oligodendrocyte can myelinate multiple axons. Take a pencil or stick (which represents an axon) and wrap the myelin sheath around its girth, repeat for each pencil/stick. Clean your hands between each color.

Using a pecan-sized ball of green clay, flatten it to be approximately one inch in diameter and an eighth of an inch thick. This will represent the ER. Place the clay on top of the soma, relatively in the center. With a toothpick, poke several small holes into the central section of the ER. These holes represent ribosomes that make proteins.

Take a peanut-sized ball of yellow clay and roll it into a ball. This will represent the nucleus of the oligodendrocyte. The nucleus houses the genetic material. Slightly flatten one side and place on top of the ER; the nucleus is not always in the center of the cell.

Finally, make four to five tic-tac-sized ovals. These are the mitochondria, which generate energy for the cell. Place throughout the cytoplasm.

Riannon C. Atwater

See also: Glia; Multiple Sclerosis; Myelin; Myelin Conduction Experiment (in Experiments and Activities Section)

Further Reading

Purves, D., Augustine, G. J., Fitzpatrick, D., Hall, W. C., LaMantia, A.-S., McNamara, J. O., & Williams, S. M. (Eds.). (2004). *Neuroscience* (3rd ed.). Sunderland, MA: Sinauer Associates.

Pinched Nerve—Building with Clay Activity

Activity Relates to Spinal Cord; Spinal Cord with Vertebra (in Experiments and Activities Section); Vertebra

The spinal roots and nerves travel within the intervertebral foramen, which is formed by the upper and lower vertebral transverse processes. Between each vertebra, there is an intervertebral disk used to cushion the bones during compression as well as to make a fibrous cartilaginous joint. This allows the spinal column to bend without letting the vertebrae slip laterally (side-to-side). Within the intervertebral disk, there are two regions: the *anulus fibrosus* and the *nucleus pulposus*. The *nucleus pulposus* is found in the middle and is very jelly-like while the *anulus fibrosus* makes up the fibrous portion of the joint. Sometimes, if the vertebrae are injured, they can damage the *anulus fibrosus* causing the *nucleus pulposus* to squeeze out. The intervertebral disk has often been referred to as a "jelly-doughnut." If the *nucleus pulposus* squeezes laterally toward the spinal nerves, it reduces the area the spinal roots travel in causing them to be "pinched."

Materials: Six colors of clay (brown, red, blue, yellow, white, and green), wax paper, tabletop, paper towels, and toothpick.

Methods:

Follow the directions in the activity *Spinal Cord with Vertebra*. Make two vertebrae so that you can see the natural space being built between the transverse processes. Now make a jelly doughnut by rolling a pecan-sized ball of white clay into a flattened pancake approximately half of an inch thick. Dig out a trough in the white clay leading to one edge with your toothpick and fingers. Fill this hole will green clay—this is the *nucleus pulposus* squeezing through the damaged *anulus fibrosus*. Place the white clay onto one of the vertebral bodies with the trough pointing toward one of the transverse processes of the vertebra. Place the other vertebra that you have built on top of the intervertebral disk. You can move the green clay to different regions to see the myriad of possible injuries.

Riannon C. Atwater

See also: Spinal Cord; Spinal Cord with Vertebra (in Experiments and Activities Section); Vertebra

Further Reading

Purves, D., Augustine, G. J., Fitzpatrick, D., Hall, W. C., LaMantia, A.-S., McNamara, J. O., & Williams, S. M. (Eds.). (2004). *Neuroscience* (3rd ed.). Sunderland, MA: Sinauer Associates.

Purkinje Cells—Building with Clay Activity

Activity Relates to Cerebellum; Neuron

Purkinje cells are responsible for inhibiting neurons within the deep cerebellar nuclei (DCN). They utilize the neurotransmitter GABA (γ-aminobutyric acid) to send inhibitory signals and contain an incredibly intricate "arbor" of dendritic processes. It is important that the brain is able to inhibit certain neural signals; otherwise, individuals would react to every signal out of millions and could not properly function. The inhibition of the DCN plays a role in coordinating movement. As most biological cells, Purkinje cells contain, but are not limited to: cell membrane, cytoplasm, nucleus, ribosomes, endoplasmic reticulum (ER), and mitochondria.

Materials: Four colors of clay (red, green, yellow, and blue), wax paper, tabletop, paper towels, and toothpick.

Methods:
Roll a walnut-sized ball of red clay; this will represent the cell membrane and cytoplasm together forming the cell body (soma). Flatten this into a quarter-inch thick, two-inch diameter "pancake." Pinch and pull one edge of the "pancake;" form this edge into a highly branched tree. This will represent the dendritic arbor of the cell. These dendrites are responsible for receiving signals from other neurons. Clean your hands each time you switch colors.

Using a pecan-sized ball of green clay, flatten it to be approximately one inch in diameter and an eighth of an inch thick. This will represent the ER. Place the clay on top of the soma, relatively in the center. With a toothpick, poke several small holes into the central section of the ER. These holes represent ribosomes, used to make proteins.

Take a peanut-sized ball of yellow clay and roll it into a ball. This will represent the nucleus of the astrocyte. The nucleus houses the genetic material. Slightly flatten one side and place on top of the ER; the nucleus is not always in the center of the cell.

Finally, make four to five tic-tac-sized ovals. These are the mitochondria, which generate energy for the cell. Place throughout the cytoplasm.

Riannon C. Atwater

See also: Cerebellum; Neuron

Further Reading

Kandel, E. R., Schwartz, J. H., Jessell, T. M., Siegelbaum, S. A., & Hudspeth, A. J. (Eds.). (2012). *Principles of neural science* (5th ed.). New York, NY: McGraw-Hill.

A Sample Immunohistochemistry Protocol with Thought Questions

Experiment Relates to **Immunuohistochemistry**

Immunohistochemistry for Frozen Sections

1. Dip a specimen prepared slide in cold acetone (three minutes). What is the purpose of this step?
2. Phosphate buffered saline (PBS) washes.
3. Dry/circle specimen.
4. Ten percent blocking solution for 30 minutes at 37°C. What could be used as a blocking solution?
5. PBS washes.
6. Primary antibody—overnight incubation at 4°C.
7. PBS washes.
8. Secondary antibody—incubate for one hour at room temperature. To what do you think this antibody is conjugated?
9. Streptavidin-FITC or Streptavidin-AMCA 10 to 15 minute room temperature incubation.
10. PBS washes. Why does this protocol have so many washes? What if you skipped these steps?
11. Water washes.
12. Eosin counterstaining.
13. Mount with coverslip and view. What considerations should be made when selecting a mounting medium?

Protocol courtesy of the Fleming Lab at Kansas State University.

See also: Immunohistochemistry

Schwann Cells—Building with Clay Activity

Activity Relates to Glia

Schwann cells are supportive cells within the peripheral nervous system (PNS). Analogous to the oligodendrocytes in the central nervous system, Schwann cells are responsible for myelinating neurons. The myelin sheaths formed by Schwann cells help increase the speed of signal conduction through a process called, *salutatory conduction*. As most biological cells, Schwann cells contain, but not limited to, cell membrane, cytoplasm, nucleus, ribosomes, endoplasmic reticulum (ER), and Golgi apparatus.

Materials: Four colors of clay (red, green, yellow, and brown), wax paper, tabletop, paper towels, and toothpick.

Methods:
Roll a walnut-sized ball of red clay; this will represent the cell membrane and cytoplasm together forming the cell body (soma). Flatten this into a quarter-inch thick, two-inch diameter "pancake." Pinch and pull the two opposite edges of the "pancake" to make the long, thin portions that wrap around the axon, making the myelin sheath. Clean your hands each time you switch colors.

Using a pecan-sized ball of green clay, flatten it to be approximately one inch in diameter and an eighth of an inch thick. This will represent the ER. Place the clay on top of the soma, relatively in the center. With a toothpick, poke several small holes into the central section of the ER. These holes represent ribosomes, used to make proteins.

Take a peanut-sized ball of yellow clay and roll it into a ball. This will represent the nucleus of the Schwann cell. The nucleus houses the genetic material. Slightly flatten one side and place on top of the ER; the nucleus is not always in the center of the cell.

Take a pea-sized ball of brown clay and form three to four small worms. Place these next to each other, between the ER and the edge of the cell body. These represent the Golgi apparatus, which packages nutrients, waste, and other chemicals to transport throughout the cell.

Riannon C. Atwater

See also: Glia; Myelin; Myelin Conduction Experiment (in Experiments and Activities Section)

Further Reading

Kandel, E. R., Schwartz, J. H., Jessell, T. M., Siegelbaum, S. A., & Hudspeth, A. J. (Eds.). (2012). *Principles of neural science* (5th ed.). New York, NY: McGraw-Hill.

Spinal Cord with Vertebra—Building with Clay Activity

Activity Relates to Lumbar Puncture; Spinal Cord; Vertebra

The spinal cord is a bundle of nervous tissue and is a part of the central nervous system. Conduction of sensory and motor information is carried by the spinal cord to and from the brain. The spinal cord is also responsible for coordination of reflexes. It extends from the *foramen magnum* (a natural large opening) in the skull to the *conus medullaris* (tapered, lower end of the spinal cord) terminating in the *filum terminale* (the end of the spinal cord that is depicted by a delicate strand of fibrous tissue that extends from the conus medullaris). The spinal cord is protected by 24 of 31 vertebrae separated into cervical (7), thoracic (12), and lumbar (5) bones. The remaining seven vertebrae do not protect the spinal cord, as the spinal cord is shorter than the entire boney spinal column. Each vertebra is separated by specialized disc of cartilaginous fibers known as an intervertebral disk.

Materials: Four colors of clay (brown, red, blue, and yellow), wax paper, tabletop, paper towels, and toothpick.

Methods:

Take an almond-sized piece of brown clay and roll it into a ball on to the wax paper to protect the tabletop. Flatten the clay into a disk approximately an eighth of an inch thick and two inches in diameter. This will represent the body of the vertebra. Next take another piece of clay and roll it into a worm shape that is an eighth of an inch in diameter and approximately five inches long. Connect this piece of clay to the disk in a loop. Roll three additional "worms," each an eighth of an inch in diameter and two inches long. Place these on the other three sides of the loop. These are the two transverse processes and the spinous process. Clean your hands each time you switch colors.

Next, form a disk from the yellow clay approximately an eighth an inch thick and one-and-a-half inches in diameter. This represents the spinal cord. With the toothpick, make a dot in the center; this is the central canal where cerebrospinal fluid flows within the spinal cord. Draw a "butterfly" in the yellow clay. Two of the "wings" are dorsal horns and two are ventral horns. Place the disk inside the loop of brown clay.

Make a long, thin "worm" out of the blue clay. Gently set one end of the worm on one of the two "wings" closest to the vertebral body, extending away; this is the motor pathway which transduces signals away from the spinal cord.

Make a second long, thin "worm" out of the red clay with a rounded enlargement approximately one-and-a-half inches from one end. Place this end gently on the "wing" furthest from the vertebral body on the same side. This represents the sensory pathway which transduces signals toward the spinal cord. The enlargement is the dorsal root ganglion, which houses the cell bodies of sensory neurons.

Riannon C. Atwater

See also: Lumbar Puncture; Spinal Cord; Vertebra

Further Reading

Kandel, E. R., Schwartz, J. H., Jessell, T. M., Siegelbaum, S. A., & Hudspeth, A. J. (Eds.). (2012). *Principles of neural science* (5th ed.). New York, NY: McGraw-Hill.

Voltage Clamp Experiment

Experiment Relates to **Action Potential; Axon; Electrophysiology Setup and Experiments (in Experiment and Activities Section)**

Electrophysiology studies the electrical impulses (synaptic activity) produced by neurons as well as the activity of membrane receptors such as the acetylcholine receptor. These recordings can identify how local circuits or single neurons work in the "normal" brain and compare that activity to brain dysfunctions. Electrophysiology is divided into two categories: extracellular and intracellular recordings. Extracellular recordings measure the synaptic activity of all the neurons located below the tip of the recording electrode. This recording is the sum of the grouped firing of action potentials, which produce population spikes and field post-synaptic potentials (fPSP). However, to identify how a single neuron or specific receptor responds to chemicals, scientists perform intracellular or whole-cell recordings.

Intracellular experiments are able to measure the membrane voltage of a neuron and its action potential activity. Specifically the tip of the electrode must enter the cell without rupturing it. This allows the electrode to act like part of the cell as long as the solution within the electrode matches the neurons' intracellular fluid concentrations. The first such recordings were performed by Alan Lloyd Hodgkin (1914–1998) and Andrew Fielding Huxley (1917–2012) in the giant squid axon. This experiment will use the hippocampus slice to measure the resting membrane potential and action potential activity of granule cells compared to pyramidal cells.

Materials:

Intracellular preamplifier
Slice chamber
Stimulator

Stimulus Isolation Unit (SIU)
Oscilloscope
Cables
Artificial cerebrospinal fluid (ACSF)
Recording electrodes

Drip chamber
Micromanipulators
Thermometer and external heater
O_2 and N_2 tanks
Fluid pump
Beaker
Air table
Microscope

Procedure:

The electrophysiological equipment setup is similar to the frog sciatic nerve setup. The hippocampal slice must be placed on the ramp of the slice chamber for about one to two hours with continual flow of ACSF and oxygen. This allows the hippocampal slice to equilibrate to its new environment. The relevant anatomy for this experiment is the hippocampal dentate gyrus, which contains the molecular layer, granule cell layer, hilus, and the CA3 pyramidal cell layer. In the figure, identify the recording and stimulating electrodes and the respective regions in which they are placed.

1 *Resting membrane potentials of different neuron types:* Before inserting the tip of the recording electrode in a granule cell, measure the electrode's resistance. Higher electrode resistances produce better recordings. Using a microscope, focus on a neuron and carefully lower the recording tip to the neuron's cell body. Enter the neuron and then measure the resting membrane potential. Repeat this step using a new electrode and a CA3 pyramidal neuron.

Q1: What is the difference between the resting membrane potential of a granule cell and a CA3 pyramidal neuron?

2. *Action potentials in granule and CA3 pyramidal neurons:* Measure the resistance of a new electrode and perform an intracellular recording from a granule cell. Carefully place a stimulating electrode in the molecular layer near the cell being recording. Stimulate the neuron and record the response. Change the location of the stimulating electrode and record the action potentials generated. Repeat this step using a new electrode and a CA3 pyramidal neuron.

Q2: What is the difference between the granule and CA3 pyramidal cell responses?

Jennifer L. Hellier

See also: Action Potential; Axon; Electrophysiology Setup and Experiments

Further Reading

ADInstruments. (2012). *Intracellular recordings*. Retrieved from http://www.adinstruments.com/solutions/research/applications/intracellular-recordings#overview

Recommended Resources

Bear, M. F., Connors, B. W., & Paradiso, M. A. (2007). *Neuroscience exploring the brain* (3rd ed.). Baltimore, MD: Lippincott Williams & Wilkins.

Chudler, E. H. (2014). *Neuroscience for kids*. Retrieved from http://faculty.washington.edu/chudler/neurok.html

Dougherty, P., & Tsuchitani, C. (1997). Somatosensory systems. In *Neuroscience Online, an electronic textbook for the neurosciences* (Chap. 2). Open-access educational resource provided by the Department of Neurobiology and Anatomy at the University of Texas Medical School at Houston. Retrieved from http://neuroscience.uth.tmc.edu/s2/chapter02.html

Kandel, E. R., Schwartz, J. H., Jessell, T. M., Siegelbaum, S. A., & Hudspeth, A. J. (Eds.). (2012). *Principles of neural science* (5th ed.). New York, NY: McGraw-Hill.

Knierim, J. (1997). Disorders of the motor system. In *Neuroscience Online, an electronic textbook for the neurosciences* (Chap. 6). Open-access educational resource provided by the Department of Neurobiology and Anatomy at the University of Texas Medical School at Houston. Retrieved from http://nba.uth.tmc.edu/neuroscience/m/s3/chapter06.html

National Institute of Neurological Disorders and Stroke (NINDS). (2014). *Disorder index*. Retrieved from http://www.ninds.nih.gov/disorders/disorder_index.htm

Nolte, J. (2009). *The human brain: An introduction to its functional anatomy with student consult online access* (6th ed.). Philadelphia, PA: Mosby-Elsevier.

Purves, D., Augustine, G. J., Fitzpatrick, D., Hall, W. C., LaMantia, A.-S., McNamara, J. O., & Williams, S. M. (Eds.). (2004). *Neuroscience* (3rd ed.). Sunderland, MA: Sinauer Associates.

About the Editor and Contributors

Editor

JENNIFER L. HELLIER, PhD, is an assistant professor in the Departments of Family Medicine and Cell and Developmental Biology, the Director of Colorado Health Professions Development (Co-HPD) program, and the Associate Director of Pre-Health Programs in the Colorado Area Health Education Centers (AHEC) Program Office. Dr. Hellier earned her doctoral degree in neuroscience from Colorado State University, Fort Collins, and completed her baccalaureate of science at the University of Southern California, Los Angeles, CA. Previous to her leadership and development of the Co-HPD pipeline programs, Dr. Hellier performed peer-reviewed scientific research in schizophrenia, olfaction, and epilepsy in a neuroscience lab on the University of Colorado-Anschutz Medical Campus. Earlier in her career, Dr. Hellier was an instructor in the neurology department at Harvard Medical School, and a postdoctoral fellow at the University of Colorado Health Science Campus.

Contributors

NICOLE AREVALO, BS, MA, is a research associate in the Rocky Mountain Taste and Smell Center at the University of Colorado Denver Anschutz Medical Campus in Denver.

CAROLYN JOHNSON ATWATER has a BA in psychology from the University of Colorado at Boulder.

RIANNON C. ATWATER is an undergraduate at the University of Colorado at Denver. She is majoring in biology with minors in multidisciplinary research methods and leadership studies.

DIANNA BARTEL, PhD, is a postdoctoral research associate in the Department of Neurosurgery at Yale University School of Medicine. Her research primarily focuses on the glial cells of the brain.

B. DNATE' BAXTER, BS, MS, is a research associate at the University of Colorado Denver Anschutz Medical Campus in Denver.

KATHRYN K. BERCURY, PhD, has spent her scientific career studying neurodegenerative diseases such as amyotrophic lateral sclerosis, Alzheimer's, Parkinson's disease, and multiple sclerosis. Her graduate work was spent investigating protein kinase signaling and its role in the development of myelination glial. Her main interest is how signaling cascades modulate neuronal-glial interactions during central nervous system development and disease.

TERRI BLEVINS, MA, ED.D. is the Director of Student and Career Development and an instructor with the Department of Family Medicine at the University of Colorado School of Medicine. She has a master's degree in counseling from the University of Iowa, and is a doctoral student at the University of Colorado Denver.

PATRICIA A. BLOOMQUIST, BS, is a retiree from AT&T and Ball Aerospace. She currently is the owner of Compass Real Estate and enjoys volunteering for different organizations.

JAMESON S. BOSWELL is an undergraduate at the University of Colorado Denver, where he is majoring in biology.

EMMA BOXER is a neuroscience student at University of Colorado Denver. She currently has an internship at the Denver Museum of Nature & Science, where she has researched the genetics of the bitter taste of PTC and PROP and is currently researching the genetics of a possible sixth taste: fatty acids.

NICHOLAS BREITNAUER, MD, is an internal medicine/pediatrics resident at the University of Colorado.

JEREMY E. BROTHERS, PharmD, is a graduate of the University of Colorado Skaggs School of Pharmacy and Pharmaceutical Sciences. Jeremy will continue his education with a residency in either psychiatry or critical care–based pharmacy. He did his undergraduate work at Virginia Tech and is originally from the Washington, D.C., area.

NICOLAS BUSQUET, PhD, is a research associate in the Center for Neuroscience at the University of Colorado. He is in charge of the Animal Behavior Core, and helps research teams design, perform, and analyze behavioral tests of animal models.

JERRICA CHERRY is an undergraduate student at Adams State University. She is majoring in clinical psychology with a focus on early childhood and adolescence.

MARGARET COOK-SHIMANEK, MD, received her medical degree from the University of North Dakota School of Medicine and Health Sciences. She is currently pursuing her master of public health at the Colorado School of Public Health while training in the Preventive Medicine Residency Program at the University of Colorado.

AN K. DANG, BA, is a predoctoral student in the Biomedical Sciences Program at Colorado State University. Her research focus is the role of calcium channels in the central nervous system.

STEPHANIE DUNLAP, PharmD, is a 2014 graduate of the University of Colorado Skaggs of Pharmacy and Pharmaceutical Sciences. She received a bachelor of arts in the field of molecular and cellular biology from the University of Illinois Champaign-Urbana in 2010.

PATRICIA ELLO is an undergraduate student at the University of Colorado Denver. She is currently studying psychology and premedicine.

CHARLES A. FERGUSON, PhD, is an associate professor in the Department of Integrative Biology at the University of Colorado Denver. While his academic interests focus on neurobiology and neurotoxicology, his primary research today focuses on the transition of high school students pursuing STEM disciplines to college.

RICHARD FERRO is a student and teaching assistant at the University of Colorado Denver. He also works as a part-time tutor and has helped teach general biology and human physiology at the university since 2012.

SARAH CHANG FOSTER, BA, is a medical student at the University of Colorado Denver. Her interests include rural primary care and emergency medicine.

PAMELA GILLEN, ND, RN, is an assistant professor in the Department of Nursing at the University of Colorado Anschutz Medical Campus in Aurora, Colorado. She has presented extensively on fetal alcohol spectrum disorders. She was the past cochair elect for the FASD Center for Excellence expert panel.

ASHLEY N. GLASSER, Colorado State University-Pueblo student, is pursuing her bachelor of science degree in biology with an emphasis on preveterinary medicine.

MATTHEW HARRINGTON is an undergraduate student at the University of Colorado Denver. He is pursuing a bachelor of science in psychology and studying premedicine.

LIZA HUBBELL, MA, is a professional educator and writer with 15 years experience enhancing literacy skills in emergent readers and writers and in mentoring teachers to better serve children of all learning profiles.

AMANDA HUGGETT is a student at Colorado State University-Pueblo completing her bachelor of science degree in biology with a premedicine emphasis and minors in chemistry and leadership studies.

RENEE JOHNSON is an undergraduate premedical student at the University of Colorado Denver. She is studying biological physics and medical physics while getting minors in biology, mathematics, and chemistry.

AARON JONES graduated from the University of Colorado Denver. He majored in biology with a minor in ethnic studies.

CYNTHIA M. JOSEPH is an undergraduate at the University of Colorado Denver. She is a student in the University Honors and Leadership Program and is majoring in biology with a minor in multidisciplinary research methods.

JONATHON KEENEY, PhD, earned his honors BA in molecular, cellular and developmental biology at the University of Colorado, Boulder, and his PhD in neuroscience from the University of Colorado, Anshutz Medical Campus. His research explores genomic mechanisms by which human brain size has increased, and how these mechanisms influence disease.

CHRISTOPHER KNOECKEL is an MD/PhD student in the Neuroscience Program at the University of Colorado Anschutz Medical Campus. His research focuses on the role of activity in the development of the peripheral nervous system.

KEVIN LEE is a graduate of Adams State University in Alamosa where he studied cellular and molecular biology and played division II soccer.

LISA M. J. LEE, PhD, is an assistant professor in the Department of Cell and Developmental Biology at University of Colorado School of Medicine. She teaches embryology, histology, and anatomy and her research focus is on educational technology and human-computer interaction.

RYAN LERCH is an undergraduate at Colorado State University-Pueblo. He is majoring in biology with minors in chemistry and psychology.

ROBERTO LOPEZ is currently a medical student at Rocky Vista University and earned his undergraduate degree from the University of Colorado Denver. Previous to medical school, Robert worked in a neuroscience research laboratory at the University of Colorado Anschutz Medical Campus. Robert is a published author in the field of olfaction and olfactory activity maps.

BRIANNA LYNCH is a current student at Biola University. She is studying pre-med/human biology with the hopes to specialize in neurology and perform professional research in addition to clinical patient care. Her most extensive areas of research are in the frontal lobe, temporal lobe, and speech production. While completing her degree, Brianna works as a certified phlebotomist for hospitals and convalescent clinics.

STEPHEN MAZURKIVICH is an undergraduate student studying biology at Fort Lewis College in Durango, CO.

SHANNEN MCNAMARA is a student at Colorado Mesa University where she is studying biology. She has played tennis for many years, and currently plays on her college team.

ROBIN MICHAELS, PhD, received her doctorate from the University of Minnesota, Minneapolis, and completed postdoctoral training at Washington University in St. Louis. She is an associate professor in the Department of Cellular and Developmental Biology at the University of Colorado School of Medicine and serves as Assistant Dean of preclinical medical curriculum.

ADAM K. MILLS, DC, is a graduate of Parker University where he received a doctorate in chiropractic and bachelor's in anatomy; in addition he received a bachelor's in biology from Colorado State University-Pueblo. He plans to practice chiropractic in rural Colorado.

HOLLIE ELIZABETH VIGIL MILLS, MD, is a 2013 graduate of the University of Colorado School of Medicine. She will complete her residency in family medicine and plans to practice family medicine in rural Colorado.

CHASA M. MOORE graduated from the University of Arizona with a degree in biology. She earned both her nurse assistant's and massage therapy certifications in 2004. Chasa was the vice president and director of U.S. Operations for two years for HEAL International, a Phoenix-based international nonprofit organization. Chasa's main priority as a director was establishing and overseeing health education outreach programs for at-risk youth.

NHUNG T. NGUYEN is an undergraduate at the University of Colorado Denver. She is majoring in biology with emphasis on predentistry.

MITCHEL L. OLTMANNS is an undergraduate student as well as a biology teaching assistant at the University of Colorado Denver. He is pursuing a major in biology with a minor in leadership studies.

CASSANDRA LYNN OSBORNE, PhD, is an associate professor of biology in the Department of Natural and Environmental Sciences at Western State Colorado

University in Gunnison, Colorado. The focus of her current research is the role that endocrine-disrupting compounds play in the early development of the neural crest in *Xenopus laevis*.

BARIS OZBAY has a bachelor's degree in electrical engineering and is currently a PhD candidate in bioengineering at the University of Colorado Denver. His current research involves using modern microscopy techniques to study the peripheral mechanisms of olfaction.

MARIO J. PEREZ is a lead research associate in the Division of Pulmonary Sciences and Critical Care Medicine at the University of Colorado Denver Anschutz Medical Campus. He will begin medical school in 2014 at the University of Colorado Anschutz Medical Campus.

ERIC W. PRINCE is an undergraduate at the University of Colorado Denver. He is majoring in chemistry with an emphasis in biochemistry.

VIDYA PUGAZHENTHI, PharmD, graduated in 2014 at the University of Colorado Skaggs School of Pharmacy and Pharmaceutical sciences. She previously studied at the University of Denver with a focus on biochemistry.

LISA A. RABE, PhD, is a lecturer in the Department of Craniofacial Biology at the University of Colorado School of Dental Medicine where she teaches medical microbiology and immunology. After conducting research for several years in the field of immunology, she now devotes her energy to teaching and sharing her passion for science.

MICHAEL ROMANI, a California native who received his bachelor of science degree in biology from California State University, Fresno, is currently a student at the University of Colorado, School of Dental Medicine. Upon graduation he will start a Colorado dental practice or continue his education and get a degree in periodontics.

ERNESTO SALCEDO, PhD, is a faculty member in the Department of Cell and Developmental Biology at the University of Colorado School of Medicine. He received his bachelor's degree from Duke University and his doctorate degree from the University of Texas Health Sciences Center at San Antonio. Dr. Salcedo serves as a research associate at the Denver Museum of Nature & Science providing talks on olfaction and neuroscience to pubic audiences.

JASON SANTIAGO, MS, is originally from the San Francisco Bay Area. He received his master of science in biology at the University of Denver in 2010. He worked as a research scientist for several years before starting medical school at the University of Colorado, where he is currently enrolled.

C. J. SAUNDERS, PhD, is a postdoctoral researcher in the Department of Oto-rhinolaryngology at the University of Pennsylvania. He is a recent graduate of the Neuroscience program at the University of Colorado, where his dissertation research focused on the role of airway chemosensory cells in mediating sensations of irritation and inflammation.

KAREN SAVOIE, RDH, BS, is a graduate of Louisiana State University Health Sciences Center and a registered dental hygienist for over 30 years. Her primary focus is on improving oral health and access to care for vulnerable populations.

ALLISON J. SCHUSTER is an undergraduate at BIOLA University. She is majoring in human biology and is a member of the Torrey Honor's Institute.

CONRAD SCLAR is an undergraduate at the University of Colorado at Boulder. He is majoring in music performance and pursuing a minor in physics.

GEETA SHARMA, PhD, is an assistant professor in the Department of Cell and Developmental Biology at University of Colorado Denver. She has published extensively on cellular effects of nicotine. Her current research focuses on role of nicotinic receptors in adult neurogenesis and addiction.

ELIZABETH SHICK, DDS, MPH, is a pediatric dentist and received her degrees in dentistry and public Health from the University of North Carolina at Chapel Hill. She specializes in infant oral health, perinatal oral health, and global oral health. She currently lives in Denver, Colorado, and is an assistant professor at the University of Colorado School of Dental Medicine.

JOSHUA R. SKEGGS is currently an undergraduate at the University of Colorado Denver studying public health, with a premedicine emphasis.

ERIN SLOCUM is a graduate of the University of Colorado at Boulder. She is currently studying nursing at the University of Northern Colorado.

LYNELLE SMITH is a research assistant in the Department of Pulmonary Science and Critical Care Medicine at the University of Colorado Denver. She is currently in medical school at the University of Colorado Anschutz Medical Campus.

JASON SMUCNY, MS, is a predoctoral graduate student in neuroscience and member of the psychiatry department at the University of Colorado Anschutz Medical Campus.

JENNIFER M. SORGATZ is an executive officer with the National Geospatial-Intelligence Agency and has degrees in music performance and music education from the University of Southern California and certificates in geographic information systems and geospatial intelligence from Pennsylvania State University.

DANIELLE STUTZMAN, PharmD, graduated in 2014 from Skaggs School of Pharmacy and Pharmaceutical Sciences, University of Colorado Anschutz Medical Campus. She is a graduate of the University of Colorado at Boulder and received a bachelor of arts in molecular cellular developmental biology and psychology.

WALDEMAR B. SWIERCZ, PhD, is an assistant in neuroscience in the Department of Neurology at Massachusetts General Hospital and Instructor in Neurology at Harvard Medical School. His main field of research is artificial neural networks applied to simulating epileptic-like activity.

MELISSA TJANDRA is a student of University of Colorado, Boulder, pursuing a degree in bachelor of arts in biochemistry.

VIVIAN VU is a recent graduate of the University of Denver. She majored in biological sciences with minors in chemistry and business administration.

SIMON WALDBAUM, PhD, has spent over a decade conducting neuroscience research, most recently at the University of Colorado Anschutz Medical Campus. His primary research focus and areas of publication have been on inhibitory synaptic signaling and illuminating the link between neuronal mitochondrial oxidative stress and the development of acquired epilepsy.

KATHRYN WELLMAN is an undergraduate at the University of Colorado, Boulder. She is pursuing a bachelor of arts in integrative physiology with a certificate in neuroscience.

ALYSSA M. WIENECKE is a prehealthcare undergraduate student at Biola University, located in La Mirada, California. She is majoring in human biology and planning to pursue a career in neurology after graduating. In her studies, she is working to better understand autism and find better treatments or therapies for the autistic.

AUDREY S. YEE, MD, earned her medical degree from the University of Kansas School of Medicine, and then completed an Adult Neurology Residency and three Fellowships—Basic Neurophysiology, Clinical Neuromuscular/Neurodiagnostics, and Clinical Research—at the University of Colorado School of Medicine. She is faculty in the University of Colorado's Department of Pediatrics.

Index

Note: Page numbers in **bold** indicate main entries.